Management of Dyslipidaemias: Enhancing Lipid Modification to Reduce Cardiovascular Risk

Management of Dyslipidaemias: Enhancing Lipid Modification to Reduce Cardiovascular Risk

Guest Editors

Daniel Gaudet
Etienne Khoury

MDPI

Basel • Beijing • Wuhan • Barcelona • Belgrade • Novi Sad • Cluj • Manchester

Guest Editors

Daniel Gaudet
Department of Medicine
Université de Montréal
Community Gene
Medicine Center
Chicoutimi
Canada

Etienne Khoury
Department of Medicine
Université de Montréal
Chicoutimi
Canada

Editorial Office
MDPI AG
Grosspeteranlage 5
4052 Basel, Switzerland

This is a reprint of the Special Issue, published open access by the journal *Journal of Clinical Medicine* (ISSN 2077-0383), freely accessible at: https://www.mdpi.com/journal/jcm/special_issues/TZ49Z25FAH.

For citation purposes, cite each article independently as indicated on the article page online and as indicated below:

Lastname, A.A.; Lastname, B.B. Article Title. *Journal Name* **Year**, *Volume Number*, Page Range.

ISBN 978-3-7258-5623-7 (Hbk)
ISBN 978-3-7258-5624-4 (PDF)
https://doi.org/10.3390/books978-3-7258-5624-4

Contents

Journal of
Clinical Medicine

MDPI

Review

The Hurdle of Access to Emerging Therapies and Potential Solutions in the Management of Dyslipidemias

Brett S. Mansfield [1,2], Farzahna Mohamed [1,2], Miriam Larouche [3] and Frederick J. Raal [1,2,*]

1 Department of Internal Medicine, University of the Witwatersrand, Johannesburg 2193, South Africa; brett.mansfield@wits.ac.za (B.S.M.); farzahna.mohamed@wits.ac.za (F.M.)
2 Carbohydrate & Lipid Metabolism Research Unit, University of the Witwatersrand, Johannesburg 2193, South Africa
3 Département de Médecine, Université de Montréal and ECOGENE-21, Montreal, QC H3T 1J4, Canada; miriam.larouche@ecogene21.org
* Correspondence: frederick.raal@wits.ac.za

Abstract: This review explores the many barriers to accessing lipid-lowering therapies (LLTs) for the prevention and management of atherosclerotic cardiovascular disease (ASCVD). Geographical, knowledge, and regulatory barriers significantly impede access to LLTs, exacerbating disparities in healthcare infrastructure and affordability. We highlight the importance of policy reforms, including pricing regulations and reimbursement policies, for enhancing affordability and streamlining regulatory processes. Innovative funding models, such as value-based pricing and outcome-based payment arrangements, have been recommended to make novel LLTs more accessible. Public health interventions, including community-based programs and telemedicine, can be utilized to reach underserved populations and improve medication adherence. Education and advocacy initiatives led by patient advocacy groups and healthcare providers play a crucial role in raising awareness and empowering patients. Despite the barriers to access, novel LLTs present a big opportunity to reduce the burden of ASCVD, emphasizing the need for collaborative efforts among policymakers, healthcare providers, industry stakeholders, and patient advocacy groups to address these barriers to improve access to LLTs globally.

Keywords: lipid-lowering therapies; dyslipidemia; access; barriers; ASCVD; public health; telemedicine

1. Introduction

Atherosclerotic cardiovascular disease (ASCVD) remains the leading cause of morbidity and mortality worldwide [1]. More than 16 million people died from coronary artery disease or stroke in 2021 [1].

With advances in therapeutics, deaths due to ASCVD have steadily declined in most high-income countries (HICs), apart from the US which has seen a resurgence in cardiovascular mortality over the past decade [1,2]. Indeed, more people died from cardiovascular disease in the US in 2020 than in any other year since 2003 [2]. Possible reasons for this resurgence include a rising prevalence of obesity, metabolic syndrome, diabetes, and hypertension [2]. The impact of the coronavirus 2019 (COVID-19) pandemic, too, has led to excess cardiovascular mortality [2].

In addition, cardiovascular mortality in low- and middle-income countries (LMICs) remains unacceptably high, being nearly twice that of HICs [1]. Indeed, 80% of all deaths due to cardiovascular disease (CVD) occur in LMICs, with the prevalence of ASCVD and the burden of risk factors expected to rise exponentially [3,4]. The projected economic burden of risk factors and the consequences of ASCVD is expected to triple over the next 30 years [5].

Dyslipidemia, in particular, elevated low-density lipoprotein cholesterol (LDL-C), is one of the major modifiable risk factors that contribute to ASCVD [6]. This review will address therapies aimed at lowering LDL-C. Statins have been the cornerstone of lipid-lowering therapy (LLT) and have been listed on the World Health Organization (WHO) Model of Essential Medicines List (EML) since 2007 [7]. Statins are recommended for ASCVD prevention globally but remain underutilized and underdosed, especially in LMICs [4,7]. In low-income countries (LICs), only 19.8% of patients receive medicines for secondary prevention of ASCVD, compared to 54.9% in upper-middle-income countries (UMICs) [8,9].

Treatment guidelines continue to recommend lower LDL-C targets, particularly for subjects with established ASCVD, resulting in the need for additional non-statin LLTs [10]. Many patients are undertreated and do not reach current guideline-directed LDL-C targets [11,12]. Furthermore, up to 30% of patients report statin-related side effects [13,14]. Although the nocebo effect of statins is well established, poor perceptions surrounding statin use contribute to poor adherence [15–17]. As such, there is a need for non-statin LLTs to bridge this treatment gap.

The United Nations has set a Sustainable Development Goal to reduce premature mortality from non-communicable diseases (NCDs) by one-third by 2030 [3,18,19]. If this goal is to be realized, then improved access to essential medicines, including novel and emerging lipid-lowering therapies (LLTs), will need to be prioritized.

Significant differences exist in access to medications in different countries and regions around the world. While it is not possible to identify the specific barriers for all countries, this review will highlight just some of the difficulties that exist in providing novel therapies to the patients who need them.

2. Novel Lipid-Lowering Therapies

Over the past few decades, a number of new drugs have been approved for LDL-C reduction.

Evolocumab (Repatha) and alirocumab (Praluent), monoclonal antibody therapies directed against proprotein convertase subtilisin/kexin type 9 (PCSK9), are administered every 2–4 weeks as subcutaneous injections. They demonstrated a 50–60% reduction in LDL-C and reduced ASCVD mortality in the FOURIER and ODYSSEY OUTCOMES trials, respectively [20,21]. PCSK9 inhibitors are recommended for patients with ASCVD or at high risk for ASCVD who cannot achieve adequate lowering of LDL-C with maximally tolerated statin therapy or for those who are statin-intolerant [22]. Likely because of cost, the uptake of PCSK9 inhibitor therapy has been poor, with most users being in the US [11,12,23].

Tafolecimab (Sintbilo), a humanized monoclonal antibody targeting PCSK9, received approval in China in August 2023 [24]. Dosed by monthly subcutaneous injection, tafolecimab led to a 57–70% reduction in LDL-C in patients with and without FH [24–26]. As many as 10% of participants developed anti-drug antibodies and 1% developed neutralizing antibodies during a 48-week trial period [26].

Inclisiran (Leqvio or Sybrava) is a small interfering RNA (siRNA) therapy directed against the hepatic synthesis of PCSK9 and leads to an approximately 50% reduction in LDL-C [27,28]. Over and above the traditional indications for PCSK9 inhibitor therapy, inclisiran can be considered in individuals with poor adherence to or adverse effects from the PCSK9 monoclonal antibodies [22]. A significant benefit of inclisiran over evolocumab and alirocumab is its 6-monthly dosing schedule.

The widespread use of inclisiran has been significantly hampered in the UK, with less than 5000 prescriptions for the drug occurring over 18 months [29]. This number falls grossly short of the National Health Services (NHS) target of 300,000 patients by October 2024 [29]. Major factors limiting the prescribing of inclisiran include uncertainty around costs, drug safety, and the bureaucratic workload of prescribing the drug [30].

Bempedoic acid is an orally administered drug that inhibits adenosine triphosphate (ATP)-citrate lyase, an enzyme located upstream of 3-hydroxy-3-methylglutaryl coenzyme A (HMG Co-A) reductase, the rate-limiting enzyme targeted by statins [31]. Bempedoic acid leads to approximately a 24% reduction in LDL-C in statin-intolerant individuals and has a low rate of myalgias [32]. When added to maximally tolerated statin therapy, bempedoic acid reduces LDL-C by between 16 and 18% [33,34]. Moreover, the CLEAR Outcomes trial demonstrated a reduction in the incidence of ASCVD in individuals who were intolerant of statins [35].

While the monthly costs of bempedoic acid (registered as Nexletol in the USA and Nilemdo in the EU) and its combination with ezetimibe (Nexlizet in the USA and Nustendi in the EU) are cheaper than PCSK9 inhibitors, because of the smaller percentage reduction in LDL-C, they are more costly per mg/dL reduction in LDL-C achieved.

Evinacumab (Evkeeza) is a monoclonal antibody that inhibits angiopoietin-like protein 3 (ANGPTL3), lowering LDL-C by LDL-receptor-independent means. Remarkably, reductions in LDL-C levels by approximately 50% in addition to maximally tolerated LLT were seen in the ELIPSE-HoFH trial [36]. The drug has been approved for the treatment of homozygous familial hypercholesterolemia (HoFH) from the age of 5 years [36,37].

Newer therapies at various stages in the research and development pipeline are likely to become available in the future.

- Lerodalcibep, a recombinant fusion protein of a PCSK9-binding domain (adnectin) with human albumin, reduced LDL-C by over 50% with monthly subcutaneous injections when administered to heterozygous FH patients over a 24-week study period [38].
- Oral PCSK9 inhibitors have shown similar reductions to the injectable PCSK9 inhibitors [39,40]. NNC0385-0434 was withdrawn for commercial reasons, while MK-0616 is currently in phase 3 clinical trials.
- The cholesterol ester transfer protein (CETP) inhibitors as high-density lipoprotein cholesterol (HDL-C)-raising therapies did not reduce atherosclerosis or cardiovascular events [41–43]. However, obicetrapib, a novel CETP inhibitor, in addition to raising HDL-C, has demonstrated a 45% reduction in median LDL-C in a randomized phase 2 study and a 63% reduction in combination with ezetimibe [44,45].
- Zodasiran is an siRNA molecule that disrupts the expression of *ANGPTL3* [46]. The ARCHES-2 trial showed that, at varying doses, zodasiran was effective in patients with mixed hyperlipidemia, leading to a 51–63% reduction in triglycerides (TGs) and 14–20% reduction in LDL-C [46].
- Solbinsiran, a GalNAC-conjugated siRNA against ANGPTL3, produced a dose-dependent reduction in TG, non-HDL-C, and apolipoprotein B in individuals with mixed hyperlipidemia [47].
- CRISPR/Cas9-based gene editing therapies directed against the *PCSK9* and *ANGPTL3* genes are entering human trials given the safety shown in preclinical models [48–50]. These are considered good targets given the lifelong absence of any health-related consequences in individuals with naturally occurring loss-of-function *PCSK9* and *ANGPTL3* mutations.
- Vaccination strategies inducing a host immune response against circulating PCSK9 or ANGPTL3 remain within the preclinical domain but have shown promising results in non-human primates and other animal models [51–54].

It remains to be seen whether these new therapies (displayed in Table 1) will reduce cardiovascular events, and further studies are awaited. Some are indeed likely to obtain regulatory approval in the future and will enter the market alongside the currently available lipid-lowering therapies. However, the question of how accessible these therapies will be to the general population is of concern, especially considering the global underutilization of many of the currently available lipid-lowering therapies, particularly within LMICs [11,12,55].

Table 1. Novel lipid-lowering therapies for LDL-C reduction.

Medication	Mechanism of Action	LDL-C Reduction	Phase of Development
Tafolecimab	Humanized mAb against PCSK9	~57–70%	Marketed
Lerodalcibep	PCSK9-binding domain (adnectin) conjugated with human albumin	~50%	Phase 3
Inclisiran	siRNA inhibition of hepatic PCSK9 synthesis	~50%	Marketed
MK-0616 (Enlicitide decanoate)	Oral PCSK9 inhibitor	~60%	Phase 3
CVI-LM001	Oral PCSK9 inhibitor	~26%	Phase 2
Cepadacursen	Long-acting ASO targeting PCSK9	Not known	Phase 2
Bempedoic acid	Inhibits ATP-citrate lyase	~24%	Marketed
Evinacumab	ANGPTL3 inhibitor	~50%	Marketed (for HoFH)
Zodasiran	siRNA targeting hepatic ANGPTL3	~20% (mixed dyslipidemia) ~48% (HoFH)	Phase 2
Solbinsiran	GalNAc-conjugated siRNA targeting hepatic ANGPTL3	36% reduction in ApoB	Phase 2b
Obicetrapib	Inhibits CETP	~45%	Phase 3
VXX-401	Anti-PCSK9 vaccine	~65% (NHPs)	Phase 1
VERVE-201	CRISPR/Cas9-based editing of *ANGPTL3*	~46% (NHPs)	Phase 1b
VERVE-101	CRISPR/Cas9-based editing of *PCSK9*	~46%	Phase 1
CTX310	CRISPR/Cas9-based editing of *ANGPTL3*	Not known	Phase 1

mAb = monoclonal antibody; PCSK9 = proprotein convertase subtilisin/kexin type 9; siRNA = small interfering RNA; ASO = antisense oligonucleotide; ANGPTL3 = angiopoietin-like protein 3; CETP = cholesterol ester transfer protein; HoFH = homozygous familial hypercholesterolemia; GalNAc = N-acetylgalactosamine; CRISPR = clustered regularly interspaced short palindromic repeats; NHP = non-human primate.

3. Barriers to Accessing Medicines

The concept of access to medicines was defined by Pechansky and Thomas in 1981 and encompasses five key dimensions: availability, accessibility, affordability, acceptability, and quality [56].

Availability ensures that medications are supplied sufficiently, while affordability focuses on making them economically accessible to all patients. Accessibility addresses the physical reachability and obtainability of medicines, and acceptability considers the cultural and personal preferences of patients. Finally, quality refers to safe and effective medicines that are of a consistently high standard [56,57]. Collectively, these dimensions form a comprehensive framework for evaluating and improving access to essential medicines globally.

The World Health Organization (WHO) defines access as "having medicines continuously available and affordable within one hour's walk from home" [8]. The United Nations' Sustainable Development Goal 3.8 proclaims "...access to safe, effective, quality and affordable essential medicines and vaccines for all" [58].

Access to therapies will be considered in terms of economic, geographical, regulatory, and knowledge barriers.

3.1. Economic Barriers: The Availability and Affordability of Medicines

Availability has been defined by the WHO as the percentage of medicine outlets or facilities having a particular medication in stock at any one time [57,59,60]. A threshold of 80% is the target set by the WHO to declare the availability of essential affordable medicines within a particular region [57,59,60]. This reflects an understanding that while 100% availability may be ideal, it is often impractical due to logistical, economic, and systemic challenges that health systems may face. This is particularly true of LMIC, and thus, 80% serves as a realistic and impactful target.

The WHO determines affordability according to the number of days' wages needed to buy a one-month supply of medicines for chronic conditions based on the daily wage of the lowest-paid unskilled government worker. Medicines are considered unaffordable if the total cost exceeds 20% of the household income [57,59].

Economic barriers significantly impact the availability and affordability of LLTs across different income regions. Despite the clinical efficacy of lipid-lowering therapies, the financial implications often hinder their widespread adoption. High-intensity statins and ezetimibe are generally available, although significant treatment gaps remain [3,12,55].

The World Heart Federation survey drew respondents from 38 countries, with most being from the US and Europe and most working in an urban setting [3]. In LICs, 40% reported that fixed-dose statin/ezetimibe combinations were not available, and 60% noted that PCSK9 inhibitors were not available [3]. These availability issues are less pronounced in UMICs and HICs, highlighting the disparities in access [3].

Generic drugs are more affordable than patented drugs as they are usually priced more closely to the cost of production [61]. Significant disparities exist both within and between countries in terms of the availability of generic medications. Up to 20% of generic medicines are available in the public sector, whereas 60% can be found in the private sector in LMICs [60]. Poor availability of medicines in the public sector often forces patients to seek more expensive options from private facilities [60].

In patients surveyed across 21 countries (HICs, UMICs, LMICs and LICs), the availability of CV medicines was found to be 50% for antihypertensives, 62.8% for anti-platelets, and 87.2% for statins [55,59]. Importantly, 29.4% of providers who were surveyed reported that while the drugs were available but not affordable, and 25.7% lacked access to all three drugs [59]. Only 51% of participants were using a lipid-lowering agent, with 80% of participants remaining with an LDL-C above the target of 100 mg/dL [62]. CV medicines are generally unaffordable in most countries, particularly in LICs, as 75% of households in LICs and 24% in MICs could not afford two antihypertensive drugs and a statin.

Post-manufacture costs, including duties, taxes, markups, and additional charges, further increase the financial burden on patients [57,59]. In LMICs, inadequate public financing limits the availability of essential CV medicines, despite the implementation of social health insurance in some areas [3,59]. Patients without insurance who pay out of pocket often find medicines unaffordable. The affordability of combination therapy for secondary prevention of CVD is also problematic, with 33% of households in LMICs and 60% in LICs being unable to afford such treatment [57,59]. Increased copayments for medicines have been shown to reduce usage, though this evidence primarily comes from HICs [57].

Significant variability has been seen in the pricing of PCSK9 inhibitors worldwide, ranging from USD 127 per standard unit (SU) in Korea to USD 949 per SU in Argentina [23].

The affordability of medicines is often compared to the international reference price. Patented medication manufacturer prices in the US are typically 20–40% more compared to other HICs, whereas generics are cheaper in the US [63]. Government-procured generics are priced 1.5 to 3 times higher than the reference prices, while the same generics cost patients approximately 15 times the reference price in the public sector and 30 times in the private sector [57]. In the public sector, a one-month supply of a generic CVD medicine costs an average of 2 days' wages, whereas an original brand costs 8.3 days' wages for the lowest-paid government worker [57,59]. Procurement prices in LMICs are significantly higher than international reference prices, averaging 17 times higher for brand medicines and 4.5 times higher for generics [59]. Patient prices are even more inflated, being 11.2 times the international reference price for generics in the public sector [59]. The disparities in access to CV medicine between the private and public sectors, and across different countries and income levels, are significant. In the private sector, these medicines are more readily available but often less affordable, highlighting the crucial role both sectors play in ensuring access to CV treatments [59].

The high cost of novel LLTs and the increasing burden of NCDs challenge the feasibility and sustainability of universal health coverage. This contributes to the increasing burden of CVD in LMICs, where more than three-quarters of CVD-related deaths occur [59].

3.2. Geographical Barriers: Disparities in Accessibility Based on Location and Healthcare Infrastructure

Geographical barriers affect accessibility based on location and the quality of healthcare infrastructure. Structural barriers, such as limited national funding, slow inclusion of CV medicines in EMLs, and supply chain inefficiencies, exacerbate the problem, making guideline-based treatment challenging [57,59,64]. Studies have shown that the inadequate presence of healthcare workers and long distances to health facilities are significant challenges to accessing medicines and healthcare in LMICs [59].

In sub-Saharan Africa, patients often travel long distances to access health facilities. Indeed, up to 35% of patients with chronic diseases in LMICs travel more than 15 min to visit health facilities [59]. Accessibility is crucial, as patients must be able to obtain medicines even if they are affordable. Inefficient transportation systems, infrastructural inadequacies, a lack of accountability, and a low density of healthcare workers are major barriers to accessing CV medicines [57,59]. High rates of absenteeism among public-sector health workers can further hinder this access [57,59].

In LMICs, geographical location greatly affects access to NCD medicines, with those living in the capital having better access than rural residents, and long travel times to health facilities significantly reducing overall access [57]. Significant disparities exist between the public and private sectors, urban and rural areas, and various income levels, with CV medicines being more available but less affordable in the private sector, highlighting the need for policy measures to ensure access across all regions, especially in low-income economies facing high CV morbidity and mortality [59].

3.3. Knowledge Barriers: Limited Awareness and Acceptability among Healthcare Providers and Patients about New Treatment Options

Low acceptability among patients and healthcare workers, compounded by physicians' preferences for non-EML brands and complex treatment regimens, leads to poor patient adherence to medications and non-compliance with local guidelines [57,59]. This results in low treatment rates and medication adherence, despite the availability of medicines. Adherence to daily LDL-C-lowering medications is hindered by patient factors like risk perception and health literacy [65].

Non-adherence by both healthcare providers and patients further reduces the acceptability of treatments. Patient beliefs about the necessity and potential side effects of medication further contribute to non-adherence [57]. The World Heart Federation survey highlighted further roadblocks and potential solutions in ASCVD management [3]. The survey found significant disparities in clinician comfort with prescribing high-potency statins, especially in LMICs, where 60% of respondents were uncomfortable with such prescriptions compared to 35% in HICs [3].

Patient perceptions play a crucial role, with many patients in LICs finding it challenging to understand the risks associated with ASCVD and the benefits of cholesterol-lowering medications, leading to low treatment acceptance and adherence [3]. Healthcare systems often focus on treating diseases in secondary and tertiary care settings rather than on primary care and health preservation, presenting a major barrier to ASCVD prevention [3]. There is also a gap between the awareness of what combination therapies to use and their correct application, indicating the need for improved education and training among healthcare providers [3]. Simplifying prescription access through electronic solutions could help, but low awareness and acceptance of new treatments like PCSK9 inhibitors and siRNA-based therapies among providers and patients remain significant barriers [65].

Overall, the acceptability of CV medicines is influenced by a range of factors, including provider and patient perceptions, the complexity of treatment regimens, and the availability of high-quality medicines. Addressing these issues is crucial for improving CV disease outcomes, particularly in LMICs. Additionally, patent laws and systemic deficiencies contribute to the burden of counterfeit drugs in LMICs [59].

3.4. Regulatory Barriers: Delays in Approval Processes, Access Restrictions, and Quality Assurance

The prevalence of substandard and counterfeit medicines presents a major challenge, particularly in Africa, where regulatory oversight is often insufficient, with a recent study indicating that 16.3% of CV medicines in Africa are of low quality, making them one of the most commonly reported substandard medicine classes in the WHO monitoring system [59]. Concerns about medicine quality are global, leading to interventions like regular quality testing by large procurement agencies to ensure a consistent supply of quality products from manufacturers or distributors [57].

The substantial financial burden incurred by novel LLTs prompts insurers to implement stringent cost-containment strategies such as prior authorization (PA) requirements and step therapy [66]. The PA process, involving extensive paperwork and data collection, causes delays and discourages access, while step therapy mandates that patients try and fail on less expensive medications before being approved for novel agents like PCSK9 inhibitors, further delaying access to effective treatment [66]. These regulatory hurdles are compounded by a burdensome appeals process, which diverts healthcare providers' time and resources away from patient care, sometimes even imposing financial burdens on physicians through filing fees for appeals [66].

Over a period of 3 years, 91% of initial claims for PSCK9 inhibitors through commercial insurers were rejected. Following an appeals process, this figure declined to 53% [66]. But, importantly, 74% of patients who were not granted access to PCSK9 inhibitors did not commence alternative LLT [66]. In people presumed to have FH who were not meeting the recommended LDL-C targets, more than 60% of applications for PCSK9 inhibitors were rejected [67].

Meeting rigorous criteria to access therapies PCSK9 is time-consuming [68]. The bureaucracy related to these regulatory difficulties can inhibit healthcare provider prescribing [29,30]. The delays and denials can have serious implications for patient outcomes, particularly for those at high risk for cardiovascular events. Timely access to PCSK9 inhibitors is crucial for optimal lipid management and reducing ASCVD risk [66].

Inconsistencies in the approval processes further complicate access, with similar clinical histories receiving different decisions, undermining trust in the system. Additionally, the administrative burden of managing these processes imposes significant costs on medical practices, straining healthcare resources and disrupting the essential patient–clinician relationship [66].

The biannual update of the WHO Model List of Essential Medicines serves as a guide for countries to create their own prioritized medication lists according to local health needs, but applying comparative cost-effectiveness on a global scale is difficult [57]. A study conducted in sub-Saharan Africa revealed that 40% of countries had not revised their EMLs in the past five years [57]. LICs generally include CVD medicines less frequently than HICs, and only about half of countries include at least one medicine from each of the four secondary prevention therapeutic groups (aspirin, beta-blocker, ACE inhibitor, and statin) on their EMLs, with statin inclusion rates of 43%, 75%, and 69% for LICs, LMICs, and HICs, respectively [57]. The availability of generic medicines for acute conditions is generally higher than that for chronic conditions in both public and private sectors [57].

HICs have stringent regulatory frameworks (e.g., FDA and EMA) that thoroughly evaluate the safety and efficacy of novel LLTs. LMICs may possess regulatory authorities that are underfunded with inadequate expertise, which leads to less rigorous or inconsistently enforced standards that result in variations in drug quality and availability. HICs can also benefit from quicker access to novel therapies with fast-track regulatory approval programs.

3.5. *Systemic Racism as a Barrier to Access*

Structural inequalities, including systemic racism, play a significant role in shaping healthcare access and outcomes [69]. Racism within healthcare systems can manifest in various forms, including unequal treatment, bias in diagnosis and treatment decisions, and disparities in access to quality care based on race or ethnicity [69–71]. Systemic racism contributes to socioeconomic disparities, lack of health insurance coverage, and limited access to healthcare facilities, exacerbating the challenges in obtaining necessary treatments [69]. Racial disparities are seen throughout the field of medicine and, no less, in the access to LLTs [71,72].

4. Barriers and Their Budget Impact on CV Outcomes

A major barrier to adequate LDL-C lowering in LICs is the lack of registration for these therapies, as 75% of respondents in LICs cited the absence of registration for fixed-dose statin/ezetimibe combinations and PCSK9 inhibitors [3]. While LMICs also face registration challenges, they are less severe, with only 10% of UMIC respondents reporting issues with PCSK9 inhibitors [3].

Regarding prescription practices, none of the four treatments (high-intensity statins, ezetimibe, fixed-dose combinations, or PCSK9 inhibitors) are universally prescribed freely in the public sector in LICs [3]. Only 50% of respondents in LICs noted that high-intensity statins could be freely prescribed, whereas approximately 75% reported that ezetimibe, fixed-dose combinations, and PCSK9 inhibitors could not be freely prescribed [3]. In contrast, HICs typically allow most LLTs, apart from PCSK9 inhibitors, to be prescribed freely in the public sector.

Raised LDL-C in young adults is linked to later life ASCVD, yet most do not receive LLT. A study, using the U.S. National Health and Nutrition Examination Survey (NHANES) database, found that initiating statin treatment for young adults with LDL-C $\geq$ 130 mg/dL is highly cost-effective in men (USD 31,000/quality-adjusted life-year [QALY]) and moderately cost-effective in women (USD 106,000/QALY), with lifestyle interventions being less effective and more costly [73].

LLTs are most cost-effective in high-risk populations. The higher the risk, the greater the absolute risk reduction when the treatment is given, making the intervention more cost-effective [74]. Since men typically have higher baseline risk and higher rates of ASCVD events, lowering risk and preventing events lead to a more significant increase in QALYs for men as compared to women [74,75]. Furthermore, women generally have a longer life expectancy than men and, although this means they may benefit from more years of treatment, it also means costs are spread over a longer period of time.

Low/moderate-intensity statins combined with ezetimibe is the most cost-effective lipid-lowering strategy, especially when initiated at age 40, with an incremental cost-effectiveness ratio of GBP 11,107 per QALY gained [76]. PCSK9 inhibitors, alirocumab and evolocumab, face significant access barriers despite their FDA approval in 2015 for lowering LDL-C in patients with FH and ASCVD [66].

A budget impact study was conducted, using a 3-year model of introducing PCSK9 inhibitors to treat adults with heterozygous FH or established ASCVD requiring additional LDL-C lowering for a hypothetical US health plan with one million members [77]. The estimated costs over three years with the maximum PCSK9 inhibitor utilization of 1–5%, were low, with a total healthcare budget impact per patient per month of USD 3.62 in year 1, USD 7.22 in year 2, and USD 10.79 in year 3 [77]. These costs are sensitive to the model's timeframe and the cost of PCSK9 inhibitors but remain modest compared to other specialty biologics. Drug cost rebates and discounts could further reduce the budget impact [77].

A cost analysis study focused on the community taxpayers' perspective in South-Eastern Italy analyzed the costs per major cardiovascular event saved using data from randomized controlled trials [78]. Individual costs per saved adverse event ranged from EUR 0.12 to EUR 0.78. For every EUR 1 spent per inhabitant annually, 2–8.3 major adverse cardiovascular events could be avoided, demonstrating that the cost per event saved with PCSK9 inhibitors can translate into very small individual costs per year [78].

In Canada, it was estimated that 51.9% of patients with ASCVD would be eligible for PCSK9 inhibitors. Although the adoption of PCSK9 inhibitors was expected to reduce primary event rates by 1.8% after three years and save USD 44 million in events, the net budget impact over three years was USD 1.5 billion [79]. Targeting high-risk subgroups could further reduce these costs and lessen the overall budgetary impact, making the adoption of PCSK9 inhibitors more economically feasible [78,79].

Inclisiran, a small interfering RNA directed against PCSK9, was found to be the least cost-effective, not being viable in any subgroup at its current price [76]. Despite being effective, inclisiran was not cost-effective in any simulation, with its current price

(GBP 3974.72) far exceeding the maximum cost-effective price (GBP 451 for men with LDL-C $\geq$ 200 mg/dL) [76]. This highlights the need for significant price reductions for inclisiran to be a viable option for primary prevention of coronary heart disease, especially considering the cost-effectiveness of statin-based strategies even with simulated non-adherence. Additionally, for secondary prevention, inclisiran would also require a substantial price reduction to be considered cost-effective compared to other PCSK9 inhibitors [76].

Cost is an even greater barrier for novel therapies such as evinacumab for the treatment of HoFH. Although clinical trials demonstrated significant LDL-C reductions, evinacumab is not cost-effective at its current price, with an Institute for Clinical and Economic Review (ICER) of USD 8,392,585 per QALY gained, far exceeding the USD 50,000 per QALY threshold. The drug costs about USD 460,839 per year per patient, highlighting the need for a significant price reduction [37]. Despite these challenges, evinacumab addresses an important unmet need, reducing morbidity and mortality in HoFH patients [80].

Despite the higher cost of novel LLTs, there is a significant benefit in their use for reducing CVEs. Acute coronary syndromes, coronary interventions, stroke, and cardiac arrest are more prevalent in patients with rejected or abandoned PCSK9 inhibitor prescriptions compared to those with paid PCSK9 inhibitor prescriptions [81]. Higher rejection rates were observed among women, racial minorities, and lower-income groups [81]. This is further reinforced by a sub-analysis of the Prospective Urban Rural Epidemiology (PURE) study, representative of different income regions, which showed that the lower availability and affordability of essential CVD medicines were associated with a higher risk of MACEs and mortality [55].

These studies highlight the critical need for improving access to these therapies to reduce CVEs globally and that, despite the initial costs, the long-term benefits of using LLTs, particularly in high-risk patients, justify their use. By preventing costly CVEs, these therapies can ultimately reduce the financial burden on healthcare systems, especially when strategic measures like targeted high-risk group treatments and cost-sharing initiatives are employed. Therefore, improving the availability and affordability of these medications should be prioritized as a cost-effective strategy to enhance CV health outcomes globally. Affordability was often lower in the private sector despite higher availability [59].

Further cost-effectiveness studies are required in a variety of contexts. Studies that evaluate lost productivity, work absenteeism, and long-term disability can also contribute to the understanding of both the economic and clinical impact of access or lack of access to LLT in different countries and regions.

5. Potential Solutions for Improving Access

5.1. Healthcare Policy Reforms

5.1.1. Pricing Regulations

Access to medications is often limited by high costs that can neither be funded by individuals nor the countries in which they live. This is a concern for patients and health systems worldwide [82].

The WHO guideline on country pharmaceutical pricing policies refers to 10 pricing policies that countries can consider when managing medicine prices.

Government intervention in pharmaceutical pricing policies can make these therapies more affordable and thus more accessible to the broader population [82].

Value-based pricing (VBP), a strategy recommended by the WHO, is an approach that considers the value and benefits of a treatment when determining its price, thereby aligning the cost of a drug with its clinical benefits and overall value to the health system [82].

Implementing a VBP system presents several challenges due to the differences in healthcare systems as well as the differences in reimbursement found across countries and regions. VBP relies on clinical outcomes and real-world evidence to determine cost-effectiveness, but these data may be inconsistent, incomplete, or unavailable [83,84]. Ongoing evaluation of drug performance can be administratively burdensome and costly, but it can lead to drug prices changing over time as new evidence emerges [83,84]. The VBP model also requires buy-in from pharmaceutical companies, who may resist lower prices which could ultimately threaten the introduction of newer therapies onto the market [83,84].

Moreover, VBP may also lead to disparities in access. Wealthier countries have the resources to conduct comprehensive cost-effectiveness analyses and have different thresholds for determining cost-effectiveness in their healthcare systems [83,84].

External reference pricing (ERP), also known as international price referencing, is a model where drug prices are set based on the prices of the same drug in other countries [85–88]. ERP can be more effective in LMICs as it allows these countries to leverage lower prices from other countries [86,87]. ERP can be easier to implement, more effective for immediate price control, and more transparent compared to internal reference pricing (IRP) [86–88]. It provides a clear framework based on observed international prices, which helps when negotiating prices with pharmaceutical companies [89,90]. Canada uses ERP to align its drug prices with those in other developed countries. This has helped to keep drug prices relatively low while maintaining access to new therapies [89,90].

By contrast, IRP involves setting the price of a new drug relative to the prices of similar drugs within a country [85]. This model encourages competition, which drives prices down but may limit the entry of novel agents if they are priced too aggressively compared to existing therapies [82,85]. IRP can encourage the introduction of generic and biosimilar drugs into the market, as manufacturers try to offer more cost-effective alternatives to reference-priced drugs [88].

If reference prices are set too low, however, it could reduce the profitability of innovative drugs, which would discourage investment in high-risk, high-reward research and development [88].

Both ERP and IRP have strengths and weaknesses, and their effectiveness can vary based on the specific economic and healthcare contexts of different countries. Many countries adopt a hybrid approach, integrating aspects of both ERP and IRP to achieve a balance between access, affordability, and innovation [88].

Countries such as Canada, Germany, the UK, Australia, and China have implemented various policy regulations which have led to lower drug prices [90–93].

Health technology assessment (HTA) is a multidisciplinary process that evaluates the medical, social, economic, and ethical implications of using a health technology (drug, medical device, or procedure) [93]. HTA aims to provide evidence-based information about efficacy, safety, and cost-effectiveness to assist with decision making regarding the reimbursement and use of a therapy within health systems [93]. HTA aims to do this in a systematic, transparent, and unbiased manner [94]. Consequently, HTA can greatly influence the cost and reimbursement status of a medication and is, thus, an important tool for prioritizing healthcare spending [82,93].

Pooled procurement, the collective purchasing of medicines by multiple entities, allows for the negotiation of better prices [82]. Purchasing and promotion of generic medicines, which are significantly cheaper than patented medicines, is another method of ensuring affordable drugs [60]. The Pan American Health Organization (PAHO) Strategic Fund, the Organisation of Eastern Caribbean States (OECS) and the Joint Procurement Agreement (JPA) by the European Union are some examples of organizations that have successfully utilized a policy of pooled procurement in order to obtain a variety of therapies at a lower cost [95–98].

Many of these policies are repeatedly assessed against their ability to contain costs, but less in terms of their ability to provide access to medications [98].

The Patented Medicine Prices Review Board (PMPRB) is a Canadian regulatory authority that performs ongoing monitoring of patented medications. If there is concern regarding pricing which is deemed to be unreasonable, then public hearings may be held, following which orders may be issued to reduce a particular medication's price [99]. Within the European Union, several countries employ strict and rigorous pricing models which have led to lower drug costs [93,94].

Collaborative approaches between regulatory authorities and pharmaceutical companies involving these pricing policy approaches and ensuring more transparency in terms of real medicine costs, research, and development will contribute towards the curtailment of high prices.

5.1.2. Reimbursement Policies

Effective reimbursement policies ensure that out-of-pocket expenses are limited and that patients can afford their medications. Public insurance programs (such as Medicare and Medicaid in the US) can provide comprehensive public access to therapies which improve medication adherence and health outcomes.

Universal health coverage systems (such as those in Canada, the UK, and France) enable the public health system to cover most medications [100].

In countries with social health insurance systems, like Germany, mandatory health insurance covers most drug costs with modest copayments. Germany has an annual cap on out-of-pocket expenses which is set at 2% of household income, or 1% for the chronically ill [100,101]. Sweden implements a high-cost threshold system where patients pay the full price up to a certain amount, following which the government covers the costs [100].

While many healthcare systems contribute towards the cost of medicines, high copayments remain an economic barrier for many patients. Subsidies or reduced copayments based on an individual's income can make medicines more affordable and improve access. Furthermore, providing exemption status for specific groups, such as children, the elderly, low-income individuals, or those with chronic conditions, can ensure that these groups have access to necessary medications [102–104].

Tiered formulary systems are often used by private insurers to manage the costs of drugs. Drugs are classified into different tiers based on efficacy and cost. For example, tier 1 would include generic drugs with no copayments. Tier 2 might comprise preferred brand-name drugs. Tier 3 would include high-cost specialty drugs where many novel lipid-lowering therapies may be found and carry higher copayments. While tiered formulary systems may improve access to affordable medications, the high out-of-pocket expenses for higher-tier medications remain a barrier for many patients [85,93].

Risk-sharing agreements are outcome-based contracts that tie reimbursement to the clinical efficacy of the therapy. This model has been applied by some insurers to PCSK9 inhibitors where reimbursement depends on specific reductions in LDL-C and cardiovascular events [68].

5.1.3. Public Funding and Subsidies

Government-allocated funds could subsidize the cost of LLTs. Public health programs can provide these medications free to eligible patients, a system seen in various national health systems globally. However, although government subsidies for novel therapies may offset some costs, this strategy is likely unsustainable for many countries, particularly LMICs due to limited resources and competing healthcare priorities.

Public–private partnerships (PPPs) can be powerful means of leveraging both sectors. Joint ventures that focus on research and development of novel therapies allow for the pooling of resources and the sharing of both the risks and the benefits. The addition of public funding can be used to "de-risk" private investments in high-risk areas of drug development. Governments can offer grants, subsidies, or tax incentives to encourage private sector participation [105,106].

The establishment of prize funds and advanced market commitments to incentivize the development of novel therapies also can help address unmet medical needs. Furthermore, offering market exclusivity for pharmaceutical companies that develop and bring novel medications to market can incentivize development [105].

Intellectual property policies that strike a balance between rewarding innovation and ensuring access [107]. This can include measures like patent pools and promoting generic competition after patents expire. Encouraging voluntary licensing agreements where the patent holders grant licenses to manufacturers in LMICs to produce and distribute affordable versions of novel LLTs can improve access in underserved regions [105,106].

5.1.4. Innovative Funding Models

The pharmaceutical industry has also recognized its own role in improving access to medications. The European Federation of Pharmaceutical Industries and Associations (EFPIA) has described the need for novel approaches to existing traditional pricing models [94]. Some of these approaches include outcome-based payments, whereby the payment for a medicine is dependent on its real-world performance and is based on measurable outcomes [94]. Over-time or staggered payments allow payers to make payments to manufacturers over a period while the patient receives therapy [94]. This mitigates the high upfront cost of medications. Subscription payments can be used to delink payment for a treatment from the number of patients who receive treatment [94].

Combination-based pricing addresses the notion that combination therapies are not necessarily the added value of medicines used separately [94].

5.2. Streamlining Regulatory Processes

While most initial claims for PCSK9 inhibitor therapy are rejected, engaging in an appeals process with insurers leads to positive outcomes in a significant number of cases [108].

The regulatory approval process can often be lengthy and complex, and streamlining this process can facilitate quicker patient access to novel therapeutics while still maintaining rigorous safety and efficacy standards.

Regulatory requirements can vary significantly between regions. Harmonizing these regulations can reduce redundancy, decrease approval times, and facilitate simultaneous launches in multiple markets.

Mutual recognition agreements (MRAs) allow regulatory agencies in different countries to rely on each other's inspection reports and regulatory decisions. This reduces duplication and speeds up the approval process. At present, the FDA has MRAs with the EU, Switzerland, and the United Kingdom.

International regulatory bodies, such as the FDA (US) and EMA (Europe), work together through initiatives like the International Council for Harmonization of Technical Requirements for Pharmaceuticals for Human Use (ICH) [109]. The ICH brings together regulatory bodies and industry to facilitate discussion on the scientific and technical aspects of drug registration. Consistent guidelines on clinical trials, manufacturing standards, and drug evaluation can simplify the approval process across different jurisdictions [109].

Expedited approval pathways can significantly reduce the time required to bring novel LLTs to market, particularly for drugs that address unmet medical needs. This is particularly relevant for rare lipid disorders such as homozygous FH.

The FDA, as an example, has a number of expedited drug approval programs. Programs like the FDA's Fast Track Designation aims to expedite the review of drugs intended to treat serious medical conditions. The Breakthrough Therapy Designation is granted by the FDA to drugs that show a marked improvement over existing therapies based on preliminary clinical evidence. The Accelerated Approval program allows for earlier approval of drugs that treat serious conditions and fill an unmet medical need [110]. Post-marketing studies are required to confirm the clinical benefits following accelerated approval [110].

Good post-market surveillance and pharmacovigilance allow regulatory bodies to monitor the safety and effectiveness of new therapies after their approval. This effectively provides a safety net that allows for earlier market access [111].

5.3. Public Health Interventions

5.3.1. Telemedicine

The utilization of telemedicine allows patients living in remote areas to access medical care [112]. Telemedicine was initially established to assist with the timely management of acute conditions such as stroke, myocardial infarction, or trauma [113,114]. It has since expanded to encompass the comprehensive care of chronic diseases such as heart failure and diabetes [112,115,116]. As a result, telemedicine has become one of the fastest-growing healthcare delivery modalities in the US [112].

Access to healthcare can be considered in terms of three core components: entry into a health system, adequate supply of services, and timely provision of care [112]. Telemedicine can effectively address many limitations encountered by each of these aspects of healthcare access.

A significant barrier to entry into a health system is transportation. Cost, geographical distance, lack of reliable transportation, and inability to drive due to patient health status are major factors limiting patient access [117]. There is a growing shortage of physicians worldwide, particularly in rural areas and in LMICs [112,118]. Healthcare provider availability significantly influences access to treatment. Waiting times, which may be considerably longer for specialists, may also be a deterrent to accessing healthcare systems [112]. Telemedicine has been found to facilitate communication and increase collaboration between specialists and community healthcare providers.

Telemedicine has demonstrated similar, and sometimes better, health outcomes compared to the traditional models of care, and this is also true for improving access to LLTs [119,120]. There are, however, limitations to telemedicine, which may create their own barriers to access. These include the inability to perform clinical examinations, the loss of a patient–provider relationship, or the inability to respond to non-verbal cues during consultations [120]. Indeed, technological dexterity may vary across patient age groups, and the technological requirements for telemedicine may present an added cost to patients [120,121].

Interventions to improve access to telemedicine services in rural areas and LMICs might include improving technology infrastructure but also tailoring systems to patients and/or healthcare facilities with different technology infrastructure capabilities. The use of social media channels to improve awareness about telemedicine, providing dedicated outreach and technical support to people with limited access or familiarity with new technologies, and expanding insurance to include coverage for telehealth consultations are all effective strategies for improving access to telemedicine services that could be employed in rural areas and LMICs [122].

Disparities related to age, ethnicity, and socioeconomic status may, however, be exacerbated by telemedicine, creating further barriers to accessing treatment [112]. Confidentiality, legal liability, and data security are also legitimate concerns affecting a broader uptake of telemedicine [121].

Telemedicine has improved the geographical barriers to medical care and access, but to a lesser extent the social and economic disparities.

5.3.2. Education and Advocacy

Addressing knowledge barriers requires multifaceted approaches. Healthcare provider behavior change is necessary [57]. Ongoing training and educational resources for healthcare providers can ensure they are equipped to prescribe novel therapies appropriately. For example, the PCSK9 Forum is a not-for-profit educational resource offered to healthcare providers at no cost [123].

Healthcare providers should also undergo training to recognize and address implicit biases, ensuring equitable treatment for all patients. Diversification of clinical trials too improves access for racial groups that are often under-represented [71]. However, addressing systemic racism requires multifaceted approaches at various levels, including policy reforms to promote health equity and anti-discrimination measures within healthcare systems [69].

For patients, forgetting to take medications is a significant barrier to adherence, particularly when polypharmacy is required to reduce ASCVD risk. Specific strategies like text reminders and fixed-dose combination (FDC) pills improve adherence [66]. Combining several CV medicines into one FDC form, or "polypill", has been suggested to increase adherence, reduce delivery costs, and ease supply-chain burdens. A statin and ezetimibe FDC significantly improved LDL-C reduction and patient compliance compared to separate pills [124]. However, only 31.5% of patients using the FDC reached recommended LDL-C levels [124]. In a phase 3 trial, the FDC of bempedoic acid and ezetimibe outperformed ezetimibe alone and bempedoic acid alone [125]. These findings highlight the potential of FDCs to enhance LLT effectiveness and patient adherence.

Educational initiatives aimed at increasing patient awareness and improving public knowledge can also improve the uptake of novel therapies.

Patient advocacy groups and professional physician societies/organizations (such as the American Heart Association (AHA), European Society of Cardiology, National Lipid Association, and Family Heart Foundation) are important in raising awareness around lipid disorders and the need for access to effective LLTs. Indeed, a number of these groups were effective in campaigning for lower costs and broader access to PCSK9 inhibitors, which eventually led to a significant price drop in these therapies [126].

In order to overcome the barriers to access to innovation for patients who need it, a new initiative called SMASH is being deployed. The goal of SMASH (System and Molecular Approaches of Severe Hyperlipidemias) is to facilitate access to accurate diagnosis and precise treatments for patients with rare or severe lipid disorders, regardless of their economic status, mobility, or living environment, including patients in remote regions or emerging economies. SMASH has several dedicated platforms, accessible to the various actors and organizations involved in the world of rare or severe lipid diseases. This initiative is described in more detail elsewhere. To raise awareness about access to diagnosis and innovative treatments for patients with rare or severe diseases, individuals and organizations are strongly invited to sign the SMASH declaration (manifesto) at www.smash-access.org.

5.3.3. Multidisciplinary Teams

Utilizing clinical services within the community pharmacy setting can also be used to reduce costs and improve access. Community pharmacists can assist with prior authorizations, the administration of drugs such as PCSK9 inhibitors, patient education, and follow-up point-of-care cholesterol testing [127].

Effective collaboration between primary care and specialist care teams can ensure that novel therapies are rolled out at the primary care level [30,127].

6. Future Directions and Recommendations

Collaboration between healthcare providers, policymakers, industry, and patient advocacy groups is important for addressing barriers to access.

Policymakers should look to implement pricing regulations and utilize innovative funding models that ensure affordability and access to LLTs for all patient populations. Streamlining regulatory processes will not only prevent delays in medication approvals but also ensure that quality standards are maintained. Investment within public health structures such as collaborative community-based programs, telemedicine, and educational initiatives for both patients and providers is recommended.

Healthcare providers should stay up to date on the latest guidelines and recommendations for the management of dyslipidemia, especially with regard to novel LLTs. Providers are important advocates for patient access to LLTs. Telemedicine and community-based services can reach underserved populations and improve medication adherence.

The pharmaceutical industry should consider novel pricing policies such as value-based pricing models and outcome-based payment arrangements which may make novel LLTs more affordable and accessible.

Patient advocacy groups should continue to advocate for policies and initiatives that promote equitable access to LLTs for all patients, regardless of socioeconomic status or geographical location; raise awareness about dyslipidemia and the importance of early detection and treatment to prevent cardiovascular events; and provide support and resources to patients navigating insurance coverage, medication affordability, and adherence to LLT regimens.

Acknowledging and addressing systemic racism as a barrier to accessing LLT will address the racial disparity that exists throughout medicine. Inclusive and diversified clinical trials that will be more representative of the population at large should be encouraged.

7. Conclusions

Statins will remain the cornerstone for lipid management for the foreseeable future. Improving access to statins and ezetimibe in LICs as a bare minimum would alleviate a major obstacle to care. However, when lifestyle interventions and statins are insufficient to meet LDL-C targets to reduce ASCVD, additional lipid-lowering therapies need to be considered. Novel lipid-lowering therapies are being developed rapidly, increasing the options to reduce the risk for ASCVD, but currently available drugs have been significantly underutilized worldwide.

While novel LLTs offer significant clinical benefits, their high costs, together with other barriers, limit their impact. Addressing these challenges through health policy interventions, insurance reforms, improved healthcare delivery, and education initiatives can improve access and ensure that more patients benefit from these advancements in dyslipidemia management.

Author Contributions: Conceptualization, B.S.M., F.M. and F.J.R.; writing—review, B.S.M., M.L. and F.M.; writing—review and editing, B.S.M. and F.J.R.; supervision, F.J.R. All authors have read and agreed to the published version of the manuscript.

Funding: This research received no external funding.

Data Availability Statement: Not applicable.

Conflicts of Interest: The authors declare no conflicts of interest. F.J.R. has received honoraria from Amgen, Sanofi-Aventis, Novartis, and LIB Therapeutics, with no conflicts of interest related to this manuscript.

References

1. Naghavi, M.; Ong, K.L.; Aali, A.; Ababneh, H.S.; Abate, Y.H.; Abbafati, C.; Abbasgholizadeh, R.; Abbasian, M.; Abbasi-Kangevari, M.; Abbastabar, H.; et al. Global burden of 288 causes of death and life expectancy decomposition in 204 countries and territories and 811 subnational locations, 1990–2021: A systematic analysis for the Global Burden of Disease Study 2021. *Lancet* **2024**, *403*, 2100–2132. [CrossRef] [PubMed]
2. Martin, S.S.; Aday, A.W.; Almarzooq, Z.I.; Anderson, C.A.M.; Arora, P.; Avery, C.L.; Baker-Smith, C.M.; Gibbs, B.B.; Beaton, A.Z.; Boehme, A.K.; et al. 2024 Heart Disease and Stroke Statistics: A Report of US and Global Data From the American Heart Association. *Circulation* **2024**, *149*, e347–e913. [CrossRef] [PubMed]
3. Ray, K.K.; Ference, B.A.; Séverin, T.; Blom, D.; Nicholls, S.J.; Shiba, M.H.; Almahmeed, W.; Alonso, R.; Daccord, M.; Ezhov, M.; et al. World Heart Federation Cholesterol Roadmap 2022. *Glob. Heart* **2022**, *17*, 75. [CrossRef] [PubMed]
4. Li, C.; Spencer, G.; Husain, M.J.; Nugent, R.; Auzenne, D.; Kostova, D.; Richter, P. Barriers to accessibility of medicines for hyperlipidemia in low- and middle-income countries. *PLoS Glob Public Health* **2024**, *4*, e0002905. [CrossRef] [PubMed]
5. Maddox, K.E.J.; Elkind, M.S.V.; Aparicio, H.J.; Commodore-Mensah, Y.; de Ferranti, S.D.; Dowd, W.N.; Hernandez, A.F.; Khavjou, O.; Michos, E.D.; Palaniappan, L.; et al. Forecasting the Economic Burden of Cardiovascular Disease and Stroke in the United States Through 2050: A Presidential Advisory from the American Heart Association. *Circulation* **2024**, *149*. [CrossRef]
6. Yusuf, S.; Joseph, P.; Rangarajan, S.; Islam, S.; Mente, A.; Hystad, P.; Brauer, M.; Kutty, V.R.; Gupta, R.; Wielgosz, A.; et al. Modifiable risk factors, cardiovascular disease, and mortality in 155 722 individuals from 21 high-income, middle-income, and low-income countries (PURE): A prospective cohort study. *Lancet* **2020**, *395*, 795–808. [CrossRef]
7. WHO Model List of Essential Medicines—23rd List. 2023. Available online: https://www.who.int/publications-detail-redirect/WHO-MHP-HPS-EML-2023.02 (accessed on 19 May 2024).
8. MDG Gap Task Force (Ed.) *Delivering on the Global Partnership for Achieving the Millennium Development Goals: Millennium Development Goal 8: MDG Gap Task Force Report 2008*; United Nations: New York, NY, USA, 2008.
9. MDG Gap Task Force Report. UNDP. Available online: https://www.undp.org/publications/mdg-gap-task-force-report (accessed on 19 May 2024).
10. Mach, F.; Baigent, C.; Catapano, A.L.; Koskinas, K.C.; Casula, M.; Badimon, L.; Chapman, M.J.; De Backer, G.G.; Delgado, V.; Ference, B.A.; et al. 2019 ESC/EAS Guidelines for the management of dyslipidaemias: Lipid modification to reduce cardiovascular risk. *Eur. Heart J.* **2020**, *41*, 111–188. [CrossRef] [PubMed]

11. Ray, K.K.; Molemans, B.; Schoonen, W.M.; Giovas, P.; Bray, S.; Kiru, G.; Murphy, J.; Banach, M.; De Servi, S.; Gaita, D.; et al. EU-Wide Cross-Sectional Observational Study of Lipid-Modifying Therapy Use in Secondary and Primary Care: The DA VINCI study. *Eur. J. Prev. Cardiol.* **2021**, *28*, 1279–1289. [CrossRef] [PubMed]
12. Ray, K.K.; Haq, I.; Bilitou, A.; Manu, M.C.; Burden, A.; Aguiar, C.; Arca, M.; Connolly, D.L.; Eriksson, M.; Ferrieres, J.; et al. Treatment gaps in the implementation of LDL cholesterol control among high- and very high-risk patients in Europe between 2020 and 2021: The multinational observational SANTORINI study. *Lancet Reg. Health Eur.* **2023**, *29*, 100624. [CrossRef]
13. Newman, C.B.; Preiss, D.; Tobert, J.A.; Jacobson, T.A.; Page II, R.L.; Goldstein, L.B.; Chin, C.; Tannock, L.R.; Miller, M.; Raghuveer, G.; et al. Statin Safety and Associated Adverse Events: A Scientific Statement from the American Heart Association. *ATVB* **2019**, *39*, e38–e81. [CrossRef]
14. Stroes, E.S.; Thompson, P.D.; Corsini, A.; Vladutiu, G.D.; Raal, F.J.; Ray, K.K.; Roden, M.; Stein, E.; Tokgözoğlu, L.; Nordestgaard, B.G.; et al. Statin-associated muscle symptoms: Impact on statin therapy—European Atherosclerosis Society Consensus Panel Statement on Assessment, Aetiology and Management. *Eur. Heart J.* **2015**, *36*, 1012–1022. [CrossRef] [PubMed]
15. Howard, J.P.; Wood, F.A.; Finegold, J.A.; Nowbar, A.N.; Thompson, D.M.; Arnold, A.D.; Rajkumar, C.A.; Connolly, S.; Cegla, J.; Stride, C.; et al. Side Effect Patterns in a Crossover Trial of Statin, Placebo, and No Treatment. *J. Am. Coll. Cardiol.* **2021**, *78*, 1210–1222. [CrossRef]
16. Wood, F.A.; Howard, J.P.; Finegold, J.A.; Nowbar, A.N.; Thompson, D.M.; Arnold, A.D.; Rajkumar, C.A.; Connolly, S.; Cegla, J.; Stride, C.; et al. N-of-1 Trial of a Statin, Placebo, or No Treatment to Assess Side Effects. *N. Engl. J. Med.* **2020**, *383*, 2182–2184. [CrossRef] [PubMed]
17. Nielsen, S.F.; Nordestgaard, B.G. Negative statin-related news stories decrease statin persistence and increase myocardial infarction and cardiovascular mortality: A nationwide prospective cohort study. *Eur. Heart J.* **2016**, *37*, 908–916. [CrossRef]
18. Raal, F.J.; Mohamed, F. Statins: Are they appropriate for all patients? *Lancet Glob. Health* **2022**, *10*, e305–e306. [CrossRef]
19. Goal 3: Good Health and Well-Being. United Nations Development Programme. Available online: https://www.undp.org/sustainable-development-goals/good-health (accessed on 18 May 2024).
20. Sabatine, M.S.; Giugliano, R.P.; Keech, A.C.; Honarpour, N.; Wiviott, S.D.; Murphy, S.A.; Kuder, J.F.; Wang, H.; Liu, T.; Wasserman, S.M.; et al. Evolocumab and Clinical Outcomes in Patients with Cardio vascular Disease. *N. Engl. J. Med.* **2017**, *376*, 1713–1722. [CrossRef] [PubMed]
21. Schwartz, G.G.; Steg, P.G.; Szarek, M.; Bhatt, D.L.; Bittner, V.A.; Diaz, R.; Edelberg, J.M.; Goodman, S.G.; Hanotin, C.; Harrington, R.A.; et al. Alirocumab and Cardiovascular Outcomes after Acute Coronary Syndrome. *N. Engl. J. Med.* **2018**, *379*, 2097–2107. [CrossRef]
22. Lloyd-Jones, D.M.; Morris, P.B.; Ballantyne, C.M.; Birtcher, K.K.; Covington, A.M.; DePalma, S.M.; Minissian, M.B.; Orringer, C.E.; Smith, S.C., Jr.; Waring, A.A.; et al. 2022 ACC Expert Consensus Decision Pathway on the Role of Nonstatin Therapies for LDL-Cholesterol Lowering in the Management of Atherosclerotic Cardiovascular Disease Risk. *J. Am. Coll. Cardiol.* **2022**, *80*, 1366–1418. [CrossRef] [PubMed]
23. Blais, J.E.; Wei, Y.; Knapp, M.; Wong, I.C.K.; Wei, L.; Chan, E.W. Trends in PCSK9 inhibitor utilization in the United States, Europe, and other countries: An analysis of international sales data. *Am. Heart J.* **2022**, *248*, 13–20. [CrossRef]
24. Keam, S.J. Tafolecimab: First Approval. *Drugs* **2023**, *83*, 1545–1549. [CrossRef]
25. Chai, M.; He, Y.; Zhao, W.; Han, X.; Zhao, G.; Ma, X.; Qiao, P.; Shi, D.; Liu, Y.; Han, W.; et al. Efficacy and safety of tafolecimab in Chinese patients with heterozygous familial hypercholesterolemia: A randomized, double-blind, placebo-controlled phase 3 trial (CREDIT-2). *BMC Med.* **2023**, *21*, 77. [CrossRef] [PubMed]
26. Huo, Y.; Chen, B.; Lian, Q.; Wang, S.; Liu, L.; Lu, D.; Qu, Y.; Zheng, G.; Li, L.; Ji, Y.; et al. Tafolecimab in Chinese patients with non-familial hypercholesterolemia (CREDIT-1): A 48-week randomized, double-blind, placebo-controlled phase 3 trial. *Lancet Reg. Health West. Pac.* **2023**, *41*, 100907. [CrossRef] [PubMed]
27. Raal, F.J.; Kallend, D.; Ray, K.K.; Turner, T.; Koenig, W.; Wright, R.S.; Wijngaard, P.L.J.; Curcio, D.; Jaros, M.J.; Leiter, L.A.; et al. Inclisiran for the Treatment of Heterozygous Familial Hypercholesterolemia. *N. Engl. J. Med.* **2020**, *382*, 1520–1530. [CrossRef] [PubMed]
28. Ray, K.K.; Wright, R.S.; Kallend, D.; Koenig, W.; Leiter, L.A.; Raal, F.J.; Bisch, J.A.; Richardson, T.; Jaros, M.; Wijngaard, P.L.J.; et al. Two Phase 3 Trials of Inclisiran in Patients with Elevated LDL Cholesterol. *N. Engl. J. Med.* **2020**, *382*, 1507–1519. [CrossRef] [PubMed]
29. Connelly, D.; Cohen, D.; McCartney, M. Fewer than 5,000 people prescribed anticholesterol drug inclisiran in primary care as of July 2023. *Pharm. J.* **2023**. [CrossRef]
30. Iacobucci, G. GP leaders advise practices not to prescribe cholesterol lowering drug inclisiran. *BMJ* **2023**, *382*, 1757. [CrossRef] [PubMed]
31. Pinkosky, S.L.; Newton, R.S.; Day, E.A.; Ford, R.J.; Lhotak, S.; Austin, R.C.; Birch, C.M.; Smith, B.K.; Filippov, S.; Groot, P.H.E.; et al. Liver-specific ATP-citrate lyase inhibition by bempedoic acid decreases LDL-C and attenuates atherosclerosis. *Nature Communications.* **2016**, *7*, 13457. [CrossRef] [PubMed]
32. Ballantyne, C.M.; Banach, M.; Mancini, G.B.J.; Lepor, N.E.; Hanselman, J.C.; Zhao, X.; Leiter, L.A. Efficacy and safety of bempedoic acid added to ezetimibe in statin-intolerant patients with hypercholesterolemia: A randomized, placebo-controlled study. *Atherosclerosis* **2018**, *277*, 195–203. [CrossRef] [PubMed]

33. Ray, K.K.; Bays, H.E.; Catapano, A.L.; Lalwani, N.D.; Bloedon, L.T.; Sterling, L.R.; Robinson, P.L.; Ballantyne, C.M. Safety and Efficacy of Bempedoic Acid to Reduce LDL Cholesterol. *N. Engl. J. Med.* **2019**, *380*, 1022–1032. [CrossRef]
34. Goldberg, A.C.; Leiter, L.A.; Stroes, E.S.G.; Baum, S.J.; Hanselman, J.C.; Bloedon, L.T.; Lalwani, N.D.; Patel, P.M.; Zhao, X.; Duell, P.B. Effect of Bempedoic Acid vs Placebo Added to Maximally Tolerated Statins on Low-Density Lipoprotein Cholesterol in Patients at High Risk for Cardiovascular Disease: The CLEAR Wisdom Randomized Clinical Trial. *JAMA* **2019**, *322*, 1780–1788. [CrossRef]
35. Nissen, S.E.; Lincoff, A.M.; Brennan, D.; Ray, K.K.; Mason, D.; Kastelein, J.J.P.; Thompson, P.D.; Libby, P.; Cho, L.; Plutzky, J.; et al. Bempedoic Acid and Cardiovascular Outcomes in Statin- Intolerant Patients. *N. Engl. J. Med.* **2023**, *388*, 1353–1364. [CrossRef] [PubMed]
36. Mohamed, F.; Mansfield, B.; Raal, F. Targeting PCSK9 and Beyond for the Management of Low-Density Lipoprotein Cholesterol. *J. Clin. Med.* **2023**, *12*, 5082. [CrossRef] [PubMed]
37. Canadian Agency for Drugs and Technologies in Health. *Evinacumab (Evkeeza): CADTH Reimbursement Recommendation*; Canadian Agency for Drugs and Technologies in Health: Ottawa, ON, Canada, 2024. Available online: https://www.ncbi.nlm.nih.gov/books/NBK602392/ (accessed on 29 May 2024).
38. Raal, F.; Fourie, N.; Scott, R.; Blom, D.; De Vries Basson, M.; Kayikcioglu, M.; Caldwell, K.; Kallend, D.; Stein, E. Long-term efficacy and safety of lerodalcibep in heterozygous familial hypercholesterolaemia: The LIBerate-HeFH trial. *Eur. Heart J.* **2023**, *44*, 4272–4280. [CrossRef] [PubMed]
39. Koren, M.J.; Descamps, O.; Hata, Y.; Hengeveld, E.M.; Hovingh, G.K.; Ikonomidis, I.; Juul Jensen, M.D.R.; Langbakke, I.H.; Martens, F.M.A.C.; Søndergaard, A.L.; et al. PCSK9 inhibition with orally administered NNC0385-0434 in hypercholesterolaemia: A randomised, double-blind, placebo-controlled and active-controlled phase 2 trial. *Lancet Diabetes Endocrinol.* **2024**, *12*, 174–183. [CrossRef] [PubMed]
40. Ballantyne, C.M.; Banka, P.; Mendez, G.; Garcia, R.; Rosenstock, J.; Rodgers, A.; Mendizabal, G.; Mitchel, Y.; Catapano, A.L. Phase 2b Randomized Trial of the Oral PCSK9 Inhibitor MK-0616. *J. Am. Coll. Cardiol.* **2023**, *81*, 1553–1564. [CrossRef] [PubMed]
41. Kastelein, J.J.P.; Van Leuven, S.I.; Burgess, L.; Evans, G.W.; Kuivenhoven, J.A.; Barter, P.J.; Revkin, J.H.; Grobbee, D.E.; Riley, W.A.; Shear, C.L.; et al. Effect of Torcetrapib on Carotid Atherosclerosis in Familial Hypercholesterolemia. *N. Engl. J. Med.* **2007**, *356*, 1620–1630. [CrossRef] [PubMed]
42. Bowman, L.; Hopewell, J.C.; Wiviott, S.D.; Sammons, E.; Chen, F.; Wallendszus, K.; Stevens, W.; Cannon, C.P.; Braunwald, E.; Collins, R.; et al. Effects of Anacetrapib in Patients with Atherosclerotic Vascular Disease. *N. Engl. J. Med.* **2017**, *377*, 1217–1227. [CrossRef]
43. Schwartz, G.G.; Olsson, A.G.; Abt, M.; Ballantyne, C.M.; Barter, P.J.; Brumm, J.; Chaitman, B.R.; Holme, I.M.; Kallend, D.; Leiter, L.A.; et al. Effects of Dalcetrapib in Patients with a Recent Acute Coronary Syndrome. *N. Engl. J. Med.* **2012**, *367*, 2089–2099. [CrossRef] [PubMed]
44. Nicholls, S.J.; Ditmarsch, M.; Kastelein, J.J.; Rigby, S.P.; Kling, D.; Curcio, D.L.; Alp, N.J.; Davidson, M.H. Lipid lowering effects of the CETP inhibitor obicetrapib in combination with high-intensity statins: A randomized phase 2 trial. *Nat. Med.* **2022**, *28*, 1672–1678. [CrossRef]
45. Ballantyne, C.M.; Ditmarsch, M.; Kastelein, J.J.; Nelson, A.J.; Kling, D.; Hsieh, A.; Curcio, D.L.; Maki, K.C.; Davidson, M.H.; Nicholls, S.J. Obicetrapib plus ezetimibe as an adjunct to high-intensity statin therapy: A randomized phase 2 trial. *J. Clin. Lipidol.* **2023**, *17*, 491–503. [CrossRef]
46. Rosenson, R.S.; Gaudet, D.; Hegele, R.A.; Ballantyne, C.M.; Nicholls, S.J.; Lucas, K.J.; San Martin, J.; Zhou, R.; Muhsin, M.; Chang, T.; et al. Zodasiran, an RNAi Therapeutic Targeting ANGPTL3, for Mixed Hyperlipidemia. *N. Engl. J. Med.* **2024**. [CrossRef] [PubMed]
47. Ray, K.K.; Ruotolo, G.; Michael, L.; Shen, X.; Ma, X.; Lim, S.; Nicholls, S.J.; Linnebjerg, H. Solbinsiran, a GalNAC-Conjugated siRNA Targeting ANGPTL3, Reduces Atherogenic Lipoproteins in Individuals with Mixed Dyslipidaemia in a Durable and Dose Dependent Manner. *J. Am. Coll. Cardiol.* **2024**, *83*, 1673. [CrossRef]
48. Musunuru, K.; Chadwick, A.C.; Mizoguchi, T.; Garcia, S.P.; DeNizio, J.E.; Reiss, C.W.; Wang, K.; Iyer, S.; Dutta, C.; Clendaniel, V.; et al. In vivo CRISPR base editing of PCSK9 durably lowers cholesterol in primates. *Nature* **2021**, *593*, 429–434. [CrossRef] [PubMed]
49. Rothgangl, T.; Dennis, M.K.; Lin, P.J.C.; Oka, R.; Witzigmann, D.; Villiger, L.; Qi, W.; Hruzova, M.; Kissling, L.; Lenggenhager, D.; et al. In vivo adenine base editing of PCSK9 in macaques reduces LDL cholesterol levels. *Nat. Biotechnol.* **2021**, *39*, 949–957. [CrossRef]
50. Lee, R.G.; Mazzola, A.M.; Braun, M.C.; Platt, C.; Vafai, S.B.; Kathiresan, S.; Rohde, E.; Bellinger, A.M.; Khera, A.V. Efficacy and Safety of an Investigational Single-Course CRISPR Base-Editing Therapy Targeting *PCSK9* in Nonhuman Primate and Mouse Models. *Circulation* **2023**, *147*, 242–253. [CrossRef]
51. Zeitlinger, M.; Bauer, M.; Reindl-Schwaighofer, R.; Stoekenbroek, R.M.; Lambert, G.; Berger-Sieczkowski, E.; Lagler, H.; Oesterreicher, Z.; Wulkersdorfer, B.; Lührs, P.; et al. A phase I study assessing the safety, tolerability, immunogenicity, and low-density lipoprotein cholesterol-lowering activity of immunotherapeutics targeting PCSK9. *Eur. J. Clin. Pharmacol.* **2021**, *77*, 1473–1484. [CrossRef]

52. Fukami, H.; Morinaga, J.; Nakagami, H.; Hayashi, H.; Okadome, Y.; Matsunaga, E.; Kadomatsu, T.; Horiguchi, H.; Sato, M.; Sugizaki, T.; et al. Efficacy and safety in mice of repeated, lifelong administration of an ANGPTL3 vaccine. *npj Vaccines* **202**3, *8*, 168. [CrossRef]
53. Vroom, M.M.; Lu, H.; Lewis, M.; Thibodeaux, B.A.; Brooks, J.K.; Longo, M.S.; Ramos, M.M.; Sahni, J.; Wiggins, J.; Boyd, J.D.; et al. VXX-401, a novel anti-PCSK9 vaccine, reduces LDL-C in cynomolgus monkeys. *J. Lipid Res.* **2024**, *65*, 100497. [CrossRef]
54. Fowler, A.; Van Rompay, K.K.A.; Sampson, M.; Leo, J.; Watanabe, J.K.; Usachenko, J.L.; Immareddy, R.; Lovato, D.M.; Schiller, J.T.; Remaley, A.T.; et al. A virus-like particle-based bivalent PCSK9 vaccine lowers LDL-cholesterol levels in non-human primates. *npj Vaccines* **2023**, *8*, 142. [CrossRef]
55. Chow, C.K.; Nguyen, T.N.; Marschner, S.; Diaz, R.; Rahman, O.; Avezum, A.; Lear, S.A.; Teo, K.; Yeates, K.E.; Lanas, F.; et al. Availability and affordability of medicines and cardiovascular outcomes in 21 high-income, middle-income and low-income countries. *BMJ Glob. Health* **2020**, *5*, e002640. [CrossRef]
56. Penchansky, R.; Thomas, J.W. The concept of access: Definition and relationship to consumer satisfaction. *Med. Care* **1981**, *1*9, 127–140. [CrossRef] [PubMed]
57. Wirtz, V.J.; Kaplan, W.A.; Kwan, G.F.; Laing, R.O. Access to Medications for Cardiovascular Diseases in Low- and Middle-Income Countries. *Circulation* **2016**, *133*, 2076–2085. [CrossRef]
58. Access to Medicines—TAC. Available online: https://www.tac.org.za/campaign/access-to-medicines/ (accessed on 5 June 2024).
59. Harrison, M.A.; Marfo, A.F.A.; Annan, A.; Ankrah, D.N.A. Access to cardiovascular medicines in low- and middle-income countries: A mini review. *Glob. Health Res. Policy* **2023**, *8*, 17. [CrossRef] [PubMed]
60. WHO Definition of Availability. Available online: https://www.who.int/data/gho/indicator-metadata-registry/imr-details/2?02 (accessed on 9 June 2024).
61. Tenni, B.; Moir, H.V.J.; Townsend, B.; Kilic, B.; Farrell, A.-M.; Keegel, T.; Gleeson, D. What is the impact of intellectual property rules on access to medicines? A systematic review. *Glob. Health* **2022**, *18*, 40. [CrossRef]
62. Oğuz, A.; Telci Çaklılı, Ö.; Tümerdem Çalık, B.; Pure Investigators. The Prospective Urban Rural Epidemiology (PURE) study: PURE Turkey. *Turk. Kardiyol. Dern. Ars.* **2018**, *46*, 613–623. [CrossRef]
63. Danzon, P.M.; Furukawa, M.F. International Prices and Availability of Pharmaceuticals in 2005. *Health Aff.* **2008**, *27*, 221–23? [CrossRef]
64. Kishore, S.P.; Kolappa, K.; Jarvis, J.D.; Park, P.H.; Belt, R.; Balasubramaniam, T.; Kiddell-Monroe, R. Overcoming Obstacles to Enable Access to Medicines for Noncommunicable Diseases in Poor Countries. *Health Aff.* **2015**, *34*, 1569–1577. [CrossRef] [PubMed]
65. Brandts, J.; Ray, K.K. Low Density Lipoprotein Cholesterol–Lowering Strategies and Population Health. *Circulation* **2020**, *14*1, 873–876. [CrossRef] [PubMed]
66. Baum, S.J.; Toth, P.P.; Underberg, J.A.; Jellinger, P.; Ross, J.; Wilemon, K. PCSK9 inhibitor access barriers-issues and recommendations: Improving the access process for patients, clinicians and payers. *Clin. Cardiol.* **2017**, *40*, 243–254. [CrossRef]
67. Knowles, J.W.; Howard, W.H.; Karayan, L.; Baum, S.J.; Wilemon, K.A.; Ballantyne, C.M.; Myers, K.D. Access to Nonstatin Lipid-Lowering Therapies in Patients at High Risk of Atherosclerotic Cardiovascular Disease. *Circulation* **2017**, *135*, 2204–220? [CrossRef]
68. Blumenthal, D.M.; Goldman, D.P.; Jena, A.B. Outcomes-Based Pricing as a Tool to Ensure Access to Novel but Expensive Biopharmaceuticals. *Ann. Intern. Med.* **2017**, *166*, 219. [CrossRef]
69. Williams, D.R.; Lawrence, J.A.; Davis, B.A. Racism and Health: Evidence and Needed Research. *Annu. Rev. Public Health* **2019**, *40*, 105–125. [CrossRef]
70. Parrinello, C.M.; Rastegar, I.; Godino, J.G.; Miedema, M.D.; Matsushita, K.; Selvin, E. Prevalence of and Racial Disparities in Risk Factor Control in Older Adults with Diabetes: The Atherosclerosis Risk in Communities Study. *Diabetes Care* **2015**, *38*, 1290–129? [CrossRef]
71. Kalra, D.K. Bridging the Racial Disparity Gap in Lipid-Lowering Therapy. *JAHA* **2021**, *10*, e019533. [CrossRef] [PubMed]
72. Daviglus, M.L.; Ferdinand, K.C.; López, J.A.G.; Wu, Y.; Monsalvo, M.L.; Rodriguez, C.J. Effects of Evolocumab on Low-Density Lipoprotein Cholesterol, Non–High Density Lipoprotein Cholesterol, Apolipoprotein B, and Lipoprotein(a) by Race and Ethnicity: A Meta-Analysis of Individual Participant Data from Double-Blind and Open-Label Extension Studies. *JAHA* **2021**, *10*, e01683? [CrossRef] [PubMed]
73. Kohli-Lynch, C.N.; Bellows, B.K.; Zhang, Y.; Spring, B.; Kazi, D.S.; Pletcher, M.J.; Vittinghoff, E.; Allen, N.B.; Moran, A.E. Cost-Effectiveness of Lipid-Lowering Treatments in Young Adults. *J. Am. Coll. Cardiol.* **2021**, *78*, 1954–1964. [CrossRef]
74. Weinstein, M.C.; Stason, W.B. Foundations of cost-effectiveness analysis for health and medical practices. *N. Engl. J. Med.* **1977**, *296*, 716–721. [CrossRef] [PubMed]
75. Lloyd-Jones, D.M.; Larson, M.G.; Beiser, A.; Levy, D. Lifetime risk of developing coronary heart disease. *Lancet* **1999**, *353*, 89–92. [CrossRef]
76. Morton, J.I.; Marquina, C.; Lloyd, M.; Watts, G.F.; Zoungas, F.; Liew, D.; Ademi, Z. Lipid-Lowering Strategies for Primary Prevention of Coronary Heart Disease in the UK: A Cost-Effectiveness Analysis. *PharmacoEconomics* **2024**, *42*, 91–107. [CrossRef]
77. Mallya, U.G.; Boklage, S.H.; Koren, A.; Delea, T.E.; Mullins, C.D. Budget Impact Analysis of PCSK9 Inhibitors for the Management of Adult Patients with Heterozygous Familial Hypercholesterolemia or Clinical Atherosclerotic Cardiovascular Disease. *PharmacoEconomics* **2018**, *36*, 115–126. [CrossRef]

78. Brunetti, N.D.; De Gennaro, L.; Tricarico, L.; Caldarola, P. Budget impact analysis of PCSK9 inhibitors costs from a community payers' perspective in Apulia, Italy. *Open Heart* **2019**, *6*, e001018. [CrossRef]
79. Ko, D.T.; Khan, A.M.; Kotrri, G.; Austin, P.C.; Wijeysundera, H.C.; Koh, M.; Chu, A.; Jackevicius, C.A.; Lawler, P.R.; Tu, J.V. Eligibility, Clinical Outcomes, and Budget Impact of PCSK9 Inhibitor Adoption: The CANHEART PCSK9 Study. *J. Am. Heart Assoc.* **2018**, *7*, e010007. [CrossRef] [PubMed]
80. Raal, F.J.; Rosenson, R.S.; Reeskamp, L.F.; Hovingh, G.K.; Kastelein, J.J.P.; Rubba, P.; Ali, S.; Banerjee, P.; Chan, K.-C.; Gipe, D.A.; et al. Evinacumab for Homozygous Familial Hypercholesterolemia. *N. Engl. J. Med.* **2020**, *383*, 711–720. [CrossRef]
81. Myers, K.D.; Farboodi, N.; Mwamburi, M.; Howard, W.; Staszak, D.; Gidding, S.; Baum, S.J.; Wilemon, K.; Rader, D.J. Effect of Access to Prescribed PCSK9 Inhibitors on Cardiovascular Outcomes. *Circ. Cardiovasc. Qual. Outcomes* **2019**, *12*, e005404. [CrossRef] [PubMed]
82. WHO Guideline on Country Pharmaceutical Pricing Policies. Available online: https://www.who.int/publications-detail-redirect/9789240011878 (accessed on 5 June 2024).
83. Garner, S.; Rintoul, A.; Hill, S.R. Value-Based Pricing: L'Enfant Terrible? *PharmacoEconomics* **2018**, *36*, 5–6. [CrossRef] [PubMed]
84. Morgan, S.G.; Daw, J.R.; Thomson, P.A. International best practices for negotiating 'reimbursement contracts' with price rebates from pharmaceutical companies. *Health Aff.* **2013**, *32*, 771–777. [CrossRef] [PubMed]
85. Vogler, S.; Zimmermann, N.; Ferrario, A.; Wirtz, V.J.; Babar, Z. Challenges and opportunities for pharmaceutical pricing and reimbursement policies. *J. Pharm. Policy Pract.* **2015**, *8*, 2052–3211. [CrossRef] [PubMed]
86. Kanavos, P.; Fontrier, A.M.; Gill, J.; Efthymiadou, O. Does external reference pricing deliver what it promises? Evidence on its impact at national level. *Eur. J. Health Econ.* **2020**, *21*, 129–151. [CrossRef] [PubMed]
87. Fontrier, A.M.; Gill, J.; Kanavos, P. International impact of external reference pricing: Should national policy- makers care? *Eur. J. Health Econ.* **2019**, *20*, 1147–1164. [CrossRef]
88. WHO. *WHO Guideline on Country Pharmaceutical Pricing Policies*; Evidence and Recommendations; World Health Organization: Geneva, Switzerland, 2020. Available online: https://www.ncbi.nlm.nih.gov/books/NBK570143/ (accessed on 27 June 2024).
89. Voehler, D.; Koethe, B.C.; Synnott, P.G.; Ollendorf, D.A. The impact of external reference pricing on pharmaceutical costs and market dynamics. *Health Policy OPEN* **2023**, *4*, 100093. [CrossRef]
90. Leopold, C.; Vogler, S.; Mantel-Teeuwisse, A.K.; de Joncheere, K.; Leufkens, H.G.; Laing, R. Differences in external price referencing in Europe: A descriptive overview. *Health Policy* **2012**, *104*, 50–60. [CrossRef]
91. Vitry, A.; Roughead, E. Managed entry agreements for pharmaceuticals in Australia. *Health Policy* **2013**, *112*, 277–283. [CrossRef]
92. Zhang, L.; Wang, X.; Yao, H.; Ding, B.; Gao, X.; Li, X. Impact of national drug price negotiation policy on the accessibility and utilization of PCSK9 inhibitors in China. *Int. J. Equity Health* **2024**, *23*, 116. [CrossRef]
93. Vogler, S.; Paris, V.; Ferrario, A.; Wirtz, V.J.; de Joncheere, K.; Schneider, P.; Pedersen, H.B.; Dedet, G.; Babar, Z. How Can Pricing and Reimbursement Policies Improve Affordable Access to Medicines? Lessons Learned from European Countries. *Appl. Health Econ. Health Policy* **2017**, *15*, 307–321. [CrossRef]
94. Novel Pricing and Payment Models (EFPIA Report) 2021. Available online: https://www.efpia.eu/ (accessed on 5 June 2024).
95. Pan American Health Organization Strategic Fund. Available online: https://www.paho.org/en/paho-strategic-fund (accessed on 28 June 2024).
96. Organization of Eastern Caribbean States. Available online: https://oecs.int/en/our-work/knowledge/library/pps (accessed on 28 June 2024).
97. The Joint Procurement Agreement. Available online: https://health.ec.europa.eu/health-security-and-infectious-diseases/preparedness-and-response-planning/signing-ceremonies-joint-procurement-agreement_en (accessed on 28 June 2024).
98. Parmaksiz, K.; Pisani, E.; Bal, R.; Kok, M.O. A systematic review of pooled procurement of medicines and vaccines—Identifying elements of success. *Glob. Health* **2022**, *18*, 59. [CrossRef]
99. Canada Patented Medicine Prices Review Board. Available online: https://www.canada.ca/en/patented-medicine-prices-review.html (accessed on 2 June 2024).
100. International Health Policy Center, The Commonwealth Fund. Available online: https://www.commonwealthfund.org/international-health-policy-center/system-profiles (accessed on 29 June 2024).
101. Barnighausen, T.; Sauerborn, R. One Hundred and Eighteen Years of the German Health Insurance System: Are There Any Lessons for Middle- and Low-Income Countries? *Soc. Sci. Med.* **2002**, *54*, 1559–1587. [CrossRef]
102. Wouters, O.J.; Kanavos, P.; McKee, M. Comparing Generic Drug Markets in Europe and the United States: Prices, Policies, and Potential Savings. *Health Aff.* **2017**, *36*, 2101–2109.
103. Sarnak, D.O.; Squires, D.; Bishop, S. Paying for Prescription Drugs around the World: Why Is the U.S. an Outlier? The Commonwealth Fund. 2017. Available online: https://www.commonwealthfund.org/publications/issue-briefs/2017/oct/paying-prescription-drugs-around-world-why-us-outlier (accessed on 28 June 2024).
104. Choudhry, N.K.; Avorn, J.; Glynn, R.J.; Antman, E.M.; Schneeweiss, S.; Toscano, M.; Reisman, L.; Fernandes, J.; Spettell, C.; Lee, J.L.; et al. Full Coverage for Preventive Medications after Myocardial Infarction. *N. Engl. J. Med.* **2011**, *365*, 2088–2097. [CrossRef]
105. Widdus, R. Public-private partnerships for health: Their main targets, their diversity, and their future directions. *Bull. World Health Organ.* **2005**, *79*, 713–720.
106. Kesselheim, A.S.; Avorn, J. The role of government in regulating drug prices and availability: Lessons from the United States. *N. Engl. J. Med.* **2013**, *367*, 1877–1879.

107. World Intellectual Property Organization (WIPO). *Licensing of Intellectual Property Rights and Competition Law*; WIPO: Geneva, Switzerland, 2020.
108. O'Neil, A.; Calderbank, S.; Brown, J.; Vandigo, J.; Yin, P.; Bratti, K.; Howell, S. Quantification of Utilization Management Barriers for Patients Initiating Therapy to Lower Lipid Levels. *JAMA Netw. Open* **2022**, *5*, e2240513. [CrossRef] [PubMed]
109. ICH Official Web Site. Available online: https://www.ich.org/ (accessed on 5 June 2024).
110. FDA. Available online: https://www.federalregister.gov/documents/2024/01/09/2024-00217/agency-information-collection-activities-proposed-collection-comment-request-expedited-programs-for (accessed on 5 June 2024).
111. Pharmacovigilance: Overview. European Medicines Agency. Available online: https://www.ema.europa.eu/en/human-regulatory-overview/pharmacovigilance-overview (accessed on 5 June 2024).
112. Barbosa, W.; Zhou, K.; Waddell, E.; Myers, T.; Dorsey, E.R. Improving Access to Care: Telemedicine Across Medical Domains. *Annu. Rev. Public Health* **2021**, *42*, 463–481. [CrossRef] [PubMed]
113. Mehta, S.; Aboushi, H.; Campos, C.M.; Botelho, R.V.; Fernandez, F.; Rodriguez, D.; Torres, M.A.; Vieria, D.; Frauenfelder, A.; Pinto, G.; et al. Impact of a telemedicine-guided, population-based, STEMI network on reperfusion strategy, efficiency, and outcomes. *Asia Interv.* **2021**, *7*, 18–26. [CrossRef]
114. Levine, S.R.; Gorman, M. "Telestroke": The Application of Telemedicine for Stroke. *Stroke* **1999**, *30*, 464–469. [CrossRef]
115. Zhai, Y.; Zhu, W.; Cai, Y.; Sun, D.; Zhao, J. Clinical- and Cost-effectiveness of Telemedicine in Type 2 Diabetes Mellitus: A Systematic Review and Meta-analysis. *Medicine* **2014**, *93*, e312. [CrossRef] [PubMed]
116. Lin, M.; Yuan, W.; Huang, T.; Zhang, H.; Mai, J.; Wang, J. Clinical Effectiveness of Telemedicine for Chronic Heart Failure: A Systematic Review and Meta-Analysis. *J. Investig. Med.* **2017**, *65*, 899–911. [CrossRef]
117. Kruzich, J.M.; Jivanjee, P.; Robinson, A.; Friesen, B.J. Family Caregivers' Perceptions of Barriers to and Supports of Participation in Their Children's Out-of-Home Treatment. *Psychiatr. Serv.* **2003**, *54*, 1513–1518. [CrossRef]
118. Saluja, S.; Rudolfson, N.; Massenburg, B.B.; Meara, J.G.; Shrime, M.G. The impact of physician migration on mortality in low and middle-income countries: An economic modelling study. *BMJ Glob. Health* **2020**, *5*, e001535. [CrossRef] [PubMed]
119. Ekeland, A.G.; Bowes, A.; Flottorp, S. Effectiveness of telemedicine: A systematic review of reviews. *Int. J. Med. Inform.* **2010**, *79*, 736–771. [CrossRef]
120. Schubert, T.J.; Clegg, K.; Karalis, D.; Desai, N.R.; Marrs, J.C.; McNeal, C.; Mintz, G.L.; Romagnoli, K.M.; Jones, L.K. Impact of telehealth on the current and future practice of lipidology: A scoping review. *J. Clin. Lipidol.* **2023**, *17*, 40–54. [CrossRef]
121. Kruse, C.S.; Karem, P.; Shifflett, K.; Vegi, L.; Ravi, K.; Brooks, M. Evaluating barriers to adopting telemedicine worldwide: A systematic review. *J. Telemed. Telecare* **2018**, *24*, 4–12. [CrossRef] [PubMed]
122. Ye, J.; He, L.; Beestrum, M. Implications for implementation and adoption of telehealth in developing countries—A systematic review of China's practices and experiences. *npj Digit. Med.* **2023**, *6*, 174. [CrossRef] [PubMed]
123. PCSK9 Forum. Education and Research Forum. Available online: https://www.pcsk9forum.org/ (accessed on 5 June 2024).
124. Katzmann, J.L.; Sorio-Vilela, F.; Dornstauder, E.; Fraas, U.; Smieszek, T.; Zappacosta, S.; Laufs, U. Non-statin lipid-lowering therapy over time in very-high-risk patients: Effectiveness of fixed-dose statin/ezetimibe compared to separate pill combination on LDL-C. *Clin. Res. Cardiol.* **2022**, *111*, 243–252. [CrossRef] [PubMed]
125. Ballantyne, C.M.; Laufs, U.; Ray, K.K.; Leiter, L.A.; Bays, H.E.; Goldberg, A.C.; Stroes, E.S.G.; MacDougall, D.; Zhao, X.; Catapano, A.L. Bempedoic acid plus ezetimibe fixed-dose combination in patients with hypercholesterolemia and high CVD risk treated with maximally tolerated statin therapy. *Eur. J. Prev. Cardiolog.* **2020**, *27*, 593–603. [CrossRef] [PubMed]
126. Navar, A.M.; Taylor, B.; Mulder, H.; Fievitz, E.; Monda, K.L.; Fievitz, A.; Maya, J.F.; López, J.A.G.; Peterson, E.D. Association of Prior Authorization and Out-of-pocket Costs with Patient Access to PCSK9 Inhibitor Therapy. *JAMA Cardiol.* **2017**, *2*, 1217–1225. [CrossRef]
127. Dixon, D.L.; Saseen, J.J. Pharmacist-administered long-acting injectable PCSK9 service: A solution to improve patient access and adherence. *J. Am. Pharm. Assoc.* **2021**, *61*, e83–e85. [CrossRef]

Journal of
Clinical Medicine

MDPI

Review

Nanotechnology and Artificial Intelligence in Dyslipidemia Management—Cardiovascular Disease: Advances, Challenges, and Future Perspectives

Ewelina Młynarska [1,*], Kinga Bojdo [1,†], Hanna Frankenstein [1,†], Natalia Kustosik [1,†], Weronika Mstowska [1,†], Aleksandra Przybylak [1,†], Jacek Rysz [2] and Beata Franczyk [1]

1 Department of Nephrocardiology, Medical University of Lodz, 90-549 Łódź, Poland
2 Department of Nephrology, Hypertension and Internal Medicine, Medical University of Lodz, 90-549 Łodz, Poland
* Correspondence: ewelina.mlynarska@umed.lodz.pl or emmlynarska@gmail.com
† These authors contributed equally to this work.

Abstract: This narrative review explores emerging technologies in dyslipidemia management, focusing on nanotechnology and artificial intelligence (AI). It examines the current treatment recommendations and contrasts them with the future prospects enabled by these innovations. Nanotechnology shows significant potential in enhancing drug delivery systems, enabling more targeted and efficient lipid-lowering therapies. In parallel, AI offers advancements in diagnostics, cardiovascular risk prediction, and personalized treatment strategies. AI-based decision support systems and machine learning algorithms are particularly promising for analyzing large datasets and delivering evidence-based recommendations. Together, these technologies hold the potential to revolutionize dyslipidemia management, improving outcomes and optimizing patient care. In addition, this review covers key topics such as cardiovascular disease biomarkers and risk factors, providing insights into the current methods for assessing cardiovascular risk. It also discusses the current understanding of dyslipidemia, including pathophysiology and clinical management. Together, these insights and technologies hold the potential to revolutionize dyslipidemia management, improving outcomes and optimizing patient care.

Keywords: dyslipidemia; cardiovascular disease; emerging lipid-lowering therapies; nanotechnology; artificial intelligence; cardiovascular risk-related biomarkers

1. Methods Section

This review aims to evaluate current therapeutic strategies for dyslipidemia, focusing on novel approaches and their clinical applications. Evidence was synthesized from the peer-reviewed literature published before January 2025. A systematic search was conducted using the PubMed, Scopus, Google Scholar, and Web of Science databases. The search terms included "dyslipidemia", "cardiovascular disease", "lipid-lowering therapies", "nanotechnology", and "artificial intelligence". The searches were limited to English-language articles. Additional articles were identified through the manual searches of the reference lists from the included studies.

The inclusion criteria focused on peer-reviewed studies, including narrative reviews, systematic reviews, meta-analyses, and clinical trials. Studies were excluded if they were not peer-reviewed (such as editorials or commentaries), focused on topics unrelated to the scope of this review, or were published in languages other than English.

2. Cardiovascular Disease—Risk Factors, Biomarkers, and Artificial Intelligence Correlation

Cardiovascular disease (CVD) is the leading group of non-communicable diseases globally, responsible for around one-third of all deaths worldwide [1]. CVD is a general term for heterogeneous conditions affecting the heart or blood vessels, mainly such as coronary artery disease (CAD) and atherosclerosis [2,3]. Inflammatory activation and endothelial dysfunction play central roles in the onset and progression of atherosclerosis, contributing to an increased risk of cardiovascular events like myocardial infarction [4]. There are several risk factors that contribute to the development of CVD like age, gender (men over 45 and women over 55, particularly after menopause), genetics factors, smoking, lack of physical activity, high blood pressure, obesity, high cholesterol and triglyceride levels, and diabetes mellitus (DM) [5]. As we know, there is a high correlation between lipid disorders and the development of CVD. An increased level of circulating apo-B-containing lipoproteins has long-been identified as a central causal risk factor for coronary heart disease [2].

We can also distinguish biomarkers that correlate with CVD. Traditional biomarkers include high-sensitivity C-reactive protein and the cardiac troponins I or T (cTns). These biomarkers, especially cTns, are released into the bloodstream when cardiac myocytes undergo necrosis. Testing for these biomarkers is critical in diagnosing, stratifying risk, and managing patients with cardiovascular disease [6]. In the seminal JUPITER trial, Ridker et al. demonstrated that healthy community-dwellers with low concentrations of low-density lipoprotein (LDL) cholesterol, but increased concentrations of CRP (>2 mg/L), strongly benefited from statin therapy, with a reduced incidence of cardiovascular events [7,8]. While cTns are considered the gold standard for diagnosing acute CVD caused by cardiomyocyte necrosis, false-positive results can present challenges [9]. Elevated cTn levels are not limited to ischemic injuries but are also observed in nonischemic myocardial damage, such as myocarditis and cardiotoxicity, as well as in other conditions involving multifactorial injuries, including congestive heart failure and pulmonary embolism [7,8]. In 2009, two landmark studies in The New England Journal of Medicine highlighted the superior diagnostic performance of high-sensitivity troponin assays compared to conventional assays, particularly in early presenters, enabling faster acute myocardial infarction (AMI) confirmation. By 2015, a single high-sensitivity cTnI measurement below 5 ng/L was validated as a reliable cutoff for ruling out AMI in low-risk emergency patients, with a 99.6% negative predictive value. These findings were consistent across age and sex subgroups and confirmed in multiple cohorts. However, diagnostic performance was less robust for patients presenting within two hours of symptom onset [9].

Creatine Kinase-MB (CK-MB) is an enzyme predominantly found in heart muscle cells, and its presence in the blood serves as a biomarker for myocardial damage, such as that caused by a heart attack. Rapid fluctuation makes CK-MB particularly useful for identifying reinfarction, or a second heart attack that occurs shortly after an initial one. However, CK-MB is less specific than cardiac troponins for detecting myocardial injury [10].

Heart-type fatty acid-binding protein (H-FABP) is a small protein rapidly released into the bloodstream within 1–3 h of myocardial injury, making it valuable for the early diagnosis of AMI. While less specific than troponins due to potential elevation in skeletal muscle injury and renal impairment, H-FABP complements troponins by enhancing early sensitivity in diagnosing AMI. Elevated H-FABP levels are also linked to worse outcomes in acute coronary syndrome (ACS) and heart failure (HF), offering both diagnostic and prognostic insights [10,11].

Another commonly used biomarker is the N-terminal prohormone of brain natriuretic peptide (NT-proBNP) that correlates to myocardial stretch. Elevated levels of NT-proBNP in a patient's blood upon arrival at the emergency room are strongly linked to an increased likelihood of a heart failure diagnosis. Additionally, higher NT-proBNP levels at the time of hospital admission are correlated with a higher risk of in-hospital mortality [7]. Despite the high predictive value of NT-proBNP, the GUIDE-IT study, a large randomized controlled trial evaluating NT-proBNP-guided therapy for heart failure with reduced ejection fraction, was terminated early due to futility, showing no outcome differences compared to the standard care and current evidence does not support NT-proBNP-guided therapy for chronic heart failure [9].

Copeptin, a precursor of arginine vasopressin, is another biomarker linked to both ischemic events and heart failure. The vasopressin system is activated after acute myocardial infarction, so copeptin levels rise shortly after an ischemic episode and are associated with an increased risk of mortality and the development of new-onset heart failure, especially in those with an elevated NTproBNP [12,13].

The biomarkers described above are classified as classical biomarkers. However, with the advancement of technology, new biomarkers are emerging, such as microRNAs (mi-RNAs). Mi-RNAs are small, non-coding RNA molecules that play an essential role in regulating gene expression. They have distinct expression patterns and release during different stages of CVDs. For AMI, miR-29b has been identified as an important biomarker, while miR-1, miR-133, and miR-328 are relevant for AMI, arrhythmias, and HF. For HF, miRNAs like miR-18, miR-37, miR-126, miR-210, miR-221, and miR-1254 have diagnostic and prognostic significance. Additionally, miR-21, miR-208, and miR-499 serve as biomarkers for both AMI and HF, enhancing the understanding of these conditions. Analyzing miRNA profiles provides deeper insights into the molecular mechanisms behind CVDs and can reveal potential targets for therapy and tools for diagnosis [7,10].

Traditionally, statistical models incorporating risk factors and biomarkers have been widely used to predict and assess the progression of CVD. However, with technological advancements, the use of AI is rapidly gaining popularity as a method for evaluating patient risk and predicting CVD outcomes. Most studies on AI in CVD have been carried out in developed countries. These studies cover various applications, including the use of machine learning (ML) for the risk stratification of CVD, employing natural language processing to extract data from clinical and pathological reports, integrating AI into clinical decision support systems, and applying AI for the prognosis and treatment of CVD [14]. One notable example is the use of ML in risk stratification, which has demonstrated improvements in identifying high-risk patients and reducing unnecessary treatments for low-risk individuals presented by Kakadiaris et al. (2018). The ML-based calculator developed in their study surpassed the traditional ACC/AHA Risk Calculator by identifying 13% more high-risk patients and reducing therapy for low-risk individuals by 25% [15]. AI-based polygenic risk score (PRS) modeling approaches have significant potential to improve personalized CVD treatments. By integrating multi-omics data (genomic, transcriptomic, proteomic, and metabolomic), these methods provide a deeper understanding of molecular pathways and enhance the accuracy of PRS models. AI techniques are particularly useful for identifying complex patterns in high-dimensional genetic data, enabling more precise connections between genetic variations and disease risk. Moreover, AI algorithms can continually learn from new data, improving their performance and offering more accurate risk assessments over time [16].

3. Dyslipidemia—Current Understanding

Dyslipidemia refers to an abnormality in the normal levels of one or more lipid components in the blood, such as triglycerides (TGs), total cholesterol (TC), high-density lipoprotein cholesterol (HDL-C), and low-density lipoprotein cholesterol (LDL-C) [17]. Cholesterol and triglycerides are water-insoluble and require transport with proteins such as lipoproteins. These complex particles consist of a core of cholesterol esters and triglycerides surrounded by free cholesterol, phospholipids, and apolipoproteins, which play key roles in lipoprotein structure, receptor binding, assembly, and enzyme regulation. Plasma lipoproteins are classified into seven types based on size, composition, and apolipoproteins: chylomicrons, chylomicron remnants, very low-density lipoproteins (VLDLs), VLDL remnants (IDL), LDL, HDL, and lipoprotein (a) (Lp(a)). Chylomicron remnants, VLDL, IDL, LDL, and Lp(a) promote atherosclerosis, while HDL has a protective role [18]. Dyslipidemia can arise from three potential causes: intrinsic, extrinsic, or a combination of genetic and environmental factors. Secondary dyslipidemias are associated with risk factors linked to other medical conditions or environmental influences, whereas primary dyslipidemias represent a varied group of disorders stemming from genetic causes, either monogenic or polygenic in nature [17]. As we know, dyslipidemia shows a high correlation with obesity and CVD risk. In individuals with adiposity, a commonly observed lipid profile is adiposopathic dyslipidemia (also referred to as "atherogenic dyslipidemia"). This pattern is characterized by elevated blood triglyceride levels, reduced HDL-C levels, increased non-HDL-C levels, elevated apolipoprotein B levels, a higher number of LDL particles, and an increase in small dense LDL particles [19]. Lipoproteins, such as chylomicrons and VLDL, play a crucial role in lipid metabolism, transporting triglycerides from the intestine and liver to tissues like adipose tissue, muscles, and the heart. Lipoprotein lipase (LPL) breaks down triglycerides, releasing free fatty acids. As triglycerides are depleted, these lipoproteins are converted into remnant lipoproteins, which are absorbed by the liver or further processed into LDL. The accumulation of LDL and remnant lipoproteins in the arterial walls contributes to atherosclerosis, a lipid-driven process that leads to atherosclerotic cardiovascular disease (ASCVD) [20–23]. Atherosclerotic plaque formation depends on LDL-C and ApoB-containing lipoproteins, and prolonged exposure to these particles increases risk [24]. Lp(a) and inflammation are linked to ASCVD risk even in statin-treated individuals [25]. Complex classifications analyzing the factors correlated with the development of dyslipidemia could more effectively and efficiently identify potential patients. Therefore, the integration of artificial intelligence in assessing risk, diagnosis, and complications is crucial.

4. Current Recommendations in Lipid-Lowering Therapies

Dyslipidemia is a major factor in atherosclerosis and CVD. The public health priority is to achieve optimal lipoprotein levels. In general, treatment starts with lifestyle changes, including a healthy diet (low in sodium, saturated fats, and alcohol) and regular physical activity instead of sedentary life. In addition to these modifications, pharmacological treatment may be necessary [26,27].

It should be emphasized that managing weight is also essential for preventing and reducing cardiovascular risks, especially for people with obesity whose body mass index (BMI) is 30 kg/m^2 or higher or those with a BMI between 25 and 29.9 kg/m^2, classified as overweight, who have two or more additional risk factors [27]. For individuals with extreme obesity or those with comorbidities, bariatric surgery and medications like orlistat, naltrexone, bupropion, or high-dose liraglutide have demonstrated significant effectiveness [28].

The Mediterranean Diet emphasizes the consumption of fruits, vegetables, whole grains, legumes, nuts, and olive oil, with a moderate intake of fish and red wine, offering significant heart health benefits [29]. Similarly, the Dietary Approaches to Stop Hypertension (DASH) diet, which focuses on fruits, vegetables, and low-fat dairy, effectively lowers blood pressure and cardiovascular risk, with a 20% reduction in disease risk linked to adherence [28,30].

It is also important to consume healthy fats, as they play a crucial role in maintaining optimal lipid profiles and supporting overall cardiovascular health. Fats are classified by origin and structure, with animal fats being rich in saturated fatty acids (SAFAs) and plant fats containing more unsaturated fatty acids like monounsaturated (MUFAs) and polyunsaturated (PUFAs) fats [31]. Omega-3 and omega-6 PUFAs, particularly Eicosapentaenoic acid (EPA) and Docosahexaenoic acid (DHA), help reduce triglycerides by 10–50% and have cardioprotective effects [32–34], with a recommended intake of 2–4 g/day for triglyceride reduction [32]. In contrast, trans fatty acids (TFAs) found in full-fat dairy and processed foods raise LDL cholesterol and lower HDL levels, worsening lipid profiles [32]. Phytosterols, plant compounds, can reduce LDL cholesterol by 6–12% at 2 g/day by decreasing cholesterol absorption [31].

4.1. *Pharmacotherapy*

4.1.1. Statins

Statins were introduced to the pharmaceutical market in 1987, starting with lovastatin. Currently, they are the leading treatment for managing high cholesterol and preventing cardiovascular diseases. Over time, six statins have become available: two semi-synthetic statins (simvastatin and pravastatin) and four synthetic statins (fluvastatin, atorvastatin, rosuvastatin, and pitavastatin) [34]. The primary mechanism of this medicine involves inhibiting the enzyme 3-hydroxy-3-methyl-glutaryl-coenzyme A reductase (HMG-CoA). By limiting this enzyme's activity, statins reduce cholesterol synthesis within liver cells, leading to lower intrahepatic cholesterol levels. This triggers an upregulation of LDL receptors (LDLRs) in liver cells, which helps remove LDL cholesterol from the bloodstream. This reduction in LDL-C by 1 mmol/L (38.6 mg/dL) has been shown to decrease the risk of cardiovascular events even by 21% [35]. High-intensity statin therapy, such as atorvastatin (40/80 mg) or rosuvastatin (20/40 mg per day), is recommended as the initial treatment to prevent cardiovascular events. In addition to lowering LDL-C, statins are also effective in reducing triglycerides in patients with hypertriglyceridemia. As with each treatment, statins can also cause side effects, which might limit their use in some patients. The most common aftermath is myalgia, affecting 1–10% of users. Other issues like myopathy, rhabdomyolysis, liver and kidney dysfunction, type 2 diabetes, and eye conditions like cataracts have also been reported. Rosuvastatin, in particular, has been linked to a slightly higher risk of new-onset diabetes compared to atorvastatin. When statin intolerance or nocebo effects occur, patients should be prescribed the highest tolerated dose as a baseline therapy [36].

4.1.2. Fibrates

Fibrates are mainly administered to TG levels, and in some cases, to heighten HDL-C levels. They are capable of reducing TG levels by 25–50% and increasing HDL-C by 5–20%. Nevertheless, their effect on LDL-C differs depending on the patient's TG levels. For patients with very high TG levels (>500 mg/dL), fibrates may paradoxically cause an increase in LDL-C. On the other hand, in cases where TG levels are not significantly high, fibrates can decrease LDL-C by 10–30%. Although they are occasionally used to raise

HDL-C levels, their main therapeutic function is to lower TG levels. For patients with extremely high TG levels, those over 500 mg/dL, fibrates are often used to lower TG and prevent complications like pancreatitis. In these situations, fibrates can be combined with omega-3 fatty acids (fish oil) to achieve better lipid management [29].

4.1.3. Niacin

Niacin, the first drug approved for dyslipidemia, is effective in severe hypertriglyceridemia (TG > 500–1000 mg/dL). It reduces total cholesterol and triglycerides by 20–50%, LDL-C, and Lp(a). It also increases HDL-C and promotes the transition to larger, less dense LDL particles. Unfortunately, niacin may increase the risk of progression to diabetes in obese people at risk of the disease. In such cases, niacin should be used with caution [29,37,38].

4.1.4. PCSK9 Inhibitors

Proprotein convertase subtilisin/kexin type 9 inhibitors (PCSK9is) are a useful therapeutic replacement, especially for patients who cannot tolerate statins or require additional LDL-C reduction. These monoclonal antibodies, such as alirocumab and evolocumab, target PCSK9, a protein that degrades LDL receptors in hepatocytes. By repressing PCSK9, these drugs preserve LDL receptors, enhancing their ability to clear LDL-C from the blood. PCSK9is are administered subcutaneously every 2–4 weeks. They fundamentally lower LDL-C, non-HDL cholesterol, apoB, and lipoprotein A levels. Moreover, they provide cardiovascular benefits like reducing inflammation and stabilizing plaques. While generally well tolerated, with mild side effects like injection-site reactions and nasopharyngitis, their high cost remains a significant barrier to widespread use in clinical practice. Frequently joined with ezetimibe, they are an effective statin alternative [26,29,38,39].

4.1.5. Inclisiran

Inclisiran is a synthetic small interfering RNA (siRNA) designed to inhibit PCSK9 production by binding to its mRNA. This mechanism enhances LDL receptor activity, leading to a significant reduction in LDL-C levels. Clinical trials, such as ORION-10 and ORION-11, assessed their effectiveness and safety in patients with CAD or other cardiovascular risk factors and elevated LDL-C levels (≥70 or ≥100 mg/dL, respectively). The studies showed that inclisiran lowered LDL-C levels by 50% compared to the placebo, with only mild and temporary injection-site reactions as side effects [40,41]. Inclisiran is given subcutaneously in a 300 mg dose. The first injection is followed by a second dose three months later. Subsequent doses are given every six months [34]. In addition to lowering LDL-C by 50–55%, inclisiran is well tolerated and offers a promising option for long-term cholesterol management in high-risk patients.

4.1.6. Bempedoic Acid

Bempedoic acid is an oral adenosine triphosphate-citrate lyase (ACL) inhibitor that reduces LDL-C levels by decreasing hepatic cholesterol synthesis. It is mainly prescribed in combination with ezetimibe for patients who are intolerant to statins. Bempedoic acid is safe. Moreover, it reduces the risk of reinfarction [26,29,38].

4.1.7. Ezetimibe

Ezetimibe inhibits cholesterol absorption in the intestines and lowers LDL-C by approximately 20%. The drug's effectiveness depends on the presence of the Niemann-Pick1-like protein. By decreasing cholesterol delivery to the liver, it enhances the liver's LDL receptors. Ezetimibe is commonly used as an adjuvant medication therapy when statin treatment alone is insufficient or in patients who cannot tolerate statins. Additionally, it has the added benefit of improving glycemic control in diabetic patients [28,36,37]. Table 1 provides a detailed comparison of lipid-lowering medications, summarizing the information discussed in Section 4.

Table 1. Comparative overview of lipid-lowering medications [26,29,34,35,42,43].

Drug/Therapy	Mechanism of Action	Half-Life	Dosing Schedule
Statins	Inhibition of HMG-CoA reductase	14–19 h	Once daily
PCSK9 inhibitors	Reduces degradation of LDL receptors	11–20 days	Every 2–4 weeks (subcutaneous)
Inclisiran (siRNA)	RNA interference inhibits the production of PCSK9	Very long term (months)	0–90–180 days and every 6 months thereafter (subcutaneous)
Ezetimibe	Inhibits the intestinal absorption of cholesterol	22 h	Once daily
Fibrates	Activates PPARα receptors	20 h	Once or twice daily

5. Nanotechnology in Lipid-Lowering Therapies

5.1. Negatively Charged Liposome Nanoparticles

The understanding and application of nanoscience through nanotechnology began to expand rapidly in the early 2000s, sparking a transformative revolution that impacted nearly every field of science. Nanoscience focuses on structures ranging in size from 1 to 100 nanometers, while nanotechnology converts this knowledge into practical applications [44]. They have revolutionized the field of medicine, significantly enhancing the precision and effectiveness of treatments. This progress is primarily driven by nanoparticles (NPs), which enable targeted drug delivery, improve bioavailability, and reduce side effects by interacting with biological systems at the molecular and cellular levels [45]. These nanoscale carriers—including liposomes, dendrimers, and polymeric nanoparticles—allow for the controlled release and precise localization of therapeutic agents, revolutionizing disease treatments such as cancer, cardiovascular conditions, and infections.

This field continues to grow, providing innovative solutions to medical challenges. Meaningful and promising advancements are currently being made in anticancer therapy [46], infectious diseases, ophthalmology [47], and hypercholesterolemia which is the primary focus of our narrative review.

The earliest drug NPs were biomimetic, mimicking the micelles and liposomes naturally present in the body [48]. Liposomes are spherical vesicles composed primarily of phospholipids—amphiphilic molecules that contain both hydrophilic (water-attracting) heads and hydrophobic (water-repelling) tails. "The ideal NP carriers should be biodegradable, stable, non-immunogenic, easy to fabricate, cost-effective, and able to release their payloads only at the target site" [48]. Liposomes, which are mainly composed of phospholipids, are biocompatible, biodegradable, and non-immunogenic, which make them ideal carriers. They can encapsulate almost any drug or complex molecule, regardless of its hydrophobic or hydrophilic nature [49].

An effective liposomal formulation, incorporating the previously mentioned characteristics, can be achieved by selecting an optimal lipid composition, applying tailored functionalization, and designing a targeted delivery strategy. The parameters include stability depending on the surface charge, lipid rigidity, and bilayer organization. Positively charged liposomes increase uptake by tissues, while slightly negative ones increase circulation times due to reduced protein binding and opsonization [45,50]. Liposomes with a neutral surface charge tend to aggregate and lose their stability and colloidal behavior [51]. Biodistribution studies of nanoliposomes have shown that their half-life after intravenous injection is several hours due to hepatic uptake [52]. However, studies have shown that liposomes containing 75–100% anionic phospholipids can associate with LDL to form complexes that are then taken up by cells via LDL receptors or macrophages. This interaction highlights the potential of liposome-based targeted delivery systems for modulating LDL-related processes in various therapeutic applications [53,54].

A 2014 study [53] investigating the effects of negatively charged liposomes on lipoproteins demonstrated several beneficial outcomes. The treatment resulted in a reduction in LDL levels, total cholesterol, and ApoB, along with a notable decrease in triglycerides. At the same time, HDL levels were increased, and the liposomes showed enhanced uptake by macrophages. Moreover, the research identified atherosclerotic plaques as key target sites for anionic liposomes. These findings are particularly relevant because changes in these lipid components are directly linked to the risk of cardiovascular diseases, including atherosclerosis [53].

Building on these findings, a 2021 examination [55] in rabbits fed a high-cholesterol diet reported similar results and demonstrated significant reductions in triglycerides, total cholesterol, and LDL cholesterol levels. In addition, an increase in HDL cholesterol was observed. These findings support the potential of interventions targeting lipid profiles to manage hyperlipidemia and reduce cardiovascular risks. A 2018 study [56] conducted on a mouse model fed a high-fat diet revealed promising effects of anionic nanoliposomes in reducing the severity of atherosclerosis. The mice treated with these nanoliposomes showed decreased macrophage presence in atherosclerotic plaques. They also exhibited increased collagen deposition within the fibrous cap of plaques in the brachiocephalic artery (BCA) compared to control groups, suggesting a conceivable plaque-stabilizing effect [56]. This stabilization may have remarkable implications for reducing events related to advanced atherosclerosis. Additionally, the administration of nanoliposomes reduced the number of pro-inflammatory monocytes in both the spleen and BCA plaques of Ldlr−/− mice. It also limited hepatic steatosis and enhanced the expression of liver genes involved in lipid metabolism. Furthermore, nanoliposomes increased the aortic expression of ABCA1 and ABCG1, the key genes involved in reverse cholesterol transport (RCT). These findings highlight the potential of nanoliposomes to modulate inflammation, improve lipid homeostasis, and stabilize atherosclerotic plaques. This makes them a promising avenue for therapeutic strategies against cardiovascular disease [56].

Research suggests that negatively charged nanoliposomes hold significant capacity for reducing the risk of cardiovascular events associated with atherosclerosis and for managing dyslipidemia. By targeting key mechanisms such as LDL reduction, macrophage uptake, and plaque stabilization, these innovative nanocarriers offer an innovative strategy in pharmacology. Their ability to improve lipid profiles and influence plaque composition positions them as a hopeful development in the treatment and prevention of cardiovascular diseases.

5.2. Enhancing Statin Delivery via Nanoparticles

Medications used to treat hyperlipidemia are categorized into several classes, each employing distinct mechanisms to manage lipid levels. Statins are a cornerstone in the treatment of hyperlipidemia, playing a key role in lowering cholesterol levels. Their use has been linked to significant reductions in both cardiovascular-related and overall mortality rates. This impact has been observed in the prevention of atherosclerotic cardiovascular disease, benefiting patients in both primary prevention (before the onset of disease) and secondary prevention (after cardiovascular events) [57].

Statins are the primary treatment for lowering LDL-C; however, long-term adherence to this therapy is often suboptimal. Approximately 10% of the statin prescriptions are discontinued, which has been linked to a higher risk of cardiovascular events. The primary reason for discontinuation is the side effects attributed to statin. Among the various adverse effects associated with statins, muscle-related symptoms are the most frequently reported, others include hepatotoxicity, diabetes mellitus, renal impairment, and central nervous system dysfunction [58]. Although statins slightly increase the risk of mild side effects in individuals without cardiovascular disease, these effects are outweighed by their benefits in reducing major cardiovascular events. The current evidence does not strongly support the need to adjust statin type or dosage in advance to mitigate potential side effects, as limited data suggest significant variation in safety profiles across different statin regimens. This highlights the favorable balance of benefits to risks for statin use in the primary prevention of cardiovascular disease. Improving statin use in primary prevention could involve a tailored approach, adjusting the type and dose to maximize benefits while minimizing risks [59].

Anti-hyperlipidemic drugs, particularly statins, face several challenges due to their pharmacokinetic and biopharmaceutical limitations. While these drugs are well absorbed, they undergo extensive hepatic first-pass metabolism, resulting in low absolute bioavailability. This metabolic process significantly reduces their systemic effectiveness. Additionally, conventional oral dosage forms are associated with several drawbacks, including poor biodistribution, low bioavailability, limited water solubility, and inadequate site-specificity. As a result, improving the delivery mechanisms of these drugs is a key area of research to enhance their clinical effectiveness and safety profile [60] (Figure 1).

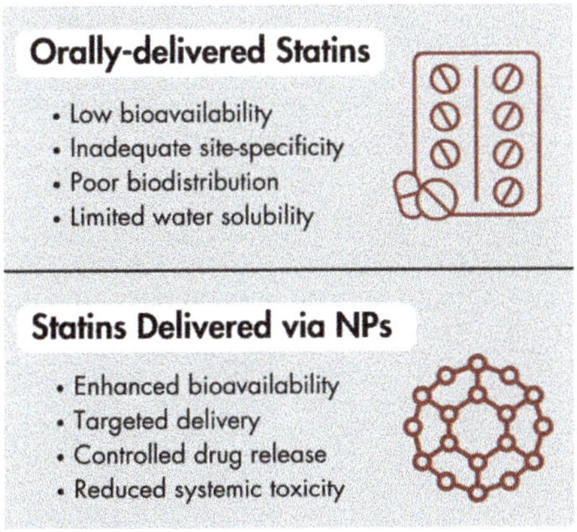

Figure 1. Comparison of orally delivered statins and statins delivered via NPs; NPs—nanoparticles [59].

As previously established, nanoparticles have the potential to address these challenges effectively. Their unique properties, such as controlled drug release, enhanced bioavailability, and targeted delivery, make them an excellent solution for overcoming the limitations of conventional drug formulations. Liposomal platforms are versatile nanocarriers used for drug delivery and molecular imaging, with ligand-functionalized liposomes specifically employed in cardiovascular imaging for targeted diagnostics [61].

In a 2021 study [62], simvastatin was encapsulated in nanoliposomes (referred to as LIPOSTAT) and tested on both 2D and 3D cell models, followed by intravenous administration. The liposomal formulation was stable, with a size of approximately 106.7 nm and a narrow size distribution. The formulation demonstrated promising therapeutic properties, including reduced inflammation and enhanced cholesterol efflux in 2D foam cells, as well as reduced inflammation in 3D spheroid models.

LIPOSTAT showed a controlled release profile, with only 10% and 20% of the drug released within the first two days, ensuring effective delivery to atherosclerotic plaques. It remained stable for at least two months and provided sustained drug release for over three weeks, enabling prolonged circulation and activity. The preliminary results highlighted its ability to regulate inflammatory and lipid accumulation pathways effectively. Specifically, LIPOSTAT significantly reduced pro-inflammatory cytokines such as IL-1α, IL-1β, and IL-18, which are key players in the early phases of inflammation. This study positions LIPOSTAT as a potential therapeutic option for targeted delivery to atherosclerotic plaques.

Another significant complication of dyslipidemia is non-alcoholic fatty liver disease (NAFLD), which can progress to fibrosis. A 2024 in vitro study [63] examined the effects of simvastatin encapsulated in nanoliposomes (SIM-LipoNPs) on fibrosis-induced liver microtissues. Simvastatin has demonstrated potential benefits in managing NAFLD, and the findings revealed that liposomal simvastatin was more effective in treating fibrosis models compared to the free drug.

The study showed that lower doses of SIM-LipoNP were as effective as higher doses of free simvastatin, likely due to the activation of the KLF2-NO signaling pathway. This suggests that liposomal formulations can overcome the challenges associated with conventional simvastatin delivery, including reducing hepatic side effects and enhancing therapeutic efficacy. The nanoliposome formulation also exhibited minimal burst release, ensuring that most of the drug payload remained intact during circulation and was efficiently delivered to the targeted liver injury site.

Despite these promising results, there remains a lack of data from in vivo studies, particularly regarding the pharmacokinetics and pharmacodynamics of SIM-LipoNP in humans. Further research is necessary to fully understand the potential of liposomal statins in treating NAFLD and to optimize their use as a targeted therapy for liver disorders.

Nanoparticles for cardiovascular diseases include gold nanoparticles, nanoliposomes, dendrimers, polymeric nanoparticles, and magnetic nanoparticles, offering unique advantages [61].

Recent studies underscore the transformative potential of nanoparticles beyond just nanoliposomes in the treatment of dyslipidemia. For instance, poly(amido)amine dendrimers (PAMAMs) were shown to significantly prolong the residence time of simvastatin and facilitate its controlled release, enhancing therapeutic outcomes [64]. Similarly, polymer vesicles loaded with pravastatin demonstrated targeted delivery and controlled release, effectively inhibiting macrophage endocytosis with reduced systemic toxicity compared to free pravastatin [65]. Additionally, poly (lactide-co-glycolic acid) (PLGA) NPs carrying atorvastatin achieved comparable efficacy to marketed formulations in hyperlipidemic rats but required a significantly lower dose, resulting in negligible myotoxicity [66].

These results emphasize the potential of nanoparticle-based systems as a game-changer for the treatment of dyslipidemia by enhancing efficacy, specificity, and safety. These innovations address many limitations of conventional therapies, offering hope for more effective and safer treatments (Figure 1). However, the lack of human trials remains a significant hurdle, requiring further research to realize their full therapeutic potential.

With continued advancements, these nanocarriers could transform cardiovascular and metabolic disease management, making them a promising focus for future pharmacological development.

It is also worth highlighting the role of nanoparticles in facilitating RNA delivery to target cells and the ORION clinical trials, which evaluate the efficacy and safety of inclisiran—a novel RNA-based therapy designed to lower LDL cholesterol. Inclisiran utilizes lipid nanoparticles for efficient RNA delivery, underscoring the critical integration of nanotechnology in modern therapeutics.

RNA-delivery technology using lipid nanoparticles plays a crucial role in the practical application of RNA-based therapies. The encapsulation of RNA into LNPs prevents degradation by RNAses in the bloodstream, enabling efficient delivery to target organs. As previously discussed, LNPs' ability to infiltrate specific hepatic cell populations contributes to the design of nanomedicines with reduced hepatotoxicity and enhanced efficacy for treating diseases originating from specific cell types [67].

Nanoparticles are essential because naked and unmodified siRNA suffers from poor stability, rapid degradation by nucleases, and potential off-target effects. Nano-delivery systems, such as LNPs, address these limitations by protecting siRNA from degradation, enhancing its stability, and improving pharmacokinetic behavior, thus facilitating its therapeutic use [68].

As previously mentioned, inclisiran, a novel siRNA drug for hypercholesterolemia, exemplifies this approach. It inhibits the production of PCSK9 in hepatocytes by silencing PCSK9 mRNA translation. This results in decreased PCSK9 synthesis, allowing more LDL receptors to clear LDL cholesterol from the bloodstream. Inclisiran received FDA approval in 2021 and EMA approval in 2020 [69], becoming the first siRNA drug approved for treating hypercholesterolemia or mixed dyslipidemia, and for patients with ASCVD or heterozygous familial hypercholesterolemia (HeFH) requiring additional LDL-C reduction [70].

The efficacy and safety of inclisiran have been evaluated in several global studies, including ORION 4, 9, 10, 11, and 18 [70]. These phase III, double-blind, randomized, placebo-controlled trials have shown that patients treated with inclisiran experienced an approximately 50% reduction in LDL cholesterol levels when administered every six months Table 2 [71,72].

Table 2. Summary of properties of inclisiran [71,72].

	INCLISIRAN
Structure	siRNA conjugated to triantennary N-acetylgalactosamine carbohydrates.
Mechanism	Inhibits the production of PCSK9 in hepatocytes by silencing the translation of PCSK9 mRNA.
FDA approval	2021
Guidelines by American College of Cardiology Expert Consensus Decision Pathway	An option for non-statin therapy in addition to maximally tolerated statin therapy in the very-high-risk ASCVD population or those with LDL-C greater than 190 mg/dL.
Dosage Regimen	Initial subcutaneous dose followed by a repeat dose at 3 months and every 6 months thereafter.
Outcomes	Consistent LDL-C lowering in the range of 44–54%.
Ongoing inclisiran cardiovascular outcome trials	ORION-4, VICTORION-2 PREVENT, and VICTORION-1 PREVENT

In summary, the integration of nanotechnology in RNA delivery, particularly through lipid nanoparticles, has revolutionized RNA-based therapeutics, enhancing their stability, efficacy, and safety. Inclisiran represents a significant advancement in this field, offering a promising therapeutic option for managing hypercholesterolemia with demonstrated clinical benefits.

5.3. Polymeric Nanoparticles—Drug Delivery

Many drugs used to treat dyslipidemia, such as statins, vibrates, or niacin, may have poor bioavailability or cause side effects due to systemic exposure. Polymeric NPs have been developed to enhance the efficacy and targeting of lipid-lowering therapies. These solid particles, typically ranging from 10 to 1000 nm, are composed of macromolecular polymers, either biodegradable or non-biodegradable. Common synthetic NPs include PLGA, polyvinyl imine (PEI), and polycaprolactone (PCL) [73].

These NPs can encapsulate macromolecules, protect them from enzymatic degradation, and change the dynamic behavior and tissue distribution of the encapsulated drugs in vivo. Drugs can not only be dissolved or encapsulated in the nanoparticles but also be bound or adsorbed on the surface of the polymer nanoparticles. Moreover, they show low toxicity, good biocompatibility, and biodegradation [73].

Polymeric nanoparticles show promise for treating type 1 diabetes-related complications, including oxidative stress mediated by iron in hemoglobin, dyslipidemia, and hyperglycemia via oral delivery. They have been extensively explored as delivery vehicles for lipid-lowering drugs to treat dyslipidemia. Despite their advantages, polymeric NPs have limitations, leading to the development of lipid–polymer hybrid nanoparticles (LPHNPs). LPHNPs feature a hydrophobic polymer core to encapsulate poorly water-soluble drugs, surrounded by a hydrophilic lipid shell and an outer lipid-PEG layer. There are two techniques for synthesizing LPHNPs: the Two-Step Method and the Single-Step Approach. In the first procedure, the polymer core and lipid shell are prepared separately and mixed, whereas in the second one, lipid and polymer are directly mixed and LPHNPs are self-assembled [74].

A study conducted in 2023 demonstrated that polymeric nanoparticles and LPHNPs play a key role in the treatment of atherosclerosis, which is a complication of hyperlipidemia. Atherosclerosis is a condition when the arteries become narrowed due to the accumulation of fatty deposits, cholesterol, cellular waste products, calcium, and fibrin known as plaques located on the inner wall of the arteries. Consequently, the blood flow is reduced. This process can lead to serious cardiovascular problems such as heart attacks and strokes. The statin therapy can reduce the chances of atherosclerotic plaque formation, but it needs to be used in higher doses due to low systemic bioavailability. It can cause side effects. To overcome these challenges, nanoparticles improving systemic drug absorption and therapeutic response have been developed. Two different types of nanoparticles were prepared such as PLGA nanoparticles (polymeric) and PLGA-DSPE-PEG-nanoparticles (polymer–lipid hybrid) for loading atorvastatin. The in vitro drug release comparison was carried out for 24 h from the nanoparticles and pure drug suspension, and the obtained release profiles. The polymeric nanoparticles showed 85% drug release after 10.3 h and hybrid nanoparticles revealed 87% drug release after 8.9 h. On the contrary, the pure drug exhibited an incomplete release profile with up to 24% discharge during the entire duration of the study period (Figure 2) [73].

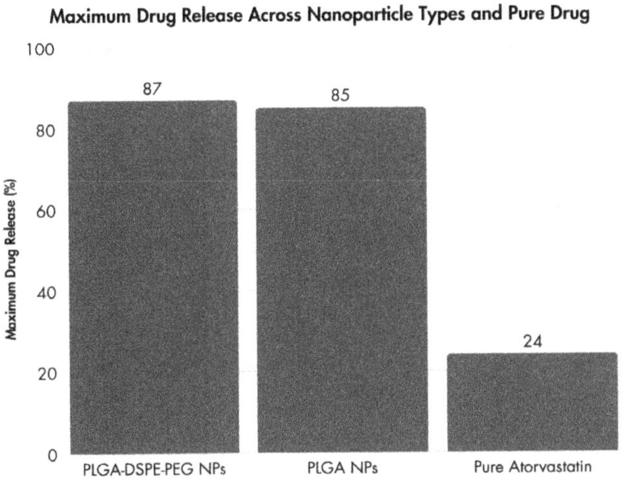

Figure 2. Maximum drug release across nanoparticle types and pure drug; PLGA NPs—poly lactide-co-glycolic acid nanoparticles; PLGA-DSPE-PEG NPs—polymer–lipid hybrid nanoparticles for loading atorvastatin [73].

The ability of nanoparticles to improve oral drug absorption has been widely discussed in the literature. Pharmacokinetic studies have shown that both polymeric and hybrid nanoparticles, due to their smaller particle size, facilitated better drug absorption through various mechanisms such as transcellular and paracellular transport. The drug-loaded nanoparticles demonstrated superior efficacy compared to the pure drug suspension. Specifically, the lipid–polymer hybrid nanoparticles resulted in a significantly greater reduction in the levels of TC (98%), LDL (78%), and TG (49%) compared to the control group ($p < 0.001$), while the polymeric nanoparticles led to reductions of 62%, 57%, and 32% in the TC, LDL, and TG levels, respectively ($p < 0.001$). In contrast, the animals treated with the pure drug suspension showed only a modest improvement in the TC (36%), LDL (28%), and TG (16%) levels compared to the control group ($p < 0.05$). HDL levels were also analyzed, showing improvements of 70%, 123%, and 257% after treatment with the pure drug, polymeric nanoparticles, and hybrid nanoparticles (Figure 3) [73].

The increase in drug levels in the body contributed to a stronger pharmacodynamic effect, as observed by the significant reduction in levels of hyperlipidemia markers, including TG, LDL, and TC, as well as an increase in HDL levels following nanoparticle treatment compared to the pure drug. High drug entrapment efficiency in nanoparticles is key to their improved efficacy. Both polymeric and hybrid nanoparticles showed over 70% drug entrapment, with sustained release profiles, evidenced by the time taken for 80% drug release. Polymeric nanoparticles had a more sustained release compared to lipid–polymer hybrids. The phospholipid in the hybrid nanoparticles likely boosted entrapment efficiency and drug absorption. In vivo studies also showed that the nanoparticles significantly improved systemic drug absorption through oral administration, with noticeable increases in Cmax and AUC compared to the pure drug [73].

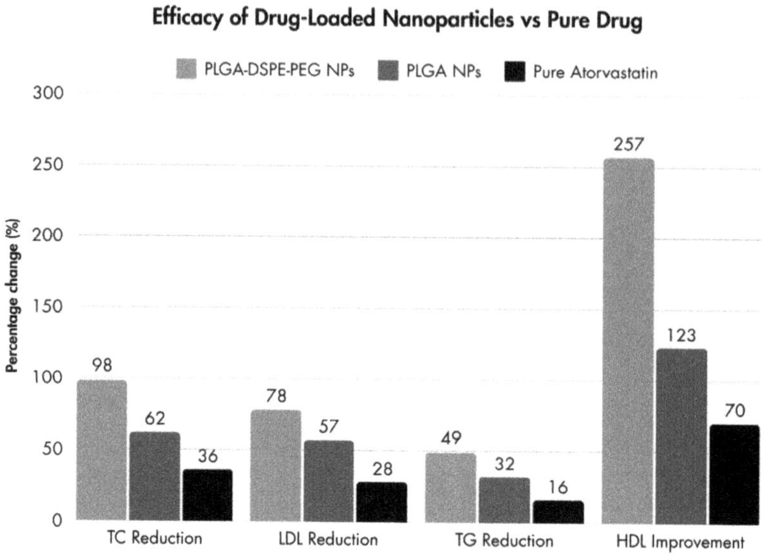

Figure 3. Efficacy of drug-loaded nanoparticles vs. pure drug; PLGA NPs—poly lactide-co-glycolic acid nanoparticles; PLGA-DSPE-PEG NPs—polymer–lipid hybrid nanoparticles for loading atorvastatin; TC—total cholesterol; LDL—low-density lipoprotein; TG—triglyceride; HDL—high-density lipoprotein [73].

5.4. Evaluating the Toxicological Impacts and Safety Strategies of Nanoparticle-Based Therapies

The potential adverse effects associated with nanoparticle-based therapies must not be overlooked. The current data on the toxicity of nanoparticles in mammalian cells and tissues underscore the need for further research to deepen our understanding of the underlying mechanisms of their toxicity. Additionally, it is imperative to develop strategies aimed at minimizing and preventing these toxic effects. Such strategies should consider both acute and chronic exposures to nanoparticles, accounting for various exposure routes and environmental contexts [74]. Below, we summarize the key side effects associated with nanoparticle-based therapies.

The toxicity of nanoparticles is influenced by their biophysical properties, including size, surface area, surface charge, and aggregation state [75]. A crucial factor in determining the efficacy or toxicity of nanoparticles is their interaction with cells. As with organ-specific toxicity, the size of nanoparticles significantly affects their cellular interactions, systemic circulation half-life, and biodistribution throughout the body [76]. The extent of endocytosis is dependent on the size of nanoparticles, with smaller nanoparticles being more readily internalized by cells, thereby increasing the likelihood of cellular toxicity. Research has also demonstrated that the shape of nanoparticles can affect their circulation time within the body, potentially delaying cellular uptake [74].

A 2018 study [77] provides a comprehensive overview of the latest findings on the side effects of nanoparticles, showing that they can accumulate in various organs, leading to different health risks. In the lungs, metal-containing nanoparticles such as cadmium-based quantum dots can induce inflammation and, in some cases, fibrosis, though recent data suggest that fibrosis may not always occur. Nanoparticles often accumulate in the liver, where they activate hepatic macrophages, contributing to liver damage. The spleen and immune system are also affected, as nanoparticles can increase cytokine levels and recruit immune cells. Small nanoparticles are typically cleared via the kidneys, but prolonged presence can lead to nephrotoxicity, including inflammation and fibrosis. Additionally, certain nanoparticles can cross the blood–brain barrier, causing hemorrhage and altering trace element levels, enzyme activity, and neurotransmitter levels after long-term exposure.

One promising approach to designing safer nanoparticles involves the development of structured nanoemulsions and solid lipid nanoparticles. These formulations utilize food-grade ingredients, generally recognized as safe (GRAS) by the FDA, such as lipids, proteins, polysaccharides, and surfactants. Research indicates that many toxic effects are associated with solid or metal-containing nanoparticles. However, further studies are necessary to assess the long-term effects and potential risks of these nanoparticles, particularly regarding their safety and side effects over extended periods [78].

5.5. Nanoliposomes vs. Polymeric Nanoparticles in Targeted Therapies

The targeted drug delivery system of nanoliposomes and polymeric nanoparticles has its advantages and disadvantages. Nanoliposomes may allow the successful entrapment of hydrophilic and hydrophobic drugs by their lipid bilayer composition to facilitate the required transport mechanism. However, they suffer from low criticality in terms of stability and increased clearance in circulation. On the other hand, polymeric nanoparticles, which are prepared from biodegradable polymers, showed better stability and enhanced drug release capabilities. That will lead to increasing the therapeutic effects of a certain drug. However, their practical application may be restricted by several factors such as complicated synthesis procedures and a possible cytotoxic effect [48,73,74].

6. Artificial Intelligence and Machine Learning in Dyslipidemia Management

With the ongoing advancements in lipid-lowering therapies, emerging technologies—such as the abovementioned nanotechnology—are reshaping the possibilities for targeted drug delivery and precision medicine. Building on these advancements, AI algorithms like ML and deep learning (DL) are probably going to revolutionize this field by enhancing the design, optimization, and application of nanomaterials [79]. The primary aim of this narrative review is to explore a novel approach to dyslipidemia management—nanotechnology. Additionally, it highlights the existing gap in the current medical approaches, specifically the potential of integrating AI with nanotechnology to enhance the dyslipidemia treatment in cardiovascular diseases.

6.1. Demystifying AI

Defining AI is challenging, as there is no universally accepted definition of the concept. However, a straightforward way to understand AI is as the simulation of human intelligence by systems or machines [80]. The primary functions of AI include perceiving, learning, planning, predicting, and decision making, among others. AI encompasses a wide range of research fields, such as search algorithms, knowledge graphs, expert systems, evolutionary algorithms, and advanced techniques like ML and DL. These fields contribute to AI's ability to analyze data, solve complex problems, and adapt to new information [81].

Physicians should develop a deeper understanding of AI applications in medicine and become familiar with related concepts, as AI holds the potential to transform medical practice in unprecedented ways. Enhanced awareness and knowledge in this area will better equip healthcare professionals to harness AI-driven innovations for improved patient care and clinical outcomes [82].

Such innovation is the use of AI in pharmacogenomics, where ML and deep learning techniques are revolutionizing personalized medicine. AI enhances the prediction of drug responses, identifies genetic markers, and refines therapeutic strategies. This integration supports the development of treatment plans, minimizes adverse effects, and advances patient-specific drug therapies, contributing to more effective and individualized care [83].

6.2. Use of AI in Dyslipidemia Management

Predicting Dyslipidemia Incident

Addressing the need for more precise and personalized approaches, AI is poised to transform dyslipidemia management by improving diagnostics and enhancing treatment strategies and cardiovascular outcomes. There was a cohort study conducted in Mexico City that investigated the application of machine learning models to identify specific characteristics connected to the factors for various types of dyslipidemia [84]. It consisted of 2621 participants aged between 20 and 50 years. These patients were men and women with and without dyslipidemia. Researchers applied the Variable Importance Measures (VIMs) of random forest (RF), XGBoost, and Gradient Boosting Machine (GBM) to enable feature selection. The study revealed that the VIM algorithm of RF and GBM identified the key risk factors of dyslipidemia the most effectively (accuracy rates up to 80%). ML techniques highlighted body mass index, elevated uric acid levels, age, sleep disorders, and anxiety as the top predictors of dyslipidemia risk [84]. Presented research demonstrates ML's ability to analyze the complex and gender-specific risk factors of dyslipidemia. Moreover, the adaptability of ML models—combined with techniques like the Synthetic Minority Oversampling Technique for dataset resampling—supports early diagnosis and personalized treatment strategies. It can make dyslipidemia management more effective and prevent cardiovascular diseases [83].

In East Azerbaijan Province, Iran, a similar study took place; it focused on predicting dyslipidemia cases using ML algorithms [85]. The used data were obtained from the Lifestyle Promotion Project. The work results highlight the effectiveness of ML—particularly the multi-layer perception (MLP) neural network—in achieving high-reliability metrics. RF also demonstrated strong predictive capabilities, as mentioned in a previous, Mexico City study [84]. These findings emphasize the value of ML in identifying key risk factors, such as waist circumference, serum vitamin D, blood pressure, and physical activity, to enhance prediction and management strategies [85].

AI can also be used to make more accurate predictions of LDL-C levels, which is crucial for assessing atherosclerotic heart disease risk. The study, based on data from the Laboratory Information Systems of Ankara Etlik City Hospital, included 60,217 patients with lipid profiles (total cholesterol, high-density cholesterol, and triglycerides). In this research, AI models such as RF and GBM demonstrated superior accuracy compared to traditional calculation formulas, showing a stronger correlation with directly measured LDL-C values. These findings underscore AI's potential to deliver both accurate and interpretable LDL-C predictions, enhancing clinical decision making and personalized patient care [86].

The provided studies highlight the potential of AI and ML in improving the accuracy of dyslipidemia diagnosis, risk factor identification, and LDL-C prediction. By leveraging these advanced technologies, healthcare providers can implement more precise, personalized, and effective strategies for preventing and managing cardiovascular diseases.

ML methods are still under evaluation, and their effectiveness may vary depending on the clinical context. Most clinical studies currently rely on the Friedewald formula (FF), which, despite being developed 50 years ago, remains widely used due to its simplicity, even though more accurate methods for estimating LDL cholesterol (LDL-C) are available [87].

A 2022 study compared the predictive performance of three ML models—random forests, XGBoost, and support vector regression (SVR)—against the traditional linear regression model and existing LDL-C calculation formulas in an eastern Indian population. The results showed that LDL-C predicted by the XGBoost and random forests models had a strong correlation with directly measured LDL-C (r = 0.98), outperforming the six commonly used formulas, including Friedewald, particularly across different triglyceride levels [88].

Additionally, a 2021 study on the Sampson formula found it to have the highest accuracy among various formulas, emphasizing its importance in avoiding the misclassification of hypercholesterolemia, which could delay treatment and lead to CVD progression [89]. Another 2022 study comparing the Friedewald, Sampson, and Martin–Hopkins formulas concluded that the extended Martin–Hopkins formula provided the most concordant results with direct LDL-C assays, especially in patients with low LDL-C levels or hypertriglyceridemia. However, it noted that the performance of these methods could vary with different assays and populations, highlighting the need for further validation [90].

In summary, while ML models show promise in providing more accurate LDL-C predictions, their effectiveness needs further validation across diverse clinical settings. Traditional formulas like Friedewald continue to be used but newer methods, such as the extended Martin–Hopkins and Sampson formulas, demonstrate potential for improved accuracy and require continued investigation to confirm their validity across various populations.

6.3. Personalized Statin Treatment Using Machine Learning

As mentioned before, AI and ML offer promising tools for personalized treatment strategies. There is research on statin therapy for individual patients that aims to enhance treatment efficacy by predicting responses and optimizing dosage based on personal risk factors. Statins are well-known and widely used medications for treating dyslipidemia. Nevertheless, they can cause side effects, such as an increased risk of diabetes mellitus, myalgia, and elevated hepatic transaminase levels [91]. This underscores the importance of personalized statin treatment.

The current guidelines provide LDL-C targets but often fail to consider individual patient responses to statins, highlighting the need for personalized therapy. In the study conducted on data sourced from patients starting statins between 2003 and 2022, a machine learning algorithm was developed using electronic health records from three tertiary hospitals (21,500 patients). The XGBoost model demonstrated the highest predictive performance, with an AUROC of 0.84 during internal validation and 0.81 during external validation, outperforming other methods like k-nearest neighbors (KNNs), support vector machine (SVM), and random forest. This model identified key factors like diabetes, baseline LDL-C, HbA1c, age, and SCORE2/SCORE2-OP as critical for predicting LDL-C target attainment. Implementing the XGB model in clinical practice could increase the likelihood of achieving LDL-C targets with initial statin prescriptions to 71–80%, offering a promising approach for personalized dyslipidemia management [92].

Another work providing a novel perspective on statin therapy explored a neural network trained to replicate National Institute for Health and Care Excellence guidelines, which was then enhanced through transfer learning using real-world outcomes from anonymized UK primary care data. The model analyzed 9675 patients receiving statin therapy and identified that for approximately 10% of the patients, smaller statin doses achieved better cholesterol reduction than higher doses recommended by guidelines. This deviation was potentially linked to improved adherence due to fewer side effects [93].

These studies highlight the potential of ML to revolutionize statin therapy by offering personalized treatment strategies that improve efficacy, optimize dosage, and enhance patient adherence through tailored care approaches.

6.4. Possible Synergy Between AI and Nanotechnology

Based on the developments in AI techniques discussed in the earlier parts of this review, it is crucial to consider the possibility of synergy between AI and nanotechnology since both techniques can be combined to enhance the efficiency and precision of the processes. The application of AI combined with nanotechnology may give new opportunities in various fields of medicine. It might improve the creation of advanced materials, devices, and systems. AI-driven computational tools and ML algorithms can enhance the design of nanomaterials [79].

6.4.1. Drug Delivery

By enabling precision drug delivery, personalized medicine, and advanced disease detection, AI-guided nanosystems enhance therapeutic efficacy and minimize side effects through targeted delivery and real-time monitoring. AI-based nanosensors are used for early disease detection and continuous monitoring, offering real-time data. These innovations provide an idea of how much AI can be combined with nanotechnology to reform healthcare [94]. AI can predict how nanoparticles interact with biological systems, including drug release and toxicity, while reducing the need for repetitive experiments. Studies demonstrate AI's potential to enhance drug delivery, analyze vascular systems, and address challenges like low nanoparticle delivery efficiency in cancer treatments [95].

While there is currently no accessible research explicitly combining nanotechnology and AI in the management of dyslipidemia, the potential for such integration is promising. To explore this possibility, insights from other medical fields, such as oncology, where the synergy between these technologies has been studied, may provide valuable guidance.

In original research from 2022, researchers have described the usage of NP delivery to tumors using ML and AI models [96]. This study applied multiple ML methods, including deep neural networks, RF, support vector machine, linear regression, and bagged models, to analyze data from the Nano-Tumor Database containing 376 datasets. To assess how NPs' physicochemical characteristics, tumor models, and cancer kinds affect the effectiveness of tumor administration, a physiologically based pharmacokinetic (PBPK) model was used.

The deep neural network model outperformed the other ML methods in predicting NP delivery efficiency, achieving an R^2 of 0.92 on the training dataset for maximum delivery efficiency and 0.70 on the test dataset. Cancer type significantly determined prediction accuracy, accounting for 19–29% of the variance.

While the model performed well on the training dataset, the R^2 values on the test dataset were notably lower for delivery efficiency at 24 h and 168 h, indicating reduced predictive power for long-term efficiency. Additionally, the study used PBPK model data, which might not accurately represent in vivo complexity.

By offering insights into enhancing tumor delivery efficiency and comprehending its underlying challenges, this work shows how combining AI with PBPK modeling can improve the design of cancer nanomedicines [96].

The Food and Administration has been actively involved in developing NP-based drug delivery systems, with notable examples like Abraxane, an albumin-based NP formulation of paclitaxel, which has shown commercial success in breast cancer treatment. Synthetic polymers, such as poly D, L-lactic-co-glycolic acid, and lipid-based formulations like Intralipid, are commonly used due to their biocompatibility, biodegradability, and ability to improve bioavailability while reducing cytotoxicity. Recent advancements include polymeric nanoparticles for controlled release and enhanced tumor localization, as seen with Vyxeos, an FDA-approved NP-based chemotherapy for acute myeloid leukemia, which improves efficacy even at lower doses. Other innovations include Myocet, a liposomal doxorubicin formulation for breast cancer metastasis, and NBTXR3, hafnium oxide nanoparticles that enhance radiotherapy by increasing tumor cell death without harming healthy tissues. Numerous NP-based drug delivery systems are currently under clinical trials, promising significant advancements in cancer treatment upon future approvals [97].

Drawing from such examples from oncology, future research could explore AI-guided nanomedical systems for precise drug delivery and the personalized treatment of dyslipidemia. This interdisciplinary approach holds promise for improving patient outcomes by tailoring therapies to individual needs.

6.4.2. NPs Design

Another important area that should be discussed is the integration of AI and nanotechnology to optimize nanoparticle design. This approach might make the applications of medicines more efficient and effective.

AI (particularly ML) has a key role in developing reproducible nanomaterials by predicting and optimizing their physical, mechanical, and chemical properties. By identifying crucial synthesis factors such as temperature, pressure, and electric current, AI tools enable the creation of tunable nanoarchitectures in dimensions like 0D, 1D, and 2D. The process begins with data cleaning and organization, followed by modeling using AI algorithms like artificial neural networks (ANNs) and deep neural networks (DNNs), allowing for reliable predictions of material properties. Although AI reduces experimental costs and time, challenges like large data requirements and computational power remain [98].

For instance, a Bayesian ML technique reduced the number of experimental runs needed to synthesize titanium nitride nanofilms to just eight. The optimized conditions predicted by the model resulted in high-quality nanofilms. The initial experimental conditions produced poor crystalline quality, but the model accurately identified accurate conditions for superior crystallinity and performance. Similarly, the synthesis of nanozeolite LTA was optimized using a complex ANN model, which identified five principal components explaining over 90% of the data variance. The model revealed relationships between key synthesis descriptors, such as temperature, pH, and pressure, and predicted the quantitative outputs of synthesis routes. This approach resulted in high-purity nanozeolite LTA, confirmed by XRD characterization. In this case, AI has not only been used to predict material properties but has also played a key role in advancing hierarchical nanostructures and self-assembling nanomaterials, showcasing its significant impact on nanotechnology [98].

The design and formulation of nanomaterials by the AI have also been successfully applied to lipid NPs, self-assembling drug–small-molecule nanoparticles, protein nanomaterials, and spherical nucleic acids. For instance, the AI-Guided Ionizable Lipid Engineering platform uses ANN to model lipid structures from the data collected by high-throughput screening large libraries of 12,000 lipid structures, identifying optimal lipid NP formulations. They were selected for their effectiveness in transfecting muscle cells, serving as a model for vaccine delivery, and macrophages, demonstrating the potential for immune cell modulation [99].

What is more, the integration of ML and high-throughput experimental data can be used to identify stable and self-assembled drug NPs. The researchers rapidly identified 100 self-assembling drug nanoparticles from 2.1 million pairings of 788 candidate drugs and 2686 approved excipients. Two nanoparticles, sorafenib–glycyrrhizin and terbinafine–

taurocholic acid, were further characterized ex vivo and in vivo. This platform has the potential to accelerate the development of safer, more effective nanoformulations with high drug-loading capacities for diverse therapeutics [99].

There is a high potential of integrating AI with nanotechnology to improve nanoparticle design and synthesis, reducing costs and time. As AI continues to develop, its applications in nanotechnology are innovative across medicine, and that opens new ways in precision engineering and therapeutic advancements.

According to the insights from oncology, where AI-guided nanotechnology has been successfully used for precision drug delivery and optimizing NPs design, similar strategies could be applied to dyslipidemia. AI models could be able to design lipid-based nanoparticles for targeted drug delivery to reduce cholesterol plaques or regulate lipid metabolism, with real-time monitoring enabling personalized treatment adjustments.

ML algorithms could be able to predict nanoparticle behavior, addressing challenges like drug release efficiency and biocompatibility. This interdisciplinary approach holds significant promise for improving therapeutic outcomes and advancing innovative solutions in dyslipidemia management and surely needs a deeper focus.

6.5. Prospects, Difficulties, and Future Developments of AI in Dyslipidemia Management

The development of advanced technologies in AI is becoming increasingly widespread in various fields of medicine, including clinical lipidology. ML techniques, particularly ensemble methods, and neural networks are being used to predict dyslipidemia with high accuracy, precision, and sensitivity. The developed algorithms demonstrate great potential in accurately diagnosing dyslipidemia, which may lead to more effective disease management strategies. ML proves to be an invaluable tool in predicting dyslipidemia and associated disorders by leveraging patient data to improve diagnostic and treatment processes [100].

However, it should be remembered that easy access to data due to digitization and the development of applications such as ML carries the risk of disclosing sensitive health information of a patient without their consent. In this context, privacy refers to protection against attacks from competitors whose main goal is to extract sensitive information from the victim, leading to an unintended data breach [100].

Large datasets have a significant impact on the digital world, as more and more companies rely on data analysis to carry out daily operations. As a result, managing how our data is stored, updated, and shared is crucial for privacy. With the growing use of powerful internet-based data analysis tools, privacy has become an important social issue. The development of AI increases the risk of privacy violations. Advanced AI methods, such as deep learning, are ideal for analyzing large datasets and represent one of the most effective ways to process huge amounts of data in an acceptable timeframe.

Most people are unaware of the amount of data generated, analyzed, or exchanged by their devices and applications, which leads to privacy violations [100].

Despite the increase in studies applying these innovative techniques, familiarizing medical personnel with new methods and introducing new tools into clinical practice remains a challenge. The key difference is that traditional statistics rely on predefined models, whereas AI and ML are data-driven, operating without a prior understanding of the relationship between data and outcomes [101].

The ethical concerns related to the use of "black-box" medical algorithms by doctors should be further developed. It is widely acknowledged that ML algorithms carry immense potential. They offer opportunities for analyzing large datasets, recognizing patterns, and making predictions, especially in the decision-making process. AI is becoming a powerful tool, delivering promising results across various applications.

However, despite the tremendous prospects of AI revolutionizing healthcare, the functioning of some advanced ML systems remains opaque. This is due to the fact that deep learning algorithms are complex structures, whose results can be difficult to understand even for researchers, as they cannot precisely determine why the algorithm produced a specific outcome.

Such a model of operation raises concerns about values like fairness, the authority of doctors, and the privacy of patient data, as the reasons behind AI-generated decisions may also be impossible for doctors to explain. Consequently, there is a significant risk that the validity of diagnoses and recommendations for medication will be questioned by patients [102].

High-dimensional data, such as multi-omics data used in personalized health, exhibit significant inter-individual variability and are strongly influenced by environmental factors and lifestyle. Studies also indicate systematic differences in the microbiome between various ethnic groups. People from different regions of the world possess unique microbial taxa that are more abundantly represented in their bodies, likely due to both genetic and environmental differences [103].

A major ML challenge is to ensure that predictive models used in personalized diets and disease management function reliably across diverse racial, ethnic, gender, cultural, and geographic groups. The risk of algorithmic bias is particularly high in personalized health, as both the source data and individual outcomes are highly heterogeneous [104].

The creation of clear regulatory frameworks for artificial intelligence in healthcare is inevitable to ensure its implementation and deployment with consideration for safety and ethical issues. These guidelines should be flexible enough to adapt to technological advancements and emerging challenges. Key to this process will be the involvement of stakeholders who will collaboratively develop principles that account for patient safety and ethical concerns related to the development and application of AI. Among the most important regulatory issues is the standardization of performance indicators, which will enable the calculation of AI efficiency and allow the comparison of different studies and applications, contributing to their transparency. Additionally, regulatory bodies should develop clear guidelines for the safe use of AI systems, including testing protocols, validation, and ongoing oversight. Furthermore, the involvement of a broad range of stakeholders, from clinicians and patients to AI developers, in the regulatory process will ensure that various viewpoints are considered when creating standards [105].

Health disparities related to ethnicity, sex, gender identity, geographic location, and socioeconomic status still exist and are often amplified by artificial intelligence. However, these studies typically treat each factor separately—race/ethnicity, sex, gender identity, socioeconomic status, abilities, etc. What is needed now are intersectional analyses in health and medical research. Intersectionality examines how overlapping or intersecting forms of discrimination related to a patient's social and cultural life course impact health outcomes. An iconic example of intersectional analysis in the context of facial recognition is a study that showed systems analyzing sex and race separately failed to capture the full extent of bias against black women. The sex analysis revealed that systems performed better on men's faces than on women's faces. The race analysis showed that systems performed better on lighter-skinned faces than on darker-skinned ones. The intersectional analysis revealed that these single axes missed the fact that systems performed much worse for black women. Further research is needed to understand how intersecting human characteristics such as sex, gender identity, race/ethnicity, socioeconomic status, and age influence health outcomes across society [106].

Currently, AI is not self-sufficient. It cannot reason in the same way that humans do. It lacks qualities such as clinical intuition and experience. Furthermore, AI does not possess developed critical thinking skills or the ability to question certain information. Instead, AI functions as a signal translator, transforming patterns from datasets. At present, AI systems are increasingly being implemented by healthcare organizations to automate time-consuming, repetitive tasks with high volumes. Additionally, significant progress has been made in applying AI to precision diagnostics (e.g., diabetic retinopathy and radiotherapy planning) [107].

The application of AI, ML, and DL in lipidology enables more accurate and clinically relevant predictions, which could significantly impact clinical practice.

Significant progress is expected in the development of powerful algorithms over the next few years, which will be efficient and capable of utilizing unstructured data as well as combining diverse data. In addition, healthcare organizations and medical practices will strive to have AI systems collaborate with technology partners in the development of new AI systems for precision therapies. However, it is crucial to understand the barriers that patients face when using lipid-lowering medications. Caution in this regard can help physicians effectively address these challenges. Moreover, in the near future, we can expect the development of improved predictive models based on lipid profiles. Additionally, innovative AI techniques could uncover previously unknown disease correlations and facilitate the implementation of precision medicine. Nonetheless, the social, methodological, and ethical complexities associated with these applications require further research and regulation.

6.6. Limitations and Challenges Associated with Nanoparticles and Artificial Intelligence: New Perspectives and Difficulties

Polymeric nanoparticles are a key tool in enhancing drug bioavailability and delivering them precisely to their site of action. Thanks to their versatility, polymers present a promising option capable of meeting the demands of various drug delivery systems used in specific therapies. With the increasing demand for nanoparticles, scaling up production processes becomes inevitable. This involves transitioning from small-scale production, such as in a laboratory, to larger-scale production suitable for industrial and commercial applications. The challenges associated with this process pertain to controlling nanoparticle properties (maintaining quality, uniformity, cost, and efficiency), as the synthesis techniques for PNPs at the laboratory scale often struggle with batch-to-batch variability. Scaling up production introduces numerous difficulties that need to be addressed to ensure efficiency and product quality control. This literature review focuses on several aspects of this problem [108].

Firstly, maintaining consistent properties (e.g., size, shape, charge, and polydispersity) of nanoparticles during mass production is more challenging. Ensuring that nanoparticle properties align with application requirements is crucial. During the scaling of laboratory techniques, reproducibility is key for real-world nanomaterial applications. Unfortunately, beneficial nanoparticle properties are sometimes lost. Particles may change over time or in response to environmental conditions. The temporal gap between analysis and application, as well as ensuring consistency or verification, is critical. A significant obstacle in this field is the diversity of the literature regarding research conducted and experimental data. However, there are ways to address this. Keeping records to identify sources and reduce particle variability, as well as implementing a "minimum standard of information" in nanoparticle research, including details of materials and experimental procedures, are recommended. Controlled replication studies are fundamental to avoiding excessive variations between systems and properly determining similarities and differences among compared systems.

Another important issue is nanotoxicology, which raises many concerns, particularly regarding toxicity and cellular uptake. The toxicity of nanoparticles depends, among other factors, on their chemical composition, shape, surface charge, aggregation, and solubility. After systemic exposure, they accumulate in the phagocytic system of parenchymal organs and cause DNA damage, cell cycle arrest, and ultimately cell death. Identifying the key physical or chemical characteristics of nanoparticles that contribute to their toxicity will help develop safer methods to minimize toxicity. However, this does not apply to polymeric nanoparticles, which are biocompatible, biodegradable, and non-toxic. This makes them safe for use in humans and improves drug bioavailability [108].

The next challenge in nanoparticle production is the need to consider environmental aspects, such as impact and safety. Currently, the production of various inorganic NPs with specific chemical compositions, sizes, and shapes is carried out using microbial fermentation (bacteria, yeasts, and fungi). Green nanotechnology, encompassing regulatory processes, purification, and remediation, supports environmental protection, waste reduction, and the use of safer solvents and renewable raw materials. Integrating the principles of green chemistry and engineering could offer an alternative to traditional NP synthesis methods. These methods rely on biological precursors and depend on parameters such as solvent, temperature, pressure, and pH.

Enhancing PNP production capacity is an unavoidable requirement for industry and human health. The transition from laboratory-scale to large-scale production, from batch systems to continuous systems, is becoming a reality. Several methods have been developed for producing nanoparticles with desirable characteristics on a large scale, including membrane extrusion, supercritical fluid technology, the use of microreactors in industry, or nanobiotechnology. Due to their numerous advantages, these methods offer hope for the development of various drug delivery systems and therapies. Nevertheless, the application of these methods to develop targeted and surface-functionalized nanoparticles on a large scale remains contentious. Nanomedicine represents a breakthrough in healthcare, and several clinical therapies are already available. Experiments that are thoroughly reported and analyzed offer hope that nanomedicine will soon transform many laboratory products into market-ready solutions for various therapies and clinical purposes [108].

AI algorithms are becoming a key component of healthcare, from diagnostics to population health management. Therefore, it is crucial to implement processes for mitigating algorithmic biases, which may lead to inequalities in care.

Addressing biases is not only about ensuring equal opportunities for optimal health outcomes but also promoting patient protection. Biased algorithms can result in situations where certain groups of patients do not receive adequate care, which can have serious consequences.

Medical institutions play a crucial role in addressing algorithmic biases. AI algorithms require evaluations in the specific context of their use, as they may be sensitive to differences between the data used during development and the data applied at the point of care for individual patients. Challenges such as algorithm drift or the emergence of new biases require continuous monitoring. Another issue is that some medical institutions are not sufficiently equipped to undertake the processes of evaluating and monitoring algorithmic biases, which may contribute to social inequalities. An alternative for those institutions without internal AI expertise is to seek assistance from developers. However, this raises concerns, as despite the best intentions, it may turn out that their algorithms lead to biased results without them realizing it [108].

To mitigate algorithmic biases, the best approach seems to be a shared responsibility model. In this model, all key partners, including medical institutions, AI developers, and regulatory bodies, take action to address the bias problem. Such an approach supports resource-limited institutions in adopting valuable AI algorithms into clinical care and ensures greater precision in controlling biases in medical institutions.

Another issue is the framework for AI algorithm transparency, which should align with the requirements of the ACA. There are already regulatory requirements for AI developers within the ONC and the FDA.

This will enable medical institutions to effectively assess and monitor algorithms, and the transparency process will build trust among patients and clinicians, fostering broader adoption. All transparency data should be stored in an open-access repository [109].

7. How AI and Nanotechnology Might Affect Healthcare?

AI offers transformative opportunities in healthcare but introduces systemic challenges and costs that require careful consideration. In the context of predictive disease models, their judicious application is vital to avoid inequitable treatment based on algorithmic predictions. As these models become integral to clinical practice, the ongoing evaluation of their performance and therapeutic impact is crucial for ensuring responsible and effective use.

To achieve fairness, training datasets must accurately represent the demographics of the target populations, integrating diverse patient data—including demographic, genetic, and environmental factors. This ensures the equitable prediction of disease progression and risk across all groups. Ethical considerations must be prioritized through informed consent, robust oversight, and comprehensive regulatory frameworks to prevent misuse or discrimination. A key advantage of AI is its potential to enhance personalized therapy, leading to reduced costs and improved patient outcomes. For example, pharmacogenomics leverages genetic information to optimize drug efficacy and minimize adverse effects, thereby advancing precision medicine [110].

Despite these benefits, implementing AI in healthcare presents significant financial and logistical challenges. By 2021, hospitals were projected to spend USD 6.6 billion annually on AI technologies, but these investments have yielded measurable benefits, such as reduced hospital readmissions, decreased emergency room visits, and improved adherence to treatment plans. For instance, Grady Hospital in Atlanta reported USD 4 million in savings over two years due to a 31% reduction in readmissions, attributed to an AI tool identifying at-risk patients [111].

However, challenges remain. Data privacy and cybersecurity risks, including unauthorized access to sensitive patient information, pose significant concerns. Ethical compliance and adherence to legal regulations are imperative to protect patient data. Additionally, AI systems developed without adequate medical expertise risk inaccuracies and misdiagnoses, compounded by a lack of transparency, errors in design, and limitations in handling unstructured data like medical imaging. The absence of standardized data further exacerbates inconsistencies across healthcare settings [112,113].

Successful AI implementation in healthcare requires addressing key issues. These include establishing ethical and secure data access processes, leveraging domain expertise to interpret data effectively, and ensuring sufficient computing power for real-time decision making, enabled by advancements in cloud computing. Rigorous research into the real-world integration of AI algorithms is essential to ensure their trustworthiness, efficacy, and seamless adoption within clinical workflows [107].

8. Conclusions

Dyslipidemia, characterized by abnormal lipid levels in the blood, is a significant risk factor for CVD and obesity-related complications. The abnormal lipid profile is commonly associated with obesity and closely linked to the development of atherosclerosis and thesubsequent cardiovascular events. Understanding the molecular mechanisms behind lipid metabolism and lipoprotein transport has paved the way for innovative therapeutic strategies, including the use of nanotechnology in drug delivery.

Nanotechnology, particularly through the development of nanoparticles like liposomes, holds promise in improving the delivery and efficacy of treatments for dyslipidemia. Liposomes, with their ability to encapsulate both hydrophilic and hydrophobic drugs, offer targeted drug delivery, potentially enhancing treatment outcomes while minimizing side effects. Negative-charged nanoliposomes, in particular, have shown potential in improving lipid profiles, stabilizing atherosclerotic plaques, and modulating inflammation, all of which are key factors in the management of cardiovascular diseases.

While statins remain the cornerstone of dyslipidemia treatment, their side effects, such as muscle pain, hepatotoxicity, and diabetes risk, limit their long-term adherence and effectiveness. Research indicates that combining statin therapy with innovative approaches like nanoliposome-based treatments could potentially enhance therapeutic outcomes, reduce side effects, and better manage cardiovascular risk.

Emerging evidence from clinical studies and the use of AI in predicting patient responses to treatments suggests that personalized approaches to statin therapy can optimize efficacy and minimize risks. ML models have demonstrated the ability to tailor statin doses and improve adherence, ultimately improving outcomes for dyslipidemia management.

In conclusion, while challenges remain in optimizing the current therapies and developing new treatments, advancements in nanotechnology, personalized medicine, and ML offer promising avenues to improve the management of dyslipidemia and reduce the risk of atherosclerotic cardiovascular diseases. Continued research and clinical trials will be crucial in determining the most effective strategies for integrating these innovations into routine clinical practice.

Integrating AI with nanotechnology offers groundbreaking possibilities, particularly in medicine, where precision and efficiency are critical. The success of AI-guided nanotechnology in oncology for precision drug delivery demonstrates its transformative potential. Extending similar approaches to dyslipidemia could revolutionize its treatment, enabling the design of lipid-based nanoparticles for targeted drug delivery, real-time monitoring, and personalized therapy.

By leveraging ML algorithms to predict and optimize nanoparticle behavior, we can address challenges like drug release efficiency and biocompatibility. This interdisciplinary synergy not only enhances therapeutic outcomes but also paves the way for innovative, cost-effective solutions in managing complex conditions like dyslipidemia. The potential is immense, warranting focused research and investment to unlock new frontiers in precision medicine.

Trials combining AI with nanotechnology could involve the AI-driven analysis of nanomaterials used for targeted drug delivery, optimizing dosage and delivery mechanisms for specific patient profiles, or AI could analyze real-time data from nanosensors, monitoring biomarkers in the bloodstream and enabling early disease detection and personalized interventions. However, this requires further research to ensure the effective and ethical integration of these technologies.

Author Contributions: Conceptualization, K.B., H.F., N.K., W.M. and A.P.; Writing—original draft preparation, K.B., H.F., N.K., W.M. and A.P.; Writing—review and editing, K.B., H.F., N.K., W.M. and A.P.; Visualization, K.B., H.F., N.K., W.M. and A.P.; Supervision, E.M., J.R. and B.F.; Project administration, E.M., J.R. and B.F.; Funding acquisition, E.M., J.R. and B.F. All authors have read and agreed to the published version of the manuscript.

Funding: This research received no external funding.

Institutional Review Board Statement: Not applicable.

Informed Consent Statement: Not applicable.

Data Availability Statement: No new data were created or analyzed in this study. Data sharing is not applicable to this article.

Conflicts of Interest: The authors declare no conflicts of interest.

Abbreviations

ACA	Affordable Care Act
ACL	adenosine triphosphate-citrate lyase
ACS	acute coronary syndrome
AI	artificial intelligence
AMI	acute myocardial infarction
ANN	artificial neural network
ASCVD	atherosclerotic cardiovascular disease
BCA	brachiocephalic artery
BMI	body mass index
CAD	coronary artery disease
CK-MB	Creatine Kinase-MB
cTns	cardiac troponins I or T
CVD	cardiovascular disease
DNN	deep neural network
DHA	Docosahexaenoic acid
DL	deep learning
DM	diabetes mellitus
EPA	Eicosapentaenoic acid
FDA	Food and Drug Administration
FFA	free fatty acid
GBM	Gradient Boosting Machine
HDL	high-density lipoprotein
HDL-C	high-density lipoprotein cholesterol
H-FABP	Heart-type fatty acid-binding protein
HMG-CoA	3-hydroxy-3-methyl-glutaryl-coenzyme A reductase
HF	heart failure
IDL	VLDL remnant
KNN	k-nearest neighbor
LDL	low-density lipoprotein
LDL-C	low-density lipoprotein cholesterol
LDLR	low-density lipoprotein receptor
Lp(a)	lipoprotein (a)
LPHNPs	lipid–polymer hybrid nanoparticles

ML	machine learning
MLP	multi-layer perception
MUFA	monounsaturated fat
NAFLD	non-alcoholic fatty liver disease
NP	nanoparticle
NT-proBNP	N-terminal prohormone of brain natriuretic peptide
ONC	Office of the National Coordinator for Health Information Technology
PAMAM	poly(amido)amine dendrimer
PBPK	physiologically based pharmacokinetic
PCL	polycaprolactone
PCSK9	Proprotein convertase subtilisin/kexin type 9
PCSK9i	PCSK9 inhibitor
PEI	polyvinyl imine
PLGA	Poly(lactic-co-glycolic) acid
PRS	polygenic risk scores
PUFA	polyunsaturated fat
RCT	reverse cholesterol transport
RF	random forest
SAFA	saturated fatty acid
SIM-LipoNP	simvastatin encapsulated in nanoliposome
siRNA	small interfering RNA
SVM	support vector machine
TC	total cholesterol
TFA	trans fatty acid
TG	triglyceride
VIM	Variable Importance Measure
VLDL	very low-density lipoprotein

References

1. Global Cardiovascular Risk Consortium; Magnussen, C.; Ojeda, F.M.; Leong, D.P.; Alegre-Diaz, J.; Amouyel, P.; Aviles-Santa, L.; De Bacquer, D.; Ballantyne, C.M.; Bernabé-Ortiz, A.; et al. Global Effect of Modifiable Risk Factors on Cardiovascular Disease and Mortality. *N. Engl. J. Med.* **2023**, *389*, 1273–1285. [CrossRef] [PubMed] [PubMed Central]
2. Shaya, G.E.; Leucker, T.M.; Jones, S.R.; Martin, S.S.; Toth, P.P. Coronary heart disease risk: Low-density lipoprotein and beyond. *Trends Cardiovasc. Med.* **2022**, *32*, 181–194. [CrossRef] [PubMed]
3. Katta, N.; Loethen, T.; Lavie, C.J.; Alpert, M.A. Obesity and Coronary Heart Disease: Epidemiology, Pathology, and Coronary Artery Imaging. *Curr. Probl. Cardiol.* **2021**, *46*, 100655. [CrossRef] [PubMed]
4. Medina-Leyte, D.J.; Zepeda-García, O.; Domínguez-Pérez, M.; González-Garrido, A.; Villarreal-Molina, T.; Jacobo-Albavera, L. Endothelial Dysfunction, Inflammation and Coronary Artery Disease: Potential Biomarkers and Promising Therapeutical Approaches. *Int. J. Mol. Sci.* **2021**, *22*, 3850. [CrossRef] [PubMed] [PubMed Central]
5. Francula-Zaninovic, S.; Nola, I.A. Management of Measurable Variable Cardiovascular Disease' Risk Factors. *Curr. Cardiol. Rev.* **2018**, *14*, 153–163. [CrossRef] [PubMed] [PubMed Central]
6. Collet, J.P.; Thiele, H.; Barbato, E.; Barthélémy, O.; Bauersachs, J.; Bhatt, D.L.; Dendale, P.; Dorobantu, M.; Edvardsen, T.; Folliguet, T.; et al. 2020 ESC Guidelines for the management of acute coronary syndromes in patients presenting without persistent ST-segment elevation. *Rev. Esp. Cardiol.* **2021**, *74*, 544. [CrossRef] [PubMed]
7. Dhingra, R.; Vasan, R.S. Biomarkers in cardiovascular disease: Statistical assessment and section on key novel heart failure biomarkers. *Trends Cardiovasc. Med.* **2017**, *27*, 123–133. [CrossRef] [PubMed] [PubMed Central]
8. Chaulin, A.M. The Importance of Cardiac Troponin Metabolism in the Laboratory Diagnosis of Myocardial Infarction (Comprehensive Review). *Biomed. Res. Int.* **2022**, *2022*, 6454467. [CrossRef] [PubMed] [PubMed Central]
9. Lyngbakken, M.N.; Myhre, P.L.; Røsjø, H.; Omland, T. Novel biomarkers of cardiovascular disease: Applications in clinical practice. *Crit. Rev. Clin. Lab. Sci.* **2019**, *56*, 33–60. [CrossRef] [PubMed]
10. Netala, V.R.; Teertam, S.K.; Li, H.; Zhang, Z. A Comprehensive Review of Cardiovascular Disease Management: Cardiac Biomarkers, Imaging Modalities, Pharmacotherapy, Surgical Interventions, and Herbal Remedies. *Cells* **2024**, *13*, 1471. [CrossRef] [PubMed] [PubMed Central]

11. Rezar, R.; Jirak, P.; Gschwandtner, M.; Derler, R.; Felder, T.K.; Haslinger, M.; Kopp, K.; Seelmaier, C.; Granitz, C.; Hoppe, U.C.; et al. Heart-Type Fatty Acid-Binding Protein (H-FABP) and its Role as a Biomarker in Heart Failure: What Do We Know So Far? *J. Clin. Med.* **2020**, *9*, 164. [CrossRef] [PubMed] [PubMed Central]
12. Khan, S.Q.; Dhillon, O.S.; O'Brien, R.J.; Struck, J.; Quinn, P.A.; Morgenthaler, N.G.; Squire, I.B.; Davies, J.E.; Bergmann, A.; Ng, L.L. C-terminal provasopressin (copeptin) as a novel and prognostic marker in acute myocardial infarction: Leicester Acute Myocardial Infarction Peptide (LAMP) study. *Circulation* **2007**, *115*, 2103–2110. [CrossRef] [PubMed]
13. Maisel, A.; Xue, Y.; Shah, K.; Mueller, C.; Nowak, R.; Peacock, W.F.; Ponikowski, P.; Mockel, M.; Hogan, C.; Wu, A.H.; et al. Increased 90-day mortality in patients with acute heart failure with elevated copeptin: Secondary results from the Biomarkers in Acute Heart Failure (BACH) study. *Circ. Heart Fail.* **2011**, *4*, 613–620. [CrossRef] [PubMed]
14. Mohd Faizal, A.S.; Thevarajah, T.M.; Khor, S.M.; Chang, S.W. A review of risk prediction models in cardiovascular disease: Conventional approach vs. artificial intelligent approach. *Comput. Methods Programs Biomed.* **2021**, *207*, 106190. [CrossRef] [PubMed]
15. Kakadiaris, I.A.; Vrigkas, M.; Yen, A.A.; Kuznetsova, T.; Budoff, M.; Naghavi, M. Machine Learning Outperforms ACC / AHA CVD Risk Calculator in MESA. *J. Am. Heart Assoc.* **2018**, *7*, e009476. [CrossRef] [PubMed] [PubMed Central]
16. Khanna, N.N.; Singh, M.; Maindarkar, M.; Kumar, A.; Johri, A.M.; Mentella, L.; Laird, J.R.; Paraskevas, K.I.; Ruzsa, Z.; Singh, N.; et al. Polygenic Risk Score for Cardiovascular Diseases in Artificial Intelligence Paradigm: A Review. *J. Korean Med. Sci.* **2023**, *38*, e395. [CrossRef] [PubMed]
17. Alqahtani, M.S.; Alzibali, K.F.; Mahdi, A.M.M.; Alharbi, O.M.A.; Harbi, R.H.A.; Alkhaldi, H.S.M.; Alsayafi, Z.A.A.; Albisher, F.H.; Buqurayn, M.H.; Alharbi, M.M. Lipid-Lowering Medications for Managing Dyslipidemia: A Narrative Review. *Cureus* **2024**, *16*, e65202. [CrossRef] [PubMed] [PubMed Central]
18. Feingold, K.R. Introduction to Lipids and Lipoproteins. 14 January 2024. In *Endotext [Internet]*; Feingold, K.R., Anawalt, B., Blackman, M.R., Boyce, A., Chrousos, G., Corpas, E., de Herder, W.W., Dhatariya, K., Dungan, K., Hofland, J., et al., Eds.; MDText.com, Inc.: South Dartmouth, MA, USA, 2000. [PubMed]
19. Bays, H.E.; Kirkpatrick, C.; Maki, K.C.; Toth, P.P.; Morgan, R.T.; Tondt, J.; Christensen, S.M.; Dixon, D.; Jacobson, T.A. Obesity, dyslipidemia, and cardiovascular disease: A joint expert review from the Obesity Medicine Association and the National Lipid Association 2024. *Obes. Pillars* **2024**, *10*, 100108. [CrossRef] [PubMed] [PubMed Central]
20. Heeren, J.; Scheja, L. Metabolic-associated fatty liver disease and lipoprotein metabolism. *Mol. Metab.* **2021**, *50*, 101238. [CrossRef] [PubMed] [PubMed Central]
21. Wu, S.A.; Kersten, S.; Qi, L. Lipoprotein Lipase and Its Regulators: An Unfolding Story. *Trends Endocrinol. Metab.* **2021**, *32*, 48–61. [CrossRef] [PubMed] [PubMed Central]
22. Choi, S.H.; Ginsberg, H.N. Increased very low density lipoprotein (VLDL) secretion, hepatic steatosis, and insulin resistance. *Trends Endocrinol. Metab.* **2011**, *22*, 353–363. [CrossRef] [PubMed] [PubMed Central]
23. Pahwa, R.; Jialal, I. Atherosclerosis. 8 August 2023. In *StatPearls [Internet]*; StatPearls Publishing: Treasure Island, FL, USA, 2024. [PubMed]
24. Mach, F.; Baigent, C.; Catapano, A.L.; Koskinas, K.C.; Casula, M.; Badimon, L.; Chapman, M.J.; De Backer, G.G.; Delgado, V.; Ference, B.A.; et al. 2019 ESC/EAS Guidelines for the management of dyslipidaemias: Lipid modification to reduce cardiovascular risk. *Eur. Heart J.* **2020**, *41*, 111–188; Erratum in *Eur. Heart J.* **2020**, *41*, 4255. https://doi.org/10.1093/eurheartj/ehz826. [CrossRef] [PubMed]
25. Hoogeveen, R.C.; Ballantyne, C.M. Residual Cardiovascular Risk at Low LDL: Remnants, Lipoprotein(a), and Inflammation. *Clin. Chem.* **2021**, *67*, 143–153. [CrossRef] [PubMed] [PubMed Central]
26. Dybiec, J.; Baran, W.; Dąbek, B.; Fularski, P.; Młynarska, E.; Radzioch, E.; Rysz, J.; Franczyk, B. Advances in Treatment of Dyslipidemia. *Int. J. Mol. Sci.* **2023**, *24*, 13288. [CrossRef] [PubMed] [PubMed Central]
27. Yang, Y.J. An Overview of Current Physical Activity Recommendations in Primary Care. *Korean J. Fam. Med.* **2019**, *40*, 135–142. [CrossRef] [PubMed] [PubMed Central]
28. Mannu, G.S.; Zaman, M.J.; Gupta, A.; Rehman, H.U.; Myint, P.K. Evidence of lifestyle modification in the management of hypercholesterolemia. *Curr. Cardiol. Rev.* **2013**, *9*, 2–14. [CrossRef] [PubMed] [PubMed Central]
29. Visseren, F.L.J.; Mach, F.; Smulders, Y.M.; Carballo, D.; Koskinas, K.C.; Bäck, M.; Benetos, A.; Biffi, A.; Boavida, J.M.; Capodanno, D.; et al. 2021 ESC Guidelines on cardiovascular disease prevention in clinical practice: Developed by the Task Force for cardiovascular disease prevention in clinical practice with representatives of the European Society of Cardiology and 12 medical societies with the special contribution of the European Association of Preventive Cardiology (EAPC). *Rev. Esp. Cardiol.* **2022**, *75*, 429. [CrossRef] [PubMed]
30. Castro-Barquero, S.; Ruiz-León, A.M.; Sierra-Pérez, M.; Estruch, R.; Casas, R. Dietary Strategies for Metabolic Syndrome: A Comprehensive Review. *Nutrients* **2020**, *12*, 2983. [CrossRef] [PubMed] [PubMed Central]

31. Chiavaroli, L.; Viguiliouk, E.; Nishi, S.K.; Blanco Mejia, S.; Rahelić, D.; Kahleová, H.; Salas-Salvadó, J.; Kendall, C.W.; Sievenpiper, J.L. DASH Dietary Pattern and Cardiometabolic Outcomes: An Umbrella Review of Systematic Reviews and Meta-Analyses. *Nutrients* **2019**, *11*, 338. [CrossRef] [PubMed] [PubMed Central]
32. Harris, W.S. Are omega-3 fatty acids the most important nutritional modulators of coronary heart disease risk? *Curr. Atheroscler. Rep.* **2004**, *6*, 447–452. [CrossRef] [PubMed]
33. Ye, X.F.; Miao, C.Y.; Zhang, W.; Ji, L.N.; Wang, J.G.; ATTEND investigators. Alcohol intake and dyslipidemia in male patients with hypertension and diabetes enrolled in a China multicenter registry. *J. Clin. Hypertens.* **2023**, *25*, 183–190. [CrossRef] [PubMed] [PubMed Central]
34. Dec, A.; Niemiec, A.; Wojciechowska, E.; Maligłówka, M.; Bułdak, Ł.; Bołdys, A.; Okopień, B. Inclisiran—A Revolutionary Addition to a Cholesterol-Lowering Therapy. *Int. J. Mol. Sci.* **2023**, *24*, 6858. [CrossRef] [PubMed] [PubMed Central]
35. Agnello, F.; Ingala, S.; Laterra, G.; Scalia, L.; Barbanti, M. Novel and Emerging LDL-C Lowering Strategies: A New Era of Dyslipidemia Management. *J. Clin. Med.* **2024**, *13*, 1251. [CrossRef] [PubMed] [PubMed Central]
36. Aguilar-Salinas, C.A.; Gómez-Díaz, R.A.; Corral, P. New Therapies for Primary Hyperlipidemia. *J. Clin. Endocrinol. Metab.* **2022**, *107*, 1216–1224. [CrossRef] [PubMed]
37. Penson, P.E.; Bruckert, E.; Marais, D.; Reiner, Ž.; Pirro, M.; Sahebkar, A.; Bajraktari, G.; Mirrakhimov, E.; Rizzo, M.; Mikhailidis, D.P.; et al. Step-by-step diagnosis and management of the nocebo/drucebo effect in statin-associated muscle symptoms patients: A position paper from the International Lipid Expert Panel (ILEP). *J. Cachexia Sarcopenia Muscle* **2022**, *13*, 1596–1622. [CrossRef] [PubMed] [PubMed Central]
38. Feingold, K.R. Obesity and Dyslipidemia. 19 June 2023. In *Endotext [Internet]*; Feingold, K.R., Anawalt, B., Blackman, M.R., Boyce, A., Chrousos, G., Corpas, E., de Herder, W.W., Dhatariya, K., Dungan, K., Hofland, J., et al., Eds.; MDText.com, Inc.: South Dartmouth, MA, USA, 2000. [PubMed]
39. Repp, M.L.; Edwards, M.D.; Burch, C.S.; Rao, A.; Chinyere, I.R. PCSK9 Inhibitors and Anthracyclines: The Future of Cardioprotection in Cardio-Oncology. *Hearts* **2024**, *5*, 375–388. [CrossRef] [PubMed] [PubMed Central]
40. Ray, K.K.; Wright, R.S.; Kallend, D.; Koenig, W.; Leiter, L.A.; Raal, F.J.; Bisch, J.A.; Richardson, T.; Jaros, M.; Wijngaard, P.L.J.; et al. Two Phase 3 Trials of Inclisiran in Patients with Elevated LDL Cholesterol. *N. Engl. J. Med.* **2020**, *382*, 1507–1519. [CrossRef] [PubMed]
41. Sucato, V.; Ortello, A.; Comparato, F.; Novo, G.; Galassi, A.R. Cholesterol-Lowering Strategies for Cardiovascular Disease Prevention: The Importance of Intensive Treatment and the Simplification of Medical Therapy. *J. Clin. Med.* **2024**, *13*, 1882. [CrossRef] [PubMed] [PubMed Central]
42. Kosoglou, T.; Statkevich, P.; Johnson-Levonas, A.O.; Paolini, J.F.; Bergman, A.J.; Alton, K.B. Ezetimibe: A review of its metabolism, pharmacokinetics and drug interactions. *Clin. Pharmacokinet.* **2005**, *44*, 467–494. [CrossRef] [PubMed]
43. Najib, J. Fenofibrate in the treatment of dyslipidemia: A review of the data as they relate to the new suprabioavailable tablet formulation. *Clin. Ther.* **2002**, *24*, 2022–2050. [CrossRef] [PubMed]
44. Bayda, S.; Adeel, M.; Tuccinardi, T.; Cordani, M.; Rizzolio, F. The History of Nanoscience and Nanotechnology: From Chemical-Physical Applications to Nanomedicine. *Molecules* **2019**, *25*, 112. [CrossRef] [PubMed] [PubMed Central]
45. Lombardo, D.; Calandra, P.; Barreca, D.; Magazù, S.; Kiselev, M.A. Soft Interaction in Liposome Nanocarriers for Therapeutic Drug Delivery. *Nanomaterials* **2016**, *6*, 125. [CrossRef] [PubMed] [PubMed Central]
46. Fan, D.; Cao, Y.; Cao, M.; Wang, Y.; Cao, Y.; Gong, T. Nanomedicine in cancer therapy. *Signal Transduct. Target. Ther.* **2023**, *8*, 293. [CrossRef] [PubMed] [PubMed Central]
47. Huang, X.; Li, L.; Chen, Z.; Yu, H.; You, X.; Kong, N.; Tao, W.; Zhou, X.; Huang, J. Nanomedicine for the Detection and Treatment of Ocular Bacterial Infections. *Adv. Mater.* **2023**, *35*, e2302431. [CrossRef] [PubMed]
48. Yu, X.; Trase, I.; Ren, M.; Duval, K.; Guo, X.; Chen, Z. Design of Nanoparticle-Based Carriers for Targeted Drug Delivery. *J. Nanomater.* **2016**, *2016*, 1087250. [CrossRef] [PubMed] [PubMed Central]
49. Cardoso, R.V.; Pereira, P.R.; Freitas, C.S.; Paschoalin, V.M.F. Trends in Drug Delivery Systems for Natural Bioactive Molecules to Treat Health Disorders: The Importance of Nano-Liposomes. *Pharmaceutics* **2022**, *14*, 2808. [CrossRef] [PubMed] [PubMed Central]
50. Liu, W.; Ye, A.; Han, F.; Han, J. Advances and challenges in liposome digestion: Surface interaction, biological fate, and GIT modeling. *Adv. Colloid. Interface Sci.* **2019**, *263*, 52–67. [CrossRef] [PubMed]
51. Jiang, Y.; Li, W.; Wang, Z.; Lu, J. Lipid-Based Nanotechnology: Liposome. *Pharmaceutics* **2023**, *16*, 34. [CrossRef] [PubMed] [PubMed Central]
52. Torchilin, V.P. Recent advances with liposomes as pharmaceutical carriers. *Nat. Rev. Drug Discov.* **2005**, *4*, 145–160. [CrossRef] [PubMed]

53. Sahebkar, A.; Badiee, A.; Ghayour-Mobarhan, M.; Goldouzian, S.R.; Jaafari, M.R. A simple and effective approach for th treatment of dyslipidemia using anionic nanoliposomes. *Colloids Surf. B Biointerfaces* **2014**, *122*, 645–652. [CrossRef] [PubMed]
54. Amin, K.; Ng, K.Y.; Brown, C.S.; Bruno, M.S.; Heath, T.D. LDL induced association of anionic liposomes with cells and delivery o contents as shown by the increase in potency of liposome dependent drugs. *Pharm. Res.* **2001**, *18*, 914–921. [CrossRef] [PubMed
55. Momtazi-Borojeni, A.A.; Abdollahi, E.; Jaafari, M.R.; Banach, M.; Watts, G.F.; Sahebkar, A. Negatively-charged Liposom Nanoparticles Can Prevent Dyslipidemia and Atherosclerosis Progression in the Rabbit Model. *Curr. Vasc. Pharmacol.* **2022**, *2C* e200821195754. [CrossRef] [PubMed]
56. Krishna, S.M.; Moxon, J.V.; Jose, R.J.; Li, J.; Sahebkar, A.; Jaafari, M.R.; Hatamipour, M.; Liu, D.; Golledge, J. Anionic nanoliposome reduced atherosclerosis progression in Low Density Lipoprotein Receptor (LDLR) deficient mice fed a high fat diet. *J. Cell Physio* **2018**, *233*, 6951–6964. [CrossRef] [PubMed]
57. Sharma, K.; Kumar, K.; Mishra, N. Nanoparticulate carrier system: A novel treatment approach for hyperlipidemia. *Drug Deli* **2016**, *23*, 684–699. [CrossRef] [PubMed]
58. Martirossian, A.N.; Goldberg, A.C. Management of patients with statin intolerance. *Best Pract. Res. Clin. Endocrinol. Metab.* **2023** *37*, 101714. [CrossRef] [PubMed] [PubMed Central]
59. Cai, T.; Abel, L.; Langford, O.; Monaghan, G.; Aronson, J.K.; Stevens, R.J.; Lay-Flurrie, S.; Koshiaris, C.; McManus, R.J.; Hobbs F.R.; et al. Associations between statins and adverse events in primary prevention of cardiovascular disease: Systematic review with pairwise, network, and dose-response meta-analyses. *BMJ* **2021**, *374*, n1537. [CrossRef] [PubMed]
60. Mathur, M.; Kusum Devi, V. Potential of novel drug delivery strategies for the treatment of hyperlipidemia. *J. Drug Target.* **2016** *24*, 916–926. [CrossRef] [PubMed]
61. Pala, R.; Anju, V.T.; Dyavaiah, M.; Busi, S.; Nauli, S.M. Nanoparticle-Mediated Drug Delivery for the Treatment of Cardiovascular Diseases. *Int. J. Nanomed.* **2020**, *15*, 3741–3769. [CrossRef] [PubMed] [PubMed Central]
62. Rakshit, M.; Darwitan, A.; Muktabar, A.; Das, P.; Nguyen, L.T.H.; Cao, Y.; Vizetto-Duarte, C.; Tang, J.; Wong, Y.S.; Venkatraman S.; et al. Anti-inflammatory potential of simvastatin loaded nanoliposomes in 2D and 3D foam cell models. *Nanomedicine* **2021**, *37*, 102434. [CrossRef] [PubMed]
63. Parsa, S.; Dousti, M.; Mohammadi, N.; Abedanzadeh, M.; Dehdari Ebrahimi, N.; Dara, M.; Sani, M.; Nekouee, M.; Abolmaali, S.S. Sani, F.; et al. The effects of simvastatin-loaded nanoliposomes on human multilineage liver fibrosis microtissue. *J. Cell. Mol. Med* **2024**, *28*, e18529. [CrossRef] [PubMed] [PubMed Central]
64. Kulhari, H.; Kulhari, D.P.; Prajapati, S.K.; Chauhan, A.S. Pharmacokinetic and pharmacodynamic studies of poly(amidoamine) dendrimer based simvastatin oral formulations for the treatment of hypercholesterolemia. *Mol. Pharm.* **2013**, *10*, 2528–2533 [CrossRef] [PubMed]
65. Broz, P.; Ben-Haim, N.; Grzelakowski, M.; Marsch, S.; Meier, W.; Hunziker, P. Inhibition of macrophage phagocytotic activity by a receptor-targeted polymer vesicle-based drug delivery formulation of pravastatin. *J. Cardiovasc. Pharmacol.* **2008**, *51*, 246–252. [CrossRef] [PubMed]
66. Meena, A.K.; Ratnam, D.V.; Chandraiah, G.; Ankola, D.D.; Rao, P.R.; Kumar, M.N. Oral nanoparticulate atorvastatin calcium is more efficient and safe in comparison to Lipicure in treating hyperlipidemia. *Lipids* **2008**, *43*, 231–241. [CrossRef] [PubMed]
67. Maeki, M.; Uno, S.; Niwa, A.; Okada, Y.; Tokeshi, M. Microfluidic technologies and devices for lipid nanoparticle-based RNA delivery. *J. Control Release* **2022**, *344*, 80–96. [CrossRef] [PubMed] [PubMed Central]
68. Hu, B.; Zhong, L.; Weng, Y.; Peng, L.; Huang, Y.; Zhao, Y.; Liang, X.J. Therapeutic siRNA: State of the art. *Signal Transduct. Target. Ther.* **2020**, *5*, 101. [CrossRef] [PubMed] [PubMed Central]
69. Zhang, J.; Chen, B.; Gan, C.; Sun, H.; Zhang, J.; Feng, L. A Comprehensive Review of Small Interfering RNAs (siRNAs): Mechanism, Therapeutic Targets, and Delivery Strategies for Cancer Therapy. *Int. J. Nanomed.* **2023**, *18*, 7605–7635. [CrossRef] [PubMed] [PubMed Central]
70. Marrs, J.C.; Anderson, S.L. Inclisiran for the treatment of hypercholesterolaemia. *Drugs Context* **2024**, *13*, 2023-12-3. [CrossRef] [PubMed] [PubMed Central]
71. Zhang, Y.; Chen, H.; Hong, L.; Wang, H.; Li, B.; Zhang, M.; Li, J.; Yang, L.; Liu, F. Inclisiran: A new generation of lipid-lowering siRNA therapeutic. *Front. Pharmacol.* **2023**, *14*, 1260921. [CrossRef] [PubMed] [PubMed Central]
72. Traber, G.M.; Yu, A.M. RNAi-Based Therapeutics and Novel RNA Bioengineering Technologies. *J. Pharmacol. Exp. Ther.* **2023**, *384*, 133–154. [CrossRef] [PubMed] [PubMed Central]
73. Liu, M.; Gao, T.; Jiang, L.; Li, S.; Shi, B.; Li, F. Enhancing the biopharmaceutical attributes of atorvastatin calcium using polymeric and lipid-polymer hybrid nanoparticles: An approach for atherosclerosis treatment. *Biomed. Pharmacother.* **2023**, *159*, 114261. [CrossRef] [PubMed]

74. Mukherjee, A.; Waters, A.K.; Kalyan, P.; Achrol, A.S.; Kesari, S.; Yenugonda, V.M. Lipid-polymer hybrid nanoparticles as a next-generation drug delivery platform: State of the art, emerging technologies, and perspectives. *Int. J. Nanomed.* **2019**, *14*, 1937–1952. [CrossRef] [PubMed] [PubMed Central]
75. Ali, M. What function of nanoparticles is the primary factor for their hyper-toxicity? *Adv. Colloid. Interface Sci.* **2023**, *314*, 102881. [CrossRef] [PubMed]
76. Sharifi, S.; Behzadi, S.; Laurent, S.; Forrest, M.L.; Stroeve, P.; Mahmoudi, M. Toxicity of nanomaterials. *Chem. Soc. Rev.* **2012**, *41*, 2323–2343. [CrossRef] [PubMed] [PubMed Central]
77. Missaoui, W.N.; Arnold, R.D.; Cummings, B.S. Toxicological status of nanoparticles: What we know and what we don't know. *Chem. Biol. Interact.* **2018**, *295*, 1–12. [CrossRef] [PubMed] [PubMed Central]
78. Mohammadpour, R.; Dobrovolskaia, M.A.; Cheney, D.L.; Greish, K.F.; Ghandehari, H. Subchronic and chronic toxicity evaluation of inorganic nanoparticles for delivery applications. *Adv. Drug Deliv. Rev.* **2019**, *144*, 112–132. [CrossRef] [PubMed] [PubMed Central]
79. Naik, G.G.; Jagtap, V.A. Two heads are better than one: Unravelling the potential Impact of Artificial Intelligence in nanotechnology. *Nano TransMed* **2024**, *3*, 100041. [CrossRef]
80. Sheikh, H.; Prins, C.; Schrijvers, E. Artificial Intelligence: Definition and Background. In *Mission AI. Research for Policy*; Springer: Cham, Switzerland, 2023. [CrossRef]
81. Xu, Y.; Liu, X.; Cao, X.; Huang, C.; Liu, E.; Qian, S.; Liu, X.; Wu, Y.; Dong, F.; Qiu, C.W.; et al. Artificial intelligence: A powerful paradigm for scientific research. *Innovation* **2021**, *2*, 100179. [CrossRef] [PubMed] [PubMed Central]
82. Malik, P.; Pathania, M.; Rathaur, V.K. Overview of artificial intelligence in medicine. *J. Family Med. Prim. Care* **2019**, *8*, 2328–2331. [CrossRef] [PubMed] [PubMed Central]
83. Taherdoost, H.; Ghofrani, A. AI's role in revolutionizing personalized medicine by reshaping pharmacogenomics and drug therapy. *Intell. Pharm.* **2024**, *2*, 643–650. [CrossRef]
84. Gutiérrez-Esparza, G.; Pulido, T.; Martínez-García, M.; Ramírez-delReal, T.; Groves-Miralrio, L.E.; Márquez-Murillo, M.F.; Amezcua-Guerra, L.M.; Vargas-Alarcón, G.; Hernández-Lemus, E. A machine learning approach to personalized predictors of dyslipidemia: A cohort study. *Front. Public Health* **2023**, *11*, 1213926. [CrossRef] [PubMed] [PubMed Central]
85. Naderian, S.; Nikniaz, Z.; Farhangi, M.A.; Nikniaz, L.; Sama-Soltani, T.; Rostami, P. Predicting dyslipidemia incidence: Unleashing machine learning algorithms on Lifestyle Promotion Project data. *BMC Public Health* **2024**, *24*, 1777. [CrossRef] [PubMed] [PubMed Central]
86. Sezer, S.; Oter, A.; Ersoz, B.; Topcuoglu, C.; İbrahim Bulbul, H.; Sagiroglu, S.; Akin, M.; Yilmaz, G. Explainable artificial intelligence for LDL cholesterol prediction and classification. *Clin. Biochem.* **2024**, *130*, 110791. [CrossRef] [PubMed]
87. Romaszko, J.; Gromadziński, L.; Buciński, A. Friedewald formula may be used to calculate non-HDL-C from LDL-C and TG. *Front. Med.* **2023**, *10*, 1247126. [CrossRef] [PubMed] [PubMed Central]
88. PP, A.; Kumari, S.; Rajasimman, A.S.; Nayak, S.; Priyadarsini, P. Machine learning predictive models of LDL-C in the population of eastern India and its comparison with directly measured and calculated LDL-C. *Ann. Clin. Biochem.* **2022**, *59*, 76–86. [CrossRef] [PubMed]
89. Piani, F.; Cicero, A.F.G.; Borghi, C.; D'Addato, S.; BLIP Study Group. Is the 2020 Sampson equation the best formula for LDL-C estimation? *Eur. J. Intern. Med.* **2021**, *83*, 99–101. [CrossRef] [PubMed]
90. Ertürk Zararsız, G.; Bolat, S.; Cephe, A.; Kochan, N.; Yerlitaş, S.İ.; Doğan, H.O.; Zararsız, G. Validation of Friedewald, Martin-Hopkins and Sampson low-density lipoprotein cholesterol equations. *PLoS ONE* **2022**, *17*, e0263860. [CrossRef] [PubMed] [PubMed Central]
91. Ruscica, M.; Ferri, N.; Banach, M.; Sirtori, C.R.; Corsini, A. Side effects of statins: From pathophysiology and epidemiology to diagnostic and therapeutic implications. *Cardiovasc. Res.* **2023**, *118*, 3288–3304. [CrossRef] [PubMed]
92. Joo, H.; Kim, E.; Kim, Y. Machine Learning-Based Personalized Statin Therapy for Dyslipidemia Management. *J. Am. Coll. Cardiol.* **2024**, *83*, 1716. [CrossRef]
93. Krentz, A.; Fournier, L.; Castiglione, T.; Curcin, V.; Haldane, C.; Liu, T.; Jaun, A. Machine learning to optimise statin therapy using real-world primary care outcomes: Can statin doses be reduced in some patients? *Atherosclerosis* **2024**, *395*, 117927. [CrossRef]
94. Olawade, D.B.; Ige, A.O.; Olaremu, A.G.; Ijiwade, J.O.; Adeola, A.O. The synergy of artificial intelligence and nanotechnology towards advancing innovation and sustainability—A mini-review. *Nano Trends* **2024**, *8*, 100052. [CrossRef]
95. Vora, L.K.; Gholap, A.D.; Jetha, K.; Thakur, R.R.S.; Solanki, H.K.; Chavda, V.P. Artificial Intelligence in Pharmaceutical Technology and Drug Delivery Design. *Pharmaceutics* **2023**, *15*, 1916. [CrossRef] [PubMed] [PubMed Central]
96. Lin, Z.; Chou, W.C.; Cheng, Y.H.; He, C.; Monteiro-Riviere, N.A.; Riviere, J.E. Predicting Nanoparticle Delivery to Tumors Using Machine Learning and Artificial Intelligence Approaches. *Int. J. Nanomed.* **2022**, *17*, 1365–1379. [CrossRef] [PubMed] [PubMed Central]

97. Das, K.P.; Chandra, J. Nanoparticles and convergence of artificial intelligence for targeted drug delivery for cancer therapy: Current progress and challenges. *Front. Med. Technol.* **2023**, *4*, 1067144. [CrossRef] [PubMed] [PubMed Central]
98. Oviedo, L.R.; Oviedo, V.R.; Martins, M.O.; Fagan, S.B.; da Silva, W.L. Nanoarchitectonics: The role of artificial intelligence in the design and application of nanoarchitectures. *J. Nanopart Res.* **2022**, *24*, 157. [CrossRef]
99. Hamilton, S.; Kingston, B.R. Applying artificial intelligence and computational modeling to nanomedicine. *Curr. Opin. Biotechnol.* **2024**, *85*, 103043. [CrossRef] [PubMed]
100. Khan, M.M.; Shah, N.; Shaikh, N.; Thabet, A.; Belkhair, S. Towards secure and trusted AI in healthcare: A systematic review of emerging innovations and ethical challenges. *Int. J. Med. Inform.* **2025**, *195*, 105780. [CrossRef]
101. Hatmal, M.M.; Alshaer, W.; Mahmoud, I.S.; Al-Hatamleh, M.A.I.; Al-Ameer, H.J.; Abuyaman, O.; Zihlif, M.; Mohamud, R.; Darras, M.; Al Shhab, M.; et al. Investigating the association of CD36 gene polymorphisms (rs1761667 and rs1527483) with T2DM and dyslipidemia: Statistical analysis, machine learning based prediction, and meta-analysis. *PLoS ONE* **2021**, *16*, e0257857. [CrossRef] [PubMed] [PubMed Central]
102. Chan, B. Black-box assisted medical decisions: AI power vs. ethical physician care. *Med. Health Care Philos.* **2023**, *26*, 285–292. [CrossRef] [PubMed] [PubMed Central]
103. Ley, C.; Martin, R.K.; Pareek, A.; Groll, A.; Seil, R.; Tischer, T. Machine learning and conventional statistics: Making sense of the differences. *Knee Surg. Sports Traumatol. Arthrosc.* **2022**, *30*, 753–757. [CrossRef] [PubMed]
104. Gupta, V.K.; Paul, S.; Dutta, C. Geography, Ethnicity or Subsistence-Specific Variations in Human Microbiome Composition and Diversity. *Front. Microbiol.* **2017**, *8*, 1162. [CrossRef] [PubMed] [PubMed Central]
105. Larson, D.B.; Harvey, H.; Rubin, D.L.; Irani, N.; Tse, J.R.; Langlotz, C.P. Regulatory Frameworks for Development and Evaluation of Artificial Intelligence-Based Diagnostic Imaging Algorithms: Summary and Recommendations. *J. Am. Coll. Radiol.* **2021**, *18*, 413–424. [CrossRef] [PubMed] [PubMed Central]
106. Zou, J.; Schiebinger, L. Ensuring that biomedical AI benefits diverse populations. *eBioMedicine* **2021**, *67*, 103358. [CrossRef] [PubMed] [PubMed Central]
107. Bajwa, J.; Munir, U.; Nori, A.; Williams, B. Artificial intelligence in healthcare: Transforming the practice of medicine. *Future Healthc. J.* **2021**, *8*, e188–e194. [CrossRef] [PubMed] [PubMed Central]
108. Herdiana, Y.; Wathoni, N.; Shamsuddin, S.; Muchtaridi, M. Scale-up polymeric-based nanoparticles drug delivery systems: Development and challenges. *OpenNano* **2022**, *7*, 100048. [CrossRef]
109. Ratwani, R.M.; Sutton, K.; Galarraga, J.E. Addressing AI Algorithmic Bias in Health Care. *JAMA* **2024**, *332*, 1051–1052. [CrossRef] [PubMed]
110. Buolamwini, J.; Gebru, T. Gender Shades: Intersectional Accuracy Disparities in Commercial Gender Classification. *Proc. Mach. Learn. Res.* **2018**, *81*, 77–91.
111. Li, Y.H.; Li, Y.L.; Wei, M.Y.; Li, G.Y. Innovation and challenges of artificial intelligence technology in personalized healthcare. *Sci. Rep.* **2024**, *14*, 18994. [CrossRef] [PubMed] [PubMed Central]
112. Lee, D.; Yoon, S.N. Application of Artificial Intelligence-Based Technologies in the Healthcare Industry: Opportunities and Challenges. *Int. J. Environ. Res. Public Health* **2021**, *18*, 271. [CrossRef] [PubMed] [PubMed Central]
113. Mudgal, S.K.; Agarwal, R.; Chaturvedi, J.; Gaur, R.; Ranjan, N. Real-world application, challenges and implication of artificial intelligence in healthcare: An essay. *Pan Afr. Med. J.* **2022**, *43*, 3. [CrossRef] [PubMed] [PubMed Central]

Journal of
Clinical Medicine

MDPI

Review

Lifestyle and Lipoprotein(a) Levels: Does a Specific Counseling Make Sense?

Federica Fogacci [1,*], Valentina Di Micoli [1], Pierre Sabouret [2], Marina Giovannini [1] and Arrigo F. G. Cicero [1,3,*]

1 Hypertension and Cardiovascular Risk Research Center, Medical and Surgical Sciences Department, Alma Mater Studiorum University of Bologna, 40100 Bologna, Italy; valentina.dimicoli2@unibo.it (V.D.M.); marina.giovannini3@unibo.it (M.G.)
2 INSERM UMRS_1166, Cardiology Institute, Pitié Salpêtrière Hospital (AP-HP), ACTION Study Group, Sorbonne University, 75013 Paris, France; cardiology.sabouret@gmail.com
3 Cardiovascular Medicine Unit, Heart, Thoracic and Vascular Department, IRCCS Azienda Ospedaliero-Universitaria di Bologna, 40100 Bologna, Italy
* Correspondence: federica.fogacci@studio.unibo.it (F.F.); arrigo.cicero@unibo.it (A.F.G.C.)

Abstract: Lipoprotein(Lp)(a) is a variant of low-density lipoprotein (LDL), bound to apolipoprotein B100, whose levels are associated with a significant increase in the risk of atherosclerosis-related cardiovascular events, but also to aortic stenosis and atrial fibrillation. Since plasma levels of Lp(a) are commonly considered resistant to lifestyle changes, we critically reviewed the available evidence on the effect of weight loss, dietary supplements, and physical activity on this risk factor. In our review, we observed that relevant body weight loss, a relatively high intake of saturated fatty acids, the consumption of red wine, and intense physical exercise seems to be associated with significantly lower plasma Lp(a) levels. On the contrary, foods rich in trans-unsaturated fatty acids are associated with increased Lp(a) levels. With regard to dietary supplements, coenzyme Q10, L-Carnitine, and flaxseed exert a mild but significant lowering effect on plasma Lp(a).

Keywords: diet; lifestyle; lipoprotein(a); nutraceuticals; physical activity

1. Introduction

It is well-known that therapeutic lifestyle changes combining physical activity, diet, and weight management usually have a positive impact on metabolic risk factors and the risk of developing CV diseases [1].

Lipoprotein(Lp)(a) is a variant of low-density lipoprotein (LDL), bound to apolipoprotein B100 and characterized by an apolipoprotein(a) (apo(a)) of a different length, whose plasma concentration is usually considered unchangeable in response to lifestyle modifications [2]. During the last decades, thanks to a number of significant epidemiological investigations, high Lp(a) plasma levels have been definitely associated not only with a significant increased risk of atherosclerosis-related CV events (namely stroke, coronary artery disease, and peripheral artery disease) [3], but also with aortic stenosis and atrial fibrillation, after adjustments for other known risk factors [4,5].

According to the findings from a recently published systematic review and meta-analysis, pooling data from 75 cohort and case-cohort studies (n = 957,253), the risk of all-cause mortality increases with progressively higher levels of Lp(a), with the hazard ratios (HRs) that compare the top vs. bottom tertiles of Lp(a) being 1.18 (95% confidence interval (CI): 1.04 to 1.34) in patients in secondary prevention for CV diseases and 1.09 (95%CI: 1.01 to 1.18) in the general population. The HRs for CV diseases mortality was 1.33 (95%CI: 1.11 to 1.58) in the general population and 1.25 (95%CI: 1.10 to 1.43) in patients in secondary prevention for CV diseases. For each 50 mg/dL rise in Lp(a) plasma levels, a 31% and 15% greater risk of CV death was also estimated, respectively, in the general population and in patients in secondary prevention for CV diseases [6].

Lp(a) plasma levels are strictly genetically determined [7], so there is poor response to both lifestyle changes and currently available pharmacological drugs [8]. The prothrombotic action of Lp(a) is partially counteracted using antiplatelets, but this effect is more evident in secondary prevention patients, who should be taking antiplatelets anyway [9]. Currently, there is ongoing development of novel lipid-lowering medications, specifically small interfering RNA (siRNA) agents, such as olpasiran, SLN360, LY3819469, and the second-generation antisense oligopeptide, pelacarsen. These drugs selectively disrupt the synthesis of Lp(a) in the liver by impeding the translation of apolipoprotein(a) mRNA [10]. The primary goal is to genetically silence the lipoprotein(a) gene (LPA), diminish apolipoprotein(a) production, and subsequently, reduce serum Lp(a) levels. Current evidence indicates that optimal results are achieved through monthly subcutaneous injections, leading to persistent and substantial reductions in Lp(a) levels of up to 95%, with the potential to reduce cardiovascular risk [11]. A relevant Lp(a)-lowering effect (up to −65%, resulting in Lp(a) plasma levels of less than 50 mg/dL in 93% of participants) has been recently shown in a phase 2 trial using muvalapalin, a small oral drug [12]. The potential of these emerging drugs under development appears highly promising, demonstrating an overall safety profile. However, their cost-effectiveness will undergo thorough evaluation as an integral component of optimizing healthcare investments in CV prevention.

However, since these drugs are currently under investigation and tested only in patients already struck by coronary artery disease with very high Lp(a) plasma levels, we have no drugs in development to manage patients in primary prevention with high Lp(a) levels.

In this context, the aim of this review is to summarize the evidence supporting the ability of lifestyle interventions to improve the Lp(a) plasma levels in the context of CV management in hyperLp(a) patients.

2. Dietary Intervention

2.1. Weight Loss and Lp(a) Levels

Low-energy diets are usually associated with a global improvement in plasma lipid concentrations [13,14]. Bariatric surgery also improves plasma lipid levels [15–17]. However, what do we know about energy restriction and the effect of bariatric surgery on Lp(a) plasma levels? The clinical evidence of different weight loss approaches on Lp(a) plasma levels are summarized in Table 1.

The study by Kiortsis et al., involved 62 healthy obese patients (21 men aged 32 ± 9.6 years and 41 women aged 37 ± 14.6 years) consuming a low-energy diet for six months. In considering the whole population, the authors observed a body weight loss of 7.5% versus baseline and a statistically significant decrease in plasma levels of total cholesterol, LDL cholesterol, and triglycerides ($p < 0.001$), while no changes in Lp(a) levels were detected. However, when considering individuals with high Lp(a) values (>20 mg/dL) at baseline, a 17.6% reduction in Lp(a) ($p < 0.05$) was observed, which was closely related with baseline Lp(a) levels ($r = 0.81$ $p < 0.001$), but not with the changes in anthropometric measurements that occurred during weight loss [18]. Therefore, a low-calorie diet that induces weight loss in individuals with obesity may have positive impacts on serum Lp(a) levels, particularly in patients with elevated pretreatment concentrations of Lp(a). However, this effect is influenced by large interindividual variability and depends on the characteristics of the patients.

Table 1. Clinical evidence of different weight loss approaches on Lp(a) plasma levels.

First Author, Year of Publication	Patients	Interventions	Main Result
Kiortsis et al., 2001 [18]	Healthy obese (n = 62)	6-week low-energy diet	17.6% Lp(a) reduction in subjects with Lp(a) > 20 mg/dL only
Berk et al., 2017 [19]	Obese and Type 2 diabetes (n = 131) Obese (n = 30) Type 2 diabetes (n = 26) Obese managed with bariatric surgery (n = 26)	4-month low-energy diet or bariatric surgery	Lp(a) increase in subjects undergoing low-energy diet, 14% Lp(a) decrease in subjects treated with bariatric surgery
Berk et al., 2022 [20]	Overweight/Obese patients (n = 293)	7-week low-energy diet followed by Roux-en-Y gastric bypass) and 52-week follow-up (surgery group) (n = 82) 59-week low-energy diet and exercise program (lifestyle group) (n = 77) 20-week low/very low energy diet (lifestyle cohort) (n = 134)	Lp(a) increase in after low/very low energy diet, 48% Lp(a) decrease after surgery
Gomez-Martin et al., 2018 [21]	40 obese women	1-year follow-up after laparoscopic Roux-en-Y gastric bypass (n = 20) or sleeve gastrectomy (n = 20) or conventional treatment with diet and exercise (n = 20)	No change in Lp(a) plasma level in any group
Paredes et al., 2020 [22]	702 obese patients (372 without metabolic syndrome)	1-year follow-up after vertical sleeve gastrectomy	10% decrease in Lp(a) levels in metabolic syndrome only
Scholl et al., 2020 [23]	Single case report of a normoweight subject	Very low carb ketogenic diet during physical training	26–39% decrease in Lp(a) levels
Ebbeling et al., 2022 [24]	164 overweight/obese subjects with mixed dyslipidaemia	20-week weight loss diet containing 20% proteins plus different amounts of carbohydrates and saturated fatty acids (20–21% vs. 40–14% vs. 60–7%)	15% decrease in Lp(a) levels in the low-carbohydrate diet group only
Cipryan et al., 2022 [25]	91 overweight subjects	High-intensity interval training program (n = 22) vs. high-intensity interval training program and very low-carb/high fat diet (n = 25) vs. very low carb/high fat (n = 22) vs. standard management	No effect of any treatment on Lp(a) plasma level)

In the study by Berk et al. [19], after a similar 3–4 month calorie-restricted diet, patients with type 2 diabetes and obesity (n = 131) experienced a significant decrease in body weight (−9.9%), while their Lp(a) plasma levels increased by 14.8 nmol/L. Obese individuals (n = 30) or type 2 diabetics (n = 26) also experienced a decrease in body weight (−7%) associated with an increase in Lp(a) (+12.7 nmol/L), while Lp(a) did not change in obese individuals (n = 26) that underwent bariatric surgery despite considerable weight loss (−14%) [19]. The same research group carried out two further independent long-term clinical trials involving 293 overweight or obese individuals. The first study was designed as a prospective two-arm clinical investigation, including 82 patients undergoing a 7-week low-energy diet followed by Roux-en-Y gastric bypass and a 52-week follow-up (surgery group), and a control cohort of 77 patients undergoing a 59-week low-energy diet and exercise program (lifestyle group). The second study included a third cohort of 134 patients undergoing a 20-week low/very low-energy diet program (lifestyle cohort). In the lifestyle group and in the lifestyle cohort, the Lp(a) plasma level [median (interquartile range)] increased by 36% [14(7–77) vs. 19(7–94) nmol/L, $p < 0.001$] and 14% [50(14–160) vs. 57(19–208) nmol/L, $p < 0.001$], respectively. In contrast, in the surgery group, the Lp(a) levels dramatically decreased by 48% after intervention [21 (7–81) vs. 11(7–56) nmol/L, $p < 0.001$]. Remarkably, arachidonic acid and total n-3 fatty acids (FA) decreased after surgery but increased after lifestyle interventions, while plasma levels of total saturated FA remained unchanged after surgery but decreased after lifestyle interventions. However, the change in Lp(a) seemed to be independent of the weight loss [20].

In 2018, Gomez-Martin et al. [21] demonstrated that vertical sleeve gastrectomy and gastric bypass have a favorable impact on serum lipids at one-year post-surgery in women with high CV risk. This effect includes a reduction in total cholesterol, triglycerides, and oxidized-LDL, although there were no associated changes in Lp(a) levels. On the other hand, in a more recent and very large study (n = 702), Paredes et al. evaluated the 1-year metabolic impact of vertical sleeve gastrectomy. According to the findings of the study by Paredes et al., patients without metabolic syndrome (n = 372) experienced a decrease in Lp(a) levels (14.7 mg/dL vs. 12.3 mg/dL, $p = 0.006$) after vertical sleeve gastrectomy, while patients with metabolic syndrome did not (13.9 mg/dL vs. 14.6 mg/dL, $p = 0.302$). The regression model showed that older age and delta HDL-C significantly predicted the change in Lp(a), while the higher the number of metabolic syndrome components and the lower the estimated body fat percentage loss, the lower the odds of Lp(a) reduction after the intervention [22].

Even if the above cited studies are relatively small and designed differently, in particular with regard to diet composition, overall we could conclude that a low-energy diet is not sufficient to significantly modify Lp(a) levels in plasma, therefore, a more dramatic intervention is needed. The diet with a metabolic impact most like that which follows bariatric surgery is the very-low carbohydrate/ketogenic diet. In a single case of a 55-year-old triathlete with a BMI of 24.9 kg/m^2, the use of a very-low carbohydrate/ketogenic diet was associated with a plasma Lp(a) decrease ranging from 26% to 39% in different dietary intervention phases [23]. In a large trial involving 164 overweight or obese patients (BMI: 32.4 $\pm$ 4.8 kg/m^2) with mixed dyslipidemia, a 20-week treatment with three different weight loss diets (one of which was a low-carbohydrate diet) exerted different effects on Lp(a). These diets were comprised of 20% protein and various contents of carbohydrates and saturated fats (low-carbohydrate diet = 20% carbohydrates, 21% saturated fats; moderate-carbohydrate diet: 40% carbohydrates, 14% saturated fats; high-carbohydrate diet: 60% carbohydrates, 7% saturated fats). At the end of the study, plasma Lp(a) was reduced by nearly 15% (−14.9%; 95% confidence interval (CI): −22.0 to −7.1) only in the group randomized to the low-carbohydrate diet. The low carbohydrate diet was also associated with a significant improvement in insulin-resistance, triglycerides, HDL-cholesterol, and adiponectin plasma levels [24]. It must be acknowledged that these findings were not confirmed in a recent 12-week randomized clinical trial examining the effect of a very low-carbohydrate/high-fat diet associated with a high-intensity interval training program in a cohort of 91 overweight individuals [25]. In this study, Lp(a) plasma levels did not change, neither in response to training (n = 22), nor diet (n = 25), nor in the training + diet combined intervention (n = 25), nor standard management (n = 19) [25].

Even if these clinical trials are relatively small and short-term, their results supported the European Society of Atherosclerosis (EAS) consensus on hyper-Lp(a) management; to follow a low carbohydrate diet to reduce the concentration of Lp(a) by ~15% [26].

2.2. Dietary Fats

Dietary patterns abundant in animal-derived proteins and fats might be linked to increased risks of CV disease and related mortality when compared to diets rich in plant-derived protein [27–29]. Once again, the evidence supporting the intake of specific fatty acids and Lp(a) plasma levels is conflicting.

In overweight and obese individuals (n = 31), a 4-week plant-based diet was associated with an improvement in inflammatory and atherogenic biomarkers, among them Lp(a) (−32 nmol/L) [30]. The existing literature indicates that replacing saturated fats with an equivalent amount of unsaturated fats leads to decreased overall mortality [31]. Including nuts in the diet is a practical strategy to boost unsaturated fat intake, as it relates to lower all-cause mortality and mortality specific to CV diseases, in particular [32]. A diet abundant in walnuts, rich in alpha-linolenic acid, polyphenols, plant sterols, and tocopherol, demonstrated an overall enhancement in the blood lipid profile [33]. However, in a randomized, prospective, controlled, crossover, clinical study involving 194 healthy volunteers, an 8-week regimen of 43 g of walnuts daily did not exert any effect on Lp(a) concentration in plasma, even if other lipid fractions (such as non-HDL-C, apoB, total cholesterol, LDL-C, very LDL (VLDL) cholesterol, and triglycerides) were improved [34]. During a 16-week randomized controlled trial, 29 participants classified as overweight or obese (with a BMI of 25–40 kg/m^2) were assigned to either consume 42.5 g/day of a mix of nuts (including cashews, almonds, macadamia nuts, Brazil nuts, pecans, pistachios, walnuts, and peanuts) or 69 g/day of isocaloric pretzels. There was no evidence that consumption of mixed nuts had an effect on LDL-C or Lp(a) throughout the intervention [35].

On the contrary, in a small study mainly enrolling Afro-Americans (n = 18/28), with a mean age of 48.3 ± 12.5 years (17 men, 11 women), Lp(a) plasma levels were negatively associated with absolute (grams/day) and relative (percentage of total calories) dietary saturated fatty acid (SFA) intake (R = −0.43, p = 0.02, SFA (% CAL): R = −0.38, p = 0.04), palmitic acid intake (R = −0.38, p = 0.05), and stearic acid intake (R = −0.40, p = 0.03) [36].

Coconut oil might also yield more favorable effects on Lp(a) concentration when compared to unsaturated oils with longer carbon chains. In a controlled crossover study involving young women and comparing two high-fat diets over a 3-week period [37], the consumption of a coconut oil-enriched diet resulted in a 17 mg/L reduction in Lp(a) levels. In contrast, the intake of highly unsaturated long-chain fatty acids led to a 25 mg/L increase in Lp(a) levels [37]. Despite being a saturated fat, it is essential to recognize that coconut oil primarily consists of medium-chain fatty acids (e.g., lauric acid), constituting 50% of its content. Consequently, it may elicit a different response in Lp(a) concentration. However, a more recent randomized, controlled, single-blinded, crossover, clinical trial that enrolled 40 healthy volunteers to investigate the short-term effect of a diet enriched in palm oil, cocoa butter, or extra virgin olive oil, with oleic acid primarily at the sn-2 position (66%, 75%, 87% sn-2 oleic acid, respectively) of the TG molecule, concluded that not one of the tested diets had a significant impact on Lp(a) levels [38].

Despite the slight benefit observed in Lp(a) levels with the consumption of coconut oil, the International guidelines advise that dietary saturated fats should constitute less than 10% of total energy intake [39,40]. This recommendation stems from the association of excess saturated fat consumption with significantly elevated morbidity and mortality rates related to cancers and CV diseases [27,31].

Trans-fatty acids are associated with adverse CV outcomes. Whether a part of this effect is mediated by an impact of trans-fatty acids on Lp(a) levels is not clear [41].

In a double-blind clinical trial involving 29 men and 29 women, the participants were randomized to eat one of four controlled diets for six weeks each, where fatty acids accounted for 39 to 40% of energy: (A) oleic (16.7% of energy as oleic acid); (B) moderate trans (3.8% of energy as trans monoenes, approximately the trans content of the U.S. diet); (C) high trans (6.6% of energy as trans monoenes); (D) saturated (16.2% of energy as lauric, myristic, and palmitic acids). The saturated diet significantly reduced Lp(a) levels from 8% to 11%. Compared with the oleic diet (A), the trans diet had no adverse effect on

Lp(a) levels in the whole cohort. However, the subgroup of individuals with higher Lp(a) levels at baseline (≥30 mg/dL) responded to the high trans diet (C) with a slight, though significant increase (+5%) in Lp(a) levels compared to the oleic (A) and moderate trans (B) diets [42].

In a small, randomized, clinical trial involving 31 young men, the consumption of hydrogenated soybean oil led to a notably higher level of Lp(a) compared to a diet primarily sourced from butter [43]. On the contrary, in a randomized, crossover study with 49 hypercholesterolemic patients following a 6-week diet rich in either butter or margarine, there was no observed change in Lp(a) [44]. Intake of meals high in specific dietary fatty acids can increase postprandial plasma lipids differently [45–48], including Lp(a) concentration. In a clinical trial enrolling healthy, young men, 16 volunteers were asked to sequentially consume five test fats dominated by (approximately 43% g/kg) stearic, palmitic, oleic, C18:1 trans, or linoleic acid incorporated into meals (1 g fat/kg body weight) after a 12-h fast, in random order on different days, separated by 3-week washout periods. Blood samples were drawn before, and 2, 4, 6, and 8 h after eating. Lp(a) plasma levels were found to increase after each supplementation, except after oleic and C18:1 trans consumption. On the contrary, oleic and C18:1 trans supplementation was associated with less area under the plasma Lp(a) concentration curve compared to those measured after stearic and palmitic acid intake ($p < 0.003$). So, long-chain stearic and palmitic acids led to significant increases in postprandial Lp(a) levels after an oral fat test in young, healthy men [49].

The clinical evidence of different dietary fatty acids on Lp(a) plasma levels have been summarized in Table 2.

Table 2. Clinical evidence of different dietary fatty acids on Lp(a) plasma levels.

First Author, Year of Publication	Patients	Interventions	Main Result
Najjar et al., 2018 [30]	31 Overweight/obese with LDL-C > 100 mg/dL	4-week plant-based diet	16% Lp(a) plasma level reduction
Bamberger et al., 2017 [34]	194 healthy subjects	8-week regimen of 43 g of walnuts daily vs. standard diet	No change in Lp(a) plasma level in any group
Nora et al., 2023 [35]	29 overweight or obese individuals	16-week consumption of either 42.5 g/day of mixed nuts (cashews, almonds, macadamia nuts, Brazil nuts, pecans, pistachios, walnuts, and peanuts) or 69 g/day isocaloric pretzels	No change in Lp(a) plasma level in any group
Mueller et al., 2003 [37]	25 healthy women	3-week coconut oil-based high fat diet vs. coconut oil-based low-fat diet vs. diet rich in mono- and polyunsaturated fatty acids	Lp(a) reduced by 17 mg/L after coconut-oil intake, but increased by 25 mg/dL after intake of unsaturated long-chain fatty acids
Loganathan et al., 2022 [38]	40 healthy women	4-week comparison of the effect of palm oil, cocoa butter, extra virgin olive oil as the main oil	No change in Lp(a) plasma level in any group
Clevidence et al., 1997 [42]	58 healthy subjects	6-week comparison of the effect of high-fat diets (fatty acids = 39–40% of total energy) characterized by oleic (16.7% of energy); trans (3.8% of energy); high trans (6.6% of energy as trans-monoenes); saturated (16.2% of energy)	8–11% decrease in Lp(a) plasma levels with high saturated fatty acids diets; 5% Lp(a) levels in subjects with higher Lp(a) at the baseline with the high trans-diet
Almendingen et al., 1995 [43]	31 young men	3-week effect of partially hydrogenated fish oil, partially hydrogenated soybean oil, and butterfat	Lp(a) plasma level increase with all diets, but larger with hydrogenated fats-enriched diets.
Chisholm, et al., 1996 [44]	49 hypercholesterolemic subjects	6-week effect of butter or an unsaturated margarine used for cooking or spreading in a reduced fat diet	No change in Lp(a) plasma level in any group
Tholstrup et al., 2004 [49]	16 young healthy men	5 test fats dominated by (approximately 43% g/kg) stearic, palmitic, oleic, C18:1 trans, or linoleic acid incorporated into meals (1 g fat/kg body weight) after a 12-h fast in random order on different days, separated by 3-week washout periods	Lp(a) plasma levels increased after each fat except oleic and C18:1 trans; oleic, C18:1 trans intake was associated with less area under the plasma Lp(a) concentration curve

In conclusion, based on the available data, mainly obtained in small and short-term clinical trials, a mild increase in plant-derived saturated fatty acids could mildly decrease the Lp(a) plasma levels, while trans-fatty acid rich foods should be avoided. The available evidence could not be translated to a suggestion to increase saturated fatty acids in a diet aiming to improve LDL-C and reduce CV risk, however, it suggests that in individuals with high Lp(a) levels, an extreme reduction of saturated fatty acids is not mandatory and probably also negative.

2.3. Popular Beverages

A variable consumption of beverages such as coffee, tea, and alcohol worldwide may be correlated with CV outcomes [50–52]. Thus, the potential effects of popular beverages on Lp(a) concentration deserves consideration.

In 15 mildly hypercholesterolemic adults (mean LDL-C = 135 mg/dL) consuming five cups/day of black tea prepared using 180 mL of water for each serving, Lp(a) decreased by 16% as compared with placebo [53]. Of course, the number of individuals enrolled in this study was too small to be conclusive with regard to the potential use of black tea as a Lp(a) lowering tool and larger long-term studies should be designed to confirm or disprove this observation. In another study, 53 volunteers with diabetes were randomly assigned to drink either black tea (n = 26) or *Hibiscus sabdarrifa* tea (n = 27), by using 2 g of tea sachet with 240 mL of boiling water for each serving, twice daily for 1 month. The Lp(a) concentrations remained unchanged from the baseline value of 26 mg/dL in both study groups [54]. Further research is needed, especially with respect to the number of commercially available tea preparations.

A rapidly increasing body of evidence recognizes the potential benefits of coffee in relation to CVD [55–58], but its effects on Lp(a) plasma levels remain unclear. Moreover, the exact mechanism by which coffee or single coffee components affect Lp(a) levels is yet to be clarified. The type of coffee and method of preparation appear to be important in determining the effect on Lp(a); in fact, coffee diterpenes present in unfiltered coffee brews are among the few dietary constituents that may modulate Lp(a) levels [59]. According to the findings of a systematic review and meta-analysis, the consumption of coffee or coffee diterpenes was associated with either a reduction in Lp(a) of 11 mg/dL (6 trials, 275 individuals), or no effect (2 trials, 56 individuals) [60]. However, it must be recognized that this metanalysis was affected by a large inter-study heterogeneity as regards study design, type of intervention, coffee source, and method of coffee processing [60].

A cross-sectional study with 309 volunteers showed that serum Lp(a) was elevated in chronic boiled coffee drinkers, who had a median Lp(a) of 13.0 mg/dL (range 0–130) compared with filter coffee drinkers who had a median Lp(a) of 7.9 mg/dL (range 0–144). The effect of coffee on Lp(a) is complex and may follow a biphasic time course, that is to say that whilst coffee may have a short-term beneficial effect in reducing Lp(a), in the longer term it may prove to be detrimental [61]. On the other hand, in the large UK Biobank database (n = 447,794 participants aged 37–73 years) no association was observed between coffee or tea intake and Lp(a) plasma levels [62].

In a cross-sectional study involving 300 middle-aged men, the Lp(a) concentrations in subgroups with low (<39 g/week), intermediate (39–132 g/week), and high (>132 g/week) ethanol intake were 137, 109, and 94 mg/L, respectively (P between groups < 0.05). Interestingly, abstainers exhibited a higher Lp(a) concentration (median, 206 mg/L) compared to drinkers [63]. However, in another cross-sectional study of 402 subjects with untreated hypertension, those with light (1–20 g/d), moderate (20–50 g/d), and heavy (>50 g/d) ethanol consumption showed 21%, 26%, and 57% lower median Lp(a) concentrations, respectively, compared to abstainers and occasional drinkers [64]. Notably, red wine consumption appears to have a greater ability to decrease Lp(a) levels than white wine. In a study involving 20 healthy male volunteers, the daily intake of 200 mL of red wine for 10 days resulted in a reduction in Lp(a) levels from 18.6 to 13.2 mg/dL ($p < 0.001$), whereas a similar effect was not observed with white wine after a 6-week washout period [65]. Of course, the study was too small and short-term to furnish strong evidence that red wine more effectively reduces Lp(a) plasma levels than white wine. In a 4-week randomized crossover study in 67 men with high estimated CV risk, Lp(a) levels were compared after the ingestion of red wine (30 g alcohol/day), the equivalent amount of dealcoholized red wine, and gin (30 g alcohol/day) [66]. The Lp(a) level fell from 54.4 mg/dL (baseline value) to 50.2 mg/dL, only after the intervention with red wine [66]. The conflicting results of the different studies suggest the need of more in depth research on larger cohorts, focusing on the different kinds of alcohol consumed (beer, red wine, white wine, shots of spirits). In any case, the adverse health effects of more than minimal alcohol intake may well outweigh any potential benefit in lowering Lp(a) levels [67,68].

3. Nutraceutical Supplementation

Several lipid-lowering nutraceuticals and functional foods have shown to significantly reduce the plasma levels of LDL-cholesterol, however, most of them have no effect on Lp(a) [69]. L-carnitine and coenzyme Q10 [70,71], are the nutraceuticals most studied for Lp(a) lowering effects, followed by flaxseed and curcumin. Of course, the available trials are small and short-term but somewhat suggestive of the positive effects of these dietary supplements.

3.1. L-Carnitine

Levo-Carnitine (L-carnitine) is an amino acid present in a number of foods, especially in meat [70]. Both oral and intravenous L-carnitine administration may provide benefits in individuals affected by CV disease [72–75], mainly because of its antioxidant and energy metabolism improvement actions [73,76]. However, the amount of L-carnitine provided by foods is much lower than that needed to achieve a reduction in Lp(a) in humans (Table 3).

Table 3. L-Carnitine contents in foods (modified from [70]).

Food Item	L-Carnitine (mg/100 gr Serving)	Food Item	L-Carnitine (mg/100 gr Serving)
Meat products		Dairy products	
Beef steak	64.6–87.5	Yogurt, regular (3.2% fat)	12.5
Pork (muscle)	13–53.5	Milk 2–4% fat	2.3–2.9
Chicken	10–10.4	Cheese	1.4–1.8
		Butter	0.85
Fish		Chicken egg	
Salmon (cooked)	5.8	Whole	Not evaluated
Cod (Atlantic)	1.8	Egg Yolk	0.8
		Egg white	0.3

A meta-analysis of data derived from seven double-blind, randomized, clinical trials (n = 300) showed a significant reduction in Lp(a) levels following L-carnitine supplementation (weighted mean difference (WMD): −8.82 mg/dL, 95% CI: −10.09, −7.55, $p < 0.001$) for 1–24 weeks. When studies were classified according to the route of administration, a significant reduction in plasma Lp(a) concentration was observed with L-carnitine by the oral route (WMD: −9.00 mg/dL, 95% CI: −10.29, −7.72, $p < 0.001$), but not by the intravenous route (WMD: −2.91 mg/dL, 95% CI: −10.22, 4.41, $p = 0.436$). The results of the meta-regression analysis showed that the pooled estimate was independent of L-carnitine dose (slope: −0.30; 95% CI: −4.19, 3.59; $p = 0.878$) and duration of therapy (slope: 0.18; 95% CI: −0.22, 0.59; $p = 0.374$) [70].

This effect was confirmed by a more recent meta-analysis evaluating the metabolic effect of L-carnitine supplementation, concluding that L-carnitine is able to reduce Lp(a) levels by a mean value of 7.13 mg/dL [95% CI: −9.82, −4.43] mg/dL; $p < 0.001$) [76].

Additionally, in individuals with mixed hyperlipidemia, Florentin et al. [77] demonstrated that the coadministration of 2 g/day of L-carnitine with 20 mg/day of simvastatin over a 12-week period resulted in a reduction of Lp(a) levels from 56 to 42 mg/dL. This benefit was not observed with simvastatin monotherapy, suggesting that the decrease in Lp(a) could be attributed to the presence of L-carnitine. The middle-term tolerability and safety of L-carnitine is high. Therefore, longitudinal studies are needed in order to provide information about whether potential benefits of L-carnitine on Lp(a) level outweigh or modulate the atherosclerotic and metabolic damage associated with increased plasma levels of trimethylamine N-oxide. In fact, L-carnitine supplementation may unfortunately raise trimethylamine N-oxide production in the liver [78–80] and thus, trimethylamine N-oxide plasma levels, which is a well-known CV risk factor [81].

3.2. Coenzyme Q10

Coenzyme Q10 (CoQ10) is a powerful antioxidant, plays an essential role in the respiratory chain as an electron carrier in mitochondrial ATP synthesis [82,83], and exerts an anti-inflammatory action [84]. Similarly to L-carnitine, coenzyme Q10 (CoQ10) supplementation may benefit individuals with CV diseases [85,86], but with dosages that cannot be reached by dietary intake (Table 4).

Table 4. Coenzyme Q10 contents in foods (modified from [82]).

Food Item	CoQ10 (mg/100 gr Serving)	Food Item	CoQ10 (mg/100 gr Serving)
Meat products		Dairy products	
Beef steak	1.61–3.65	Yogurt, regular (3.2% fat)	0.07–0.11
Pork (muscle)	2.43–4.11	Milk 2–4% fat	0.07–0.12
Chicken	1.4–2.1	Cheese	0.12–0.13
		Butter	0.71
Fish		Chicken egg	
Salmon (cooked)	0.43–0.76	Whole	0.07–0.37
Cod (Atlantic)	0.37	Egg Yolk	Not evaluated
		Egg white	0.52

A meta-analysis of seven double-blind, randomized, clinical trials found that CoQ10 supplementation was accompanied by a slight but significant reduction in plasma Lp(a) levels (WMD: −3.54 mg/dL, 95% CI: −5.50, −1.58; $p < 0.001$), an effect more robust in studies with higher baseline Lp(a) levels (slope: −0.44; 95% CI: −0.80, −0.08; $p = 0.018$). The reduction in plasma Lp(a) levels was consistent with different doses of CoQ10, with an inverse association between the dose of CoQ10 administered and the reduction in Lp(a) (slope: 0.04; 95% CI: 0.01, 0.07; $p = 0.004$) [87]. The positive effect of CoQ10 supplementation on Lp(a) plasma levels was not confirmed in a later, but smaller meta-analysis focusing only on patients affected by coronary artery disease [88], or in a further double-blind, randomized, clinical trial more recently carried out in 60 type 2 diabetics [89].

CoQ10 supplementation is tolerable and safe. Its efficacy as a Lp(a) lowering agent is mild and the identification of its most cost-effective daily dose deserves further research.

3.3. Flaxseeds

Flaxseed (*Linum usitatissimum* L.) is a rich source of alpha-linolenic acid, whose supplementation has been demonstrated to mildly, but significantly decrease plasma Lp(a) levels (standardized mean difference: −0.22, 95% CI: −0.41 to −0.04, $p = 0.017$) in a meta-analysis of six double-blind, randomized, placebo-controlled clinical trials [89].

The effect is small, the trials are few and mainly short-term, so that further evidence is needed to support supplementation with flaxseed in hyperLp(a) patients.

3.4. Curcumin

Some clinical trials suggest a positive impact of turmeric extracts on Lp(a) levels.

The first evidence came from a double blind, placebo-controlled clinical trial carried out on 100 Iranian patients affected by metabolic syndrome and randomized to assume curcuminoids (1000 mg/day plus piperine 10 mg/day; n = 50) or placebo (n = 50) for eight weeks [90], with between-group changes of 4.55 mg/dL (−5.00 to 0.00, $p < 0.001$). The same research group confirmed the results in a cohort of 118 type 2 diabetes patients randomized to be treated with curcuminoids (1000 mg/day plus piperine 10 mg/day) or placebo on top of standard care. Beyond a global positive impact on the plasma lipid patterns, Lp(a) decreased by -1.5 ± 1.6 in the active treatment group versus -0.3 ± 1.7 in the placebo treated group ($p = 0.001$) [91].

Finally, these results have been recently confirmed in a double-blind, placebo-controlled clinical trial on type 2 diabetic patients (n = 64), and mild to moderate coronary artery disease (<70% stenosis in angiography), randomized to receive nanosomal-curcumin (80 mg/day) or placebo on top of optimal medications for 90 days [92].

4. Physical Activity

It is well-known that physical activity is associated with a reduced risk of CV disease [93]. Since regular exercise is associated with favorable changes in blood lipoproteins, in particular to an increase in HDL-cholesterolemia and a decrease in triglyceridemia, the question was raised whether there might be any correlation between serum Lp(a) levels and physical activity [94]. Population and cross-sectional studies usually show a lack of association between serum Lp(a) levels and regular and moderate physical activity [95].

An exception is a large Finnish study carried out on children and young adults aged 9, 12, 15, 18, 21, and 24 years (n = 2464, where the Lp(a) ranged from <2 to 90.8 mg/dL) [96]. A physical activity index was specifically calculated for this study, where the serum Lp(a) concentration was significantly correlated with the physical activity level, independently from age and gender, and elevated Lp(a) levels (>25 mg/dL) were less frequent in more physically active subjects.

In a further small cross-sectional study carried out on 80 young patients affected by type 1 diabetes, physical activity was assessed using pedometers measuring the total number of steps per week. Here, a habitual intermediated intensity physical activity was associated with lower Lp(a) plasma levels [97].

However, some cross-sectional studies suggest that serum Lp(a) levels increase in response to intense load training (2–3 h per day), such as distance running or weight-lifting, over several months or years. These changes usually range between a 10 and 15 percent increase [98]. It is unclear whether increased serum Lp(a) levels after intense training or whether physical activity associated with favorable Lp(a) levels have clinical relevance, or whether possibly some isoforms of Lp(a) are more sensitive to the effects of training [98].

Based on the available evidence, it is hard to draw any conclusion on the relationship between Lp(a) plasma levels and different kinds of physical activities or training, because of the large heterogeneity of the available studies, the different methodologies used to record or estimate physical activity, the lack of data on different ethnicities, and on the measure of the different apo(a) isoforms.

Overall, there is inconclusive evidence that standard physical activity improves Lp(a) plasma concentrations, but some intensive training could be suggested in patients able to afford it. However, this evidence also is mainly based on the results of small and short-term trials.

5. Discussion

Hyperlipoproteinemia(a) is largely prevalent in the general population [99]. Statins have no effect on Lp(a) plasma levels, even if partly balancing the negative effect of Lp(a) on CV risk when plasma Lp(a) concentrations are less than 50 mg/dL [100]. Slow-release nicotinic acid is the only drug able to reduce Lp(a) by 20–30%, but it is not well-tolerated and its long-term safety has been questioned [101]. Mipomersen, an anti-sense oligonucleotide directed against apolipoprotein-B 100 mRNA in the liver, is also able to reduce Lp(a) levels, but its liver safety has been seriously questioned as well [102]. The cholesteryl ester transfer protein (CETP) inhibitors increase the HDL fraction while decreasing the atherogenic non-HDL particles, such as Lp(a) [103]. A meta-analysis of ten randomized clinical studies (34,781 patients overall) found that anacetrapib significantly lowers plasma Lp(a) level by a weighted mean difference of −13.35 (95%CI: −18.31 to −8.39) [104]. Another CETP inhibitor, evacetrapib has been shown to reduce Lp(a) by 30–40% over a period of 12 weeks [105]. However, once again, not one of these drugs has been associated with a CVD risk reduction.

In cohort studies, plasma proprotein convertase subtilisin/kexin type 9 (PCSK9) relates with Lp(a) plasma levels [106]. On the other hand, the PCSK9 inhibitors have been shown to significantly, though mildly, reduce Lp(a) plasma levels [107,108]. A recent network meta-analysis of 41 randomized controlled trials with 17,601 participants concluded that the available PCSK9 inhibitors are able to significantly reduce Lp(a) plasma levels (by up to 25.1%), more evidently with Evolocumab and Alirocumab than with Inclisiran [109,110]. However, they are expensive and their use is limited to patients with high-to-very high CV risk.

In our review, we observed that relevant body weight loss, a relatively high intake of saturated fatty acids, the consumption of red wine, and intense physical exercise seems to be associated with significantly lower plasma Lp(a) levels. On the contrary, foods rich in trans-unsaturated fatty acids are associated with increased Lp(a) levels. As regards dietary supplements, coenzyme Q10, L-Carnitine, and flaxseed exert a mild but significant lowering effect on plasma Lp(a).

Of course, other bioactive compounds have been supposed to exert a Lp(a) lowering effect, but their efficacy is even more questionable. For instance, different experimental models suggest that Vitamin C can modulate Lp(a) synthesis [111]. However, two randomized clinical trials did not show any Lp(a)-reducing effect of Vitamin C supplementation. The first one tested the effect of eight months of supplementation with 1 g/day vitamin C in healthy subjects [112], while the second one investigated the effect of 12 weeks of supplementation of 4.5 g/day vitamin C in patients affected by premature CV disease [113]. On the other hand, vitamin B3 (nicotinic acid) exerts a significant Lp(a) lowering effect, but at pharmacological dosages, i.e., at least 30 times the maximum daily dosage recommended as a dietary supplement (35 mg), that are also usually associated with disturbing side effects [114].

Beyond a small study carried out on 40 patients treated with peritoneal hemodialysis, in which 100 mg of soy isoflavones were associated to a significant reduction in Lp(a) levels (up to 10%) after eight weeks of intake [115], a meta-analysis of ten trials involving 973 subjects concluded that isoflavone supplementation had no effect on reducing Lp(a) levels [116].

Dietary factors other than those considered in this review could be associated with Lp(a) plasma levels. For instance, a recent cross-sectional study carried out on 7662 US adults showed a positive correlation between plasma Lp(a) and serum carotenoids (lycopene, lutein, beta-cryptoxanthin), beta-carotene, and alfa-carotene, but a negative association with serum vitamin B12 and folate, whose clinical significance has yet to be clarified [117].

Overall, a healthy diet is suggested for patients with high Lp(a) levels. Body weight reduction seems to be advisable. The most cost-effective way to quickly achieve the optimal body weight in these patients seems to be the ketogenic diet, but its chronic use should not be recommended [118], because of its possible negative affect on LDL-cholesterolemia. The dietary pattern change should be associated with intensification of physical activity. Among the potentially useful and safe dietary supplements, coenzyme Q10 and flaxseed could be considered. It could be argued that different life-style approaches should be considered for the management of high Lp(a) plasma levels in patients with pure hyperLp(a) and in those with high Lp(a) associated with hypercholesterolemia or mixed hyperlipidemia (Table 5). Of course, this is only a speculative suggestion. In fact, for the most part, currently available evidence supporting specific life-style interventions to reduce plasma Lp(a) levels come from cross-sectional studies and small intervention trials. There is a total lack of evidence that Lp(a)-induced changes by dietary and behavioral habits are also related to specific CV outcomes.

Table 5. Lifestyle suggestions for patients with pure isolated hyperLp(a), high plasma Lp(a) associated with hypercholesterolemia, and high Lp(a) associated with mixed hyperlipidemia.

	High Lp(a) Only	**High Lp(a) + High LDL**	**High Lp(a) + High LDL + High TG**
Cigarette smoking stop	↓↓	↓↓	↓↓
Physical activity	Intense	Moderate	Moderate-to-Intense
Body weight	↓↓	↓	↓↓
Alcohol intake	↑	↓	↓↓
Saturated fatty acids	↑	↓	↓
Unsaturated fatty acids	-	↑	↑
Trans fatty acids	↓↓	↓↓	↓↓
Ultraprocessed foods	↓↓	↓↓	↓↓
Whole foods	↑	↑	↑
Vegetables	↑	↑	↑
Dietary supplements	Coenzyme Q10, flaxseed, curcumin		

↓↓ = Clinically significant reduction; ↓ = Mild reduction, ↑ = Mild increase.

We also acknowledge some main limitations of this review. First, a relevant part of the available literature is relatively old. This is probably since Lp(a) has been classified as a non-modifiable risk factor, which has slowed the research on the factors that are possibly related to its modification until recent years. Second, the available evidence is related to a few epidemiological trials and to small short-term clinical trials, whose methodology is not always of high quality.

6. Conclusions

A low-energy, relatively high in saturated fatty acid diet, intense physical activity, and some dietary supplements have a mild but significant effect on plasma Lp(a) levels. Further studies are needed to confirm the available evidence and to test an Lp(a) reduction lifestyle and its impact on the risk of developing CV diseases.

Author Contributions: Conceptualization, A.F.G.C. and F.F.; methodology, V.D.M. and F.F.; writing—original draft preparation, V.D.M., F.F. and M.G.; writing—review and editing, P.S. and A.F.G.C. All authors have read and agreed to the published version of the manuscript.

Funding: This research received no external funding.

Institutional Review Board Statement: Not applicable.

Informed Consent Statement: Not applicable.

Data Availability Statement: Not applicable.

Conflicts of Interest: The authors declare no conflicts of interest.

References

1. Visseren, F.L.J.; Mach, F.; Smulders, Y.M.; Carballo, D.; Koskinas, K.C.; Bäck, M.; Benetos, A.; Biffi, A.; Boavida, J.M.; Capo-danno, D.; et al. 2021 ESC Guidelines on cardiovascular disease prevention in clinical practice: Developed by the Task Force for cardiovascular disease prevention in clinical practice with representatives of the European Society of Cardiology and 12 medical societies With the special contribution of the European Association of Preventive Cardiology (EAPC). *Rev. Esp. Cardiol. (Engl. Ed.)* **2022**, *75*, 429. [CrossRef] [PubMed]
2. Tada, H.; Yamagami, K.; Sakata, K.; Usui, S.; Kawashiri, M.A.; Takamura, M. Healthy lifestyle, lipoprotein (a) levels and the risk of coronary artery disease. *Eur. J. Clin. Investig.* **2023**, *54*, e14093. [CrossRef] [PubMed]
3. Koschinsky, M.L.; Kronenberg, F. The long journey of lipoprotein (a) from cardiovascular curiosity to therapeutic target. *Atherosclerosis* **2022**, *349*, 1–6. [CrossRef] [PubMed]
4. Arsenault, B.J.; Kamstrup, P.R. Lipoprotein (a) and cardiovascular and valvular diseases: A genetic epidemiological perspec-tive. *Atherosclerosis* **2022**, *349*, 7–16. [CrossRef] [PubMed]
5. Singh, S.; Baars, D.P.; Desai, R.; Singh, D.; Pinto-Sietsma, S.J. Association between Lipoprotein (a) and risk of atrial fibrillation: A Systematic Review and Meta-analysis of Mendelian Randomization Studies. *Curr. Probl. Cardiol.* **2023**, *49 Pt A*, 102024. [CrossRef]
6. Amiri, M.; Raeisi-Dehkordi, H.; Verkaar, A.J.C.F.; Wu, Y.; van Westing, A.C.; Berk, K.A.; Bramer, W.M.; Aune, D.; Voortman, T. Circulating lipoprotein (a) and all-cause and cause-specific mortality: A systematic review and dose-response meta-analysis. *Eur. J. Epidemiol.* **2023**, *38*, 485–499. [CrossRef] [PubMed]
7. Fogacci, F.; Di Micoli, V.; Avagimyan, A.; Giovannini, M.; Imbalzano, E.; Cicero, A.F.G. Assessment of Apolipoprotein (a) Isoform Size Using Phenotypic and Genotypic Methods. *Int. J. Mol. Sci.* **2023**, *24*, 13886. [CrossRef]
8. Banach, M. Lipoprotein (a): The enemy that we still don't know how to defeat. *Eur. Heart J. Open* **2023**, *3*, oead080. [CrossRef]
9. Sukkari, M.H.; Al-Bast, B.; Al Tamimi, R.; Giesing, W.; Siddique, M. Is there a benefit of aspirin therapy for primary prevention to reduce the risk of atherosclerotic cardiovascular disease in patients with elevated Lipoprotein (a)—A review of the evidence. *Am. J. Prev. Cardiol.* **2023**, *15*, 100579. [CrossRef]
10. Alhomoud, I.S.; Talasaz, A.; Mehta, A.; Kelly, M.S.; Sisson, E.M.; Bucheit, J.D.; Brown, R.; Dixon, D.L. Role of lipoprotein (a) in atherosclerotic cardiovascular disease: A review of current and emerging therapies. *Pharmacotherapy* **2023**, *43*, 1051–1063. [CrossRef]
11. Kosmas, C.E.; Bousvarou, M.D.; Papakonstantinou, E.J.; Tsamoulis, D.; Koulopoulos, A.; Echavarria Uceta, R.; Guzman, E.; Rallidis, L.S. Novel Pharmacological Therapies for the Management of Hyperlipoproteinemia(a). *Int. J. Mol. Sci.* **2023**, *24*, 13622. [CrossRef] [PubMed]
12. Nicholls, S.J.; Nissen, S.E.; Fleming, C.; Urva, S.; Suico, J.; Berg, P.H.; Linnebjerg, H.; Ruotolo, G.; Turner, P.K.; Michael, L.F. Muvalaplin, an Oral Small Molecule Inhibitor of Lipoprotein (a) Formation: A Randomized Clinical Trial. *J. Am. Med. Assoc.* **2023**, *330*, 1042–1053. [CrossRef]
13. Christensen, P.; Larsen, T.M.; Westerterp-Plantenga, M.; Macdonald, I.; Martinez, J.A.; Handjiev, S.; Poppitt, S.; Hansen, S.; Ritz, C.; Astrup, A.; et al. Men and women respond differently to rapid weight loss: Metabolic outcomes of a multi-centre intervention study after a low-energy diet in 2500 overweight, individuals with pre-diabetes (PREVIEW). *Diabetes Obes. Metab.* **2018**, *20*, 2840–2851. [CrossRef] [PubMed]
14. Harder, H.; Dinesen, B.; Astrup, A. The effect of a rapid weight loss on lipid profile and glycemic control in obese type 2 diabetic patients. *Int. J. Obes. Relat. Metab. Disord.* **2004**, *28*, 180–182. [CrossRef]
15. Heffron, S.P.; Parikh, A.; Volodarskiy, A.; Ren-Fielding, C.; Schwartzbard, A.; Nicholson, J.; Bangalore, S. Changes in lipid profile of obese patients following contemporary bariatric surgery: A meta-analysis. *Am. J. Med.* **2016**, *129*, 952–959. [CrossRef] [PubMed]
16. Spivak, H.; Sakran, N.; Dicker, D.; Rubin, M.; Raz, I.; Shohat, T.; Blumenfeld, O. Different effects of bariatric surgical procedures on dyslipidemia: A registry-based analysis. *Surg. Obes. Relat. Dis.* **2017**, *13*, 1189–1194. [CrossRef]
17. Mulla, C.M.; Middelbeek, R.J.W.; Patti, M.-E. Mechanisms of weight loss and improved metabolism following bariatric sur-gery. *Ann. N. Y. Acad. Sci.* **2018**, *1411*, 53–64. [CrossRef]
18. Kiortsis, D.N.; Tzotzas, T.; Giral, P.; Bruckert, E.; Beucler, I.; Valsamides, S.; Turpin, G. Changes in lipoprotein (a) levels and hormonal correlations during a weight reduction program. *Nutr. Metab. Cardiovasc. Dis.* **2001**, *11*, 153–157.

19. Berk, K.A.; Yahya, R.; Verhoeven, A.J.M.; Touw, J.; Leijten, F.P.; van Rossum, E.F.; Wester, V.L.; Lips, M.A.; Pijl, H.; Timma R.; et al. Effect of diet-induced weight loss on lipopro-tein(a) levels in obese individuals with and without type 2 diabete *Diabetologia* **2017**, *60*, 989–997. [CrossRef]
20. Berk, K.A.; Borgeraas, H.; Narverud, I.; Mulder, M.T.; Øyri, L.K.L.; Verhoeven, A.J.M.; Småstuen, M.C.; Bogsrud, M.P.; Omlanc T.; Hertel, J.K.; et al. Differential effects of bariatric surgery and lifestyle interventions on plasma levels of Lp(a) and fatty acid *Lipids Health Dis.* **2022**, *21*, 145. [CrossRef]
21. Gómez-Martin, J.M.; Balsa, J.A.; Aracil, E.; Cuadrado-Ayuso, M.; Rosillo, M.; De la Peña, G.; Lasunción, M.A.; Escobar-Morreal H.F.; Botella-Carretero, J.I. Beneficial changes on plasma apolipoproteins A and B, high density lipoproteins and oxidized lov density lipoproteins in obese women after bariatric surgery: Comparison between gastric bypass and sleeve gastrectomy. *Lipid Health Dis.* **2018**, *17*, 145. [CrossRef]
22. Paredes, S.; Alves, M.; Lopes Pereira, M.; Marques, O.; Ribeiro, L. Lipoprotein (a) Change After Sleeve Gastrectomy Is Affected b the Presence of Metabolic Syndrome. *Obes. Surg.* **2020**, *30*, 545–552. [CrossRef]
23. Scholl, J.G. Does a ketogenic diet lower a very high Lp(a)? A striking experiment in a male physician. *BMJ Nutr. Prev. Health* **202** *3*, 413–415. [CrossRef] [PubMed]
24. Ebbeling, C.B.; Knapp, A.; Johnson, A.; Wong, J.M.W.; Greco, K.F.; Ma, C.; Mora, S.; Ludwig, D.S. Effects of a low-carbohydrat diet on insulin-resistant dyslipoproteinemia-a randomized controlled feeding trial. *Am. J. Clin. Nutr.* **2022**, *115*, 154–16 [CrossRef] [PubMed]
25. Cipryan, L.; Litschmannova, M.; Maffetone, P.B.; Plews, D.J.; Dostal, T.; Hofmann, P.; Laursen, P.B. Very Low-Carbohydrate High Fat Diet Improves Risk Markers for Cardiometabolic Health More Than Exercise in Men and Women with Overfat Constitution Secondary Analysis of a Randomized Controlled Clinical Trial. *Front. Nutr.* **2022**, *9*, 867690. [CrossRef]
26. Kronenberg, F.; Mora, S.; Stroes, E.S.G.; Ference, B.A.; Arsenault, B.J.; Berglund, L.; Dweck, M.R.; Koschinsky, M.; Lambert, G Mach, F.; et al. Lipoprotein (a) in atherosclerotic cardiovascular disease and aortic stenosis: A European Atherosclerosis Societ consensus statement. *Eur. Heart J.* **2022**, *43*, 3925–3946. [CrossRef] [PubMed]
27. Seidelmann, S.B.; Claggett, B.; Cheng, S.; Henglin, M.; Shah, A.; Steffen, L.M.; Folsom, A.R.; Rimm, E.B.; Willett, W.C.; Solomon S.D. Dietary carbohydrate intake and mortality: A prospective cohort study and meta-analysis. *Lancet Public Health* **2018**, *3* e419–e428. [CrossRef] [PubMed]
28. Richter, C.K.; Skulas-Ray, A.C.; Champagne, C.M.; Kris-Etherton, P.M. Plant protein and animal proteins: Do they differen-tially affect cardiovascular disease risk? *Adv. Nutr.* **2015**, *6*, 712–728. [CrossRef]
29. Ros, E.; Martínez-González, M.A.; Estruch, R.; Salas-Salvadó, J.; Fitó, M.; Martínez, J.A.; Corella, D. Mediterranean diet and cardiovascular health: Teachings of the PREDIMED study. *Adv. Nutr.* **2014**, *5*, 330S–336S. [CrossRef]
30. Najjar, R.S.; Moore, C.E.; Montgomery, B.D. Consumption of a defined, plant-based diet reduces lipoprotein (a), inflammation and other atherogenic lipoproteins and particles within 4 weeks. *Clin. Cardiol.* **2018**, *41*, 1062–1068. [CrossRef]
31. Wang, D.D.; Li, Y.; Chiuve, S.E.; Stampfer, M.J.; Manson, J.E.; Rimm, E.B.; Willett, W.C.; Hu, F.B. Association of specific dietary fats with total and cause-specific mortality. *JAMA Intern. Med.* **2016**, *176*, 1134–1145. [CrossRef]
32. Chen, G.-C.; Zhang, R.; Martínez-González, M.A.; Zhang, Z.-L.; Bonaccio, M.; van Dam, R.B.; Qin, L.-Q. Nut consumption in relation to all-cause and cause-specific mortality: A meta-analysis 18 prospective studies. *Food Funct.* **2017**, *8*, 3893–3905. [CrossRef]
33. Guasch-Ferré, M.; Li, J.; Hu, F.B.; Salas-Salvadó, J.; Tobias, D.K. Effects of walnut consumption on blood lipids and other cardiovascular risk factors: An updated meta-analysis and systematic review of controlled trials. *Am. J. Clin. Nutr.* **2018**, *108*, 174–187. [CrossRef]
34. Bamberger, C.; Rossmeier, A.; Lechner, K.; Wu, L.; Waldmann, E.; Stark, R.G.; Altenhofer, J.; Henze, K.; Parhofer, K.G. A walnut-enriched diet reduces lipids in healthy Caucasian subjects, independent of recommended macronutrient replacement and time point of consumption: A prospective, randomized, controlled trial. *Nutrients* **2017**, *9*, 1097. [CrossRef]
35. Nora, C.L.; Zhang, L.; Castro, R.J.; Marx, A.; Carman, H.B.; Lum, T.; Tsimikas, S.; Hong, M.Y. Effects of mixed nut consumption on LDL cholesterol, lipoprotein (a), and other cardiometabolic risk factors in overweight and obese adults. *Nutr. Metab. Car-Diovasc. Dis.* **2023**, *33*, 1529–1538. [CrossRef] [PubMed]
36. Matveyenko, A.; Seid, H.; Kim, K.; Ramakrishnan, K.; Thomas, T.; Matienzo, N.; Reyes-Soffer, G. Association of free-living diet composition with plasma lipoprotein (a) levels in healthy adults. *Lipids Health Dis.* **2023**, *22*, 144. [CrossRef] [PubMed]
37. Müller, H.; Lindman, A.S.; Blomfeldt, A.; Seljeflot, I.; Pedersen, J.I. A diet rich in coconut oil reduces diurnal postprandial variations in circulating tissue plasminogen activator antigen and fasting lipoprotein (a) compared with a diet rich in un-saturated fat in women. *J. Nutr.* **2003**, *133*, 3422–3427. [CrossRef] [PubMed]
38. Loganathan, R.; Nagapan, G.; Teng, K.T.; Voon, P.T.; Yap, S.Y.; Ng, Y.T.; Ng, T.K.W.; Choo, Y.M.; Ong, A.S.H.; Ong, S.H.; et al. Diets enriched with palm olein, cocoa butter, and extra virgin olive oil exhibited similar lipid response: A randomized controlled study in young healthy adults. *Nutr. Res.* **2022**, *105*, 113–125. [CrossRef] [PubMed]
39. Harcombe, Z. US dietary guidelines: Is saturated fat a nutrient of concern? *Br. J. Sports Med.* **2018**, *53*, 1393–1396. [CrossRef] [PubMed]
40. Sacks, F.M.; Lichtenstein, A.H.; Wu, J.H.Y.; Appel, L.J.; Creager, M.A.; Kris-Etherton, P.M.; Miller, M.; Rimm, E.B.; Rudel, L.L.; Robinson, J.G.; et al. Dietary fats and cardiovascular disease: A presidential advisory from the American Heart Association. *Circulation* **2017**, *136*, e1–e23. [CrossRef] [PubMed]

41. Lichtenstein, A.L. Trans fatty acids and blood lipid levels, Lp(a), parameters of cholesterol metabolism, and hemostatic factors. *J. Nutr. Biochem.* **1998**, *9*, 244–248. [CrossRef]
42. Clevidence, B.A.; Judd, J.T.; Schaefer, E.J.; Jenner, J.L.; Lichtenstein, A.H.; Muesing, R.A.; Wittes, J.; Sunkin, M.E. Plasma lipo-protein (a) levels in men and women consuming diets enriched in saturated, cis-, or trans-monounsaturated fatty acids. *Arterioscler. Thromb. Vasc. Biol.* **1997**, *17*, 1657–1661. [CrossRef]
43. Almendingen, K.; Jordal, O.; Kierulf, P.; Sandstad, B.; Pedersen, J.I. Effects of partially hydrogenated fish oil, partially hydrogenated soybean oil, and butter on serum lipoproteins and Lp[a] in men. *J. Lipid Res.* **1995**, *36*, 1370–1384. [CrossRef]
44. Chisholm, A.; Mann, J.; Sutherland, W.; Duncan, A.; Skeaff, M.; Frampton, C. Effect on lipoprotein profile of replacing butter with margarine in a low fat diet: Randomised crossover study with hypercholesterolemic subjects. *BMJ* **1996**, *312*, 931–934. [CrossRef]
45. Bozzetto, L.; De Natale, C.; Di Capua, L.; Della Corte, G.; Patti, L.; Maione, S.; Riccardi, G.; Rivellese, A.A.; Annuzzi, G. The association of hs-CRP with fasting and postprandial plasma lipids in patients with type 2 diabetes is disrupted by dietary monounsaturated fatty acids. *Acta Diabetol.* **2013**, *50*, 273–276. [CrossRef] [PubMed]
46. Higgins, V.; Adeli, K. Postprandial dyslipidemia: Pathophysiology and cardiovascular disease risk assessment. *eJIFCC* **2017**, *28*, 168–184. [PubMed]
47. Paniagua, J.A.; de la Sacristana, A.G.; Sánchez, E.; Romero, I.; Vidal-Puig, A.; Berral, F.J.; Escribano, A.; Moyano, M.J.; Peréz-Martinez, P.; López-Miranda, J.; et al. A MUFA-rich diet improves postprandial glucose, lipid and GLP-1 responses in insulin-resistant subjects. *J. Am. Coll. Nutr.* **2007**, *26*, 434–444. [CrossRef] [PubMed]
48. Tsofliou, F.; Fyfe, C.L.; Matheson, I.; Jackson, D.M.; Horgan, G.W.; Wahle, K.W.J.; Ahren, B.; Williams, L.M.; Sneddon, A.A. Modulation of fasted and postprandial plasma lipids in healthy volunteers by a dietary mixture of omega-3 fatty acids and conjugated linoleic acid. *J. Food Lipids* **2009**, *16*, 499–513. [CrossRef]
49. Tholstrup, T.; Samman, S. Postprandial lipoprotein (a) is affected differently by specific individual dietary fatty acids in healthy young men. *J. Nutr.* **2004**, *134*, 2550–2555. [CrossRef] [PubMed]
50. Brunkwall, L.; Almgren, P.; Hellstrand, S.; Orho-Melander, M.; Ericson, U. Commonly consumed beverages associate with different lifestyle and dietary intakes. *Int. J. Food Sci. Nutr.* **2019**, *70*, 88–97. [CrossRef] [PubMed]
51. Khan, N.; Mukhtar, H. Tea and health: Studies in humans. *Curr. Pharm. Des.* **2013**, *19*, 6141–6147. [CrossRef]
52. Nova, E.; Baccan, G.C.; Veses, A.; Zapatera, B.; Marcos, A. Potential health benefits of moderate alcohol consumption: Current perspectives in research. *Proc. Nutr. Soc.* **2012**, *71*, 307–315. [CrossRef] [PubMed]
53. Davies, M.J.; Judd, J.T.; Baer, D.J.; Clevidence, B.A.; Paul, D.R.; Edwards, A.J.; Wiseman, S.A.; Muesing, R.A.; Chen, S.C. Black tea consumption reduces total and LDL cholesterol in mildly hypercholesterolemic adults. *J. Nutr.* **2003**, *133*, 3298S–3302S. [CrossRef]
54. Mozaffari-Khosravi, H.; Jalali-Khanabadi, B.-A.; Afkhami-Ardekani, M.; Fatehi, F. Effects of sour tea (*Hibiscus sabdariffa*) on lipid profile and lipoproteins in patients with type II diabetes. *J. Altern. Complement. Med.* **2009**, *15*, 899–903. [CrossRef]
55. Miranda, A.M.; Steluti, J.; Goulart, A.C.; Benseñor, I.M.; Lotufo, P.A.; Marchioni, D.M. Coffee consumption and coronary artery calcium score: Cross-sectional results of ELSA-Brasil (Brazilian Longitudinal Study of Adult Health). *J. Am. Heart Assoc.* **2018**, *7*, e007155. [CrossRef]
56. Pang, J.; Zhang, Z.; Zheng, T.-Z.; Bassig, B.A.; Mao, C.; Liu, X.; Zhu, Y.; Shi, K.; Ge, J.; Yang, Y.-J.; et al. Green tea consumption and risk of cardiovascular and ischemic related diseases: A meta-analysis. *Int. J. Cardiol.* **2016**, *202*, 967–974. [CrossRef] [PubMed]
57. Xie, C.; Cui, L.; Zhu, J.; Wang, K.; Sun, N.; Sun, C. Coffee consumption and risk of hypertension: A systematic review and dose-response meta-analysis of cohort studies. *J. Hum. Hypertens.* **2018**, *32*, 83–93. [CrossRef]
58. Zhang, C.; Qin, Y.-Y.; Wei, X.; Yu, F.-F.; Zhou, Y.-H.; He, J. Tea consumption and risk of cardiovascular outcomes and total mortality: A systematic review and meta-analysis of prospective observational studies. *Eur. J. Epidemiol.* **2015**, *30*, 103–113. [CrossRef] [PubMed]
59. Urgert, R.; Weusten-van der Wouw, M.P.; Hovenier, R.; Meyboom, S.; Beynen, A.C.; Katan, M.B. Diterpenes from coffee beans decrease serum levels of lipoprotein (a) in humans: Results from four randomised controlled trials. *Eur. J. Clin. Nutr.* **1997**, *51*, 431–436. [CrossRef]
60. Penson, P.; Serban, M.-C.; Ursoniu, S.; Banach, M.; the Lipid and Blood Pressure Meta-analysis Collaboration (LBPMC) Group. Does coffee consumption alter plasma lipoprotein (a) concentrations? A systematic review. *Crit. Rev. Food Sci. Nutr.* **2018**, *58*, 1706–1714. [CrossRef]
61. Urgert, R.; Weusten-van der Wouw, M.P.; Hovenier, R.; Lund-Larsen, P.G.; Katan, M.B. Chronic consumers of boiled coffee have elevated serum levels of lipoprotein (a). *J. Intern. Med.* **1996**, *240*, 367–371. [CrossRef]
62. Cornelis, M.C.; van Dam, R.M. Habitual Coffee and Tea Consumption and Cardiometabolic Biomarkers in the UK Biobank: The Role of Beverage Types and Genetic Variation. *J. Nutr.* **2020**, *150*, 2772–2788. [CrossRef]
63. Paassilta, M.; Kervinen, K.; Rantala, A.O.; Savolainen, M.J.; Lilja, M.; Reunanen, A.; Kesäniemi, Y.A. Social alcohol consumption and low Lp(a) lipoprotein concentrations in middle aged Finnish men: Population based study. *BMJ* **1998**, *316*, 594–595. [CrossRef]
64. Catena, C.; Novello, M.; Dotto, L.; De Marchi, S.; Sechi, L.A. Serum lipoprotein (a) concentrations and alcohol consumption in hypertension: Possible relevance for cardiovascular damage. *J. Hypertens.* **2003**, *21*, 281–288. [CrossRef] [PubMed]
65. Sharpe, P.C.; McGrath, L.T.; McClean, E.; Young, I.S.; Archbold, G.P. Effect of red wine consumption on lipoprotein (a) and other risk factors for atherosclerosis. *QJM Int. J. Med.* **1995**, *88*, 101–108.

66. Chiva-Blanch, G.; Urpi-Sarda, M.; Ros, E.; Valderas-Martinez, P.; Casas, R.; Arranz, S.; Guillén, M.; Lamuela-Raventós, R.M.; Llorach, R.; Andres-Lacueva, C.; et al. Effects of red wine polyphenols and alcohol on glucose metabolism and the lipid profile: A randomized clinical trial. *Clin. Nutr.* **2013**, *32*, 200–206. [CrossRef]
67. GBD 2016 Alcohol and Drug Use Collaborators. The global burden of disease attributable to alcohol and drug use in 195 countries and territories, 1990–2016: A systematic analysis for the Global Burden of Disease Study 2016. *Lancet Psychiatry* **2018**, *5*, 987–1012. [CrossRef] [PubMed]
68. Wood, A.W.; Kaptoge, S.; Butterworth, A.S.; Willeit, P.; Warnakula, S.; Bolton, T.; Paige, E.; Paul, D.S.; Sweeting, M.; Burgess, S.; et al. Risk thresholds for alcohol consumption: Combined analysis of individual-participant data for 599 912 current drinkers in 83 prospective studies. *Lancet* **2018**, *391*, 1513–1523. [CrossRef]
69. Cicero, A.F.G.; Fogacci, F.; Stoian, A.P.; Vrablik, M.; Al Rasadi, K.; Banach, M.; Toth, P.P.; Rizzo, M. Nutraceuticals in the Management of Dyslipidemia: Which, When, and for Whom? Could Nutraceuticals Help Low-Risk Individuals with Non-optimal Lipid Levels? *Curr. Atheroscler. Rep.* **2021**, *23*, 57. [CrossRef] [PubMed]
70. Serban, M.-C.; Sahebkar, A.; Mikhailidis, D.P.; Toth, P.P.; Jones, S.R.; Muntner, P.; Blaha, M.J.; Andrica, F.; Martin, S.S.; Borza, C.; et al. Impact of L-carnitine on plasma lipoprotein (a) concentrations: A sys-tematic review and meta-analysis of randomized controlled trials. *Sci. Rep.* **2016**, *6*, 19188. [CrossRef]
71. Pekala, J.; Patkowska-Sokoła, B.; Bodkowski, R.; Jamroz, D.; Nowakowski, P.; Lochyński, S.; Librowski, T. L-carnitine met-abolic functions and meaning in humans life. *Curr. Drug Metab.* **2011**, *12*, 667–678. [CrossRef]
72. Jing, Z.-C.; Wu, B.-X.; Peng, J.-Q.; Li, X.-L.; Pan, L.; Zhao, S.P.; Li, D.Y.; Yu, Z.X.; Gong, J.B.; Zhao, Q.Y.; et al. Effect of intravenous L-carnitine in Chinese patients with chronic heart failure. *Eur. Heart J. Suppl.* **2016**, *18* (Suppl. A), A27–A36. [CrossRef]
73. Lee, B.-J.; Lin, J.-S.; Lin, Y.-C.; Lin, P.-T. Effects of l-carnitine supplementation on lipid profiles in patients with coronary artery disease. *Lipids Health Dis.* **2016**, *15*, 107. [CrossRef]
74. Lee, B.-J.; Lin, J.-S.; Lin, Y.-C.; Lin, P.-T. Effects of l-carnitine supplementation on oxidative stress and antioxidant enzymes ac-tivities in patients with coronary artery disease: A randomized, placebo- controlled trial. *Nutr. J.* **2014**, *13*, 79. [CrossRef]
75. Asadi, M.; Rahimlou, M.; Shishehbor, F.; Mansoori, A. The effect of l-carnitine supplementation on lipid profile and glycaemic control in adults with cardiovascular risk factors: A systematic review and meta-analysis of randomized controlled clinical trials. *Clin. Nutr.* **2020**, *39*, 110–122. [CrossRef]
76. Florentin, M.; Elisaf, M.S.; Rizos, C.V.; Nikolaou, V.; Bilianou, E.; Pitsavos, C.; Liberopoulos, E.N. L-carnitine/simvastatin reduces lipoprotein (a) levels compared with simvastatin monotherapy: A randomized double-blind placebo- controlled study. *Lipids* **2017**, *52*, 1–9. [CrossRef] [PubMed]
77. Vallance, H.D.; Koochin, A.; Branov, J.; Rosen-Heath, A.; Bosdet, T.; Wang, Z.; Hazen, S.L.; Horvath, G. Marked elevation in plasma trimethylamine-N-oxide (TMAO) in patients with mitochondrial disorders treated with oral L-carnitine. *Mol. Genet. Metab. Rep.* **2018**, *15*, 130–133. [CrossRef]
78. Fukami, K.; Yamagishi, S.-I.; Sakai, K.; Kaida, Y.; Yokoro, M.; Ueda, S.; Wada, Y.; Takeuchi, M.; Shimizu, M.; Yamazaki, H.; et al. Oral L-carnitine supplementation increases trimethylamine-N-oxide but reduces markers of vascular injury in hemodialysis patients. *J. Cardiovasc. Pharmacol.* **2015**, *65*, 289–295. [CrossRef] [PubMed]
79. Miller, M.J.; Bostwick, B.L.; Kennedy, A.D.; Donti, T.R.; Sun, Q.; Sutton, V.R.; Elsea, S.H. Chronic oral L-carnitine supple-mentation drives marked plasma TMAO elevations in patients with organic acidemias despite dietary meat restrictions. *JIMD Rep.* **2016**, *30*, 39–44. [CrossRef] [PubMed]
80. Qi, J.; You, T.; Li, J.; Pan, T.; Xiang, L.; Han, Y.; Zhu, L. Circulating trimethylamine N-oxide and the risk of cardiovascular diseases: A systematic review and meta-analysis of 11 prospective cohort studies. *J. Cell Mol. Med.* **2018**, *22*, 185–194. [CrossRef] [PubMed]
81. Deichmann, R.; Lavie, C.; Andrews, S. Coenzyme Q10 and statin-induced mitochondrial dysfunction. *Ochsner J.* **2010**, *10*, 16–21. [PubMed]
82. Liu, H.-T.; Huang, Y.-C.; Cheng, S.-B.; Huang, Y.-T.; Lin, P.-T. Effects of coenzyme Q10 supplementation on antioxidant capacity and inflammation in hepatocellular carcinoma patients after surgery: A randomized, placebo-controlled trial. *Nutr. J.* **2016**, *15*, 85. [CrossRef] [PubMed]
83. Zhao, M.; Tian, Z.; Zhao, D.; Liang, Y.; Dai, S.; Xu, Y.; Hou, S.; Yang, Y. L-shaped association between dietary coenzyme Q10 intake and high-sensitivity C-reactive protein in Chinese adults: A national cross-sectional study. *Food Funct.* **2023**, *14*, 9815–9824. [CrossRef] [PubMed]
84. Fotino, A.D.; Thompson-Paul, A.; Bazzano, L.A. Effect of coenzyme Q10 supplementation on heart failure: A meta-analysis. *Am. J. Clin. Nutr.* **2013**, *97*, 268–275. [CrossRef]
85. Lei, L.; Liu, Y. Efficacy of coenzyme Q10 in patients with cardiac failure: A meta-analysis of clinical trials. *BMC Cardiovasc. Disord.* **2017**, *17*, 196. [CrossRef]
86. Jorat, M.V.; Tabrizi, R.; Mirhosseini, N.; Lankarani, K.B.; Akbari, M.; Heydari, S.T.; Mottaghi, R.; Asemi, Z. The effects of co-enzyme Q10 supplementation on lipid profiles among patients with coronary artery disease: A systematic review and me-ta-analysis of randomized controlled trials. *Lipids Health Dis.* **2018**, *17*, 230. [CrossRef] [PubMed]
87. Sahebkar, A.; Simental-Mendía, L.E.; Stefanutti, C.; Pirro, M. Supplementation with coenzyme Q10 reduces plasma lipopro-tein(a) concentrations but not other lipid indices: A systematic review and meta-analysis. *Pharmacol. Res.* **2016**, *105*, 198–209. [CrossRef]

88. Mirhashemi, S.M.; Najafi, V.; Raygan, F.; Asemi, Z. The effects of coenzyme Q10 supplementation on cardiometabolic markers in overweight type 2 diabetic patients with stable myocardial infarction: A randomized, double-blind, placebo-controlled trial. *ARYA Atheroscler.* **2016**, *12*, 158–165.
89. Sahebkar, A.; Katsiki, N.; Ward, N.; Reiner, Ž. Flaxseed Supplementation Reduces Plasma Lipoprotein (a) Levels: A Me-ta-Analysis. *Altern. Ther. Health Med.* **2021**, *27*, 50–53.
90. Panahi, Y.; Khalili, N.; Hosseini, M.S.; Abbasinazari, M.; Sahebkar, A. Lipid-modifying effects of adjunctive therapy with curcuminoids-piperine combination in patients with metabolic syndrome: Results of a randomized controlled trial. *Complement. Ther. Med.* **2014**, *22*, 851–857. [CrossRef]
91. Panahi, Y.; Khalili, N.; Sahebi, E.; Namazi, S.; Reiner, Ž.; Majeed, M.; Sahebkar, A. Curcuminoids modify lipid profile in type 2 diabetes mellitus: A randomized controlled trial. *Complement. Ther. Med.* **2017**, *33*, 1–5. [CrossRef]
92. Dastani, M.; Rahimi, H.R.; Askari, V.R.; Jaafari, M.R.; Jarahi, L.; Yadollahi, A.; Rahimi, V.B. Three months of combination therapy with nano-curcumin reduces the inflammation and lipoprotein (a) in type 2 diabetic patients with mild to moderate coronary artery disease: Evidence of a randomized, double-blinded, placebo-controlled clinical trial. *Biofactors* **2023**, *49*, 108–118. [CrossRef]
93. Sulague, R.M.; Suan, N.N.M.; Mendoza, M.F.; Lavie, C.J. The associations between exercise and lipid biomarkers. *Prog. Car-Diovasc Dis.* **2022**, *75*, 59–68. [CrossRef]
94. Mackinnon, L.T.; Hubinger, L.; Lepre, F. Effects of physical activity and diet on lipoprotein (a). *Med. Sci. Sports Exerc.* **1997**, *29*, 1429–1436. [CrossRef] [PubMed]
95. Hubinger, L.; Mackinnon, L.T.; Lepre, F. Lipoprotein (a) [Lp(a)] levels in middle-aged male runners and sedentary controls. *Med. Sci. Sports Exerc.* **1995**, *27*, 490–496. [CrossRef] [PubMed]
96. Taimela, S.; Viikari, J.S.; Porkka, K.V.; Dahlen, G.H. Lipoprotein (a) levels in children and young adults: The influence of physical activity. The Cardiovascular Risk in Young Finns Study. *Acta Paediatr.* **1994**, *83*, 1258–1263. [CrossRef]
97. Kaza, M.; Tsentidis, C.; Vlachopapadopoulou, E.; Karanasios, S.; Sakou, I.I.; Mastorakos, G.; Karavanaki, K. The Role of Exercise on Cardiometabolic Profile and Body Composition in Youth with Type 1 Diabetes. *Children* **2022**, *9*, 1840. [CrossRef]
98. Mackinnon, L.T.; Hubinger, L.M. Effects of exercise on lipoprotein (a). *Sports Med.* **1999**, *28*, 11–24. [CrossRef] [PubMed]
99. Cicero, A.F.G.; Fogacci, F.; Giovannini, M.; Grandi, E.; D'Addato, S.; Borghi, C. Estimating the Prevalence and Characteristics of Patients Potentially Eligible for Lipoprotein (a)-Lowering Therapies in a Real-World Setting. *Biomedicines* **2023**, *11*, 3289. [CrossRef]
100. Willeit, P.; Ridker, P.M.; Nestel, P.J.; Simes, J.; Tonkin, A.M.; Pedersen, T.R.; Schwartz, G.G.; Olsson, A.G.; Colhoun, H.M.; Kronenberg, F.; et al. Baseline and on-statin treatment lipoprotein (a) levels for prediction of cardiovascular events: Individual patient-data meta-analysis of statin outcome trials. *Lancet* **2018**, *392*, 1311–1320. [CrossRef]
101. Schandelmaier, S.; Briel, M.; Saccilotto, R.; Olu, K.K.; Arpagaus, A.; Hemkens, L.G.; Nordmann, A.J. Niacin for primary and secondary prevention of cardiovascular events. *Cochrane Database Syst. Rev.* **2017**, *6*, CD009744. [CrossRef]
102. Fogacci, F.; Ferri, N.; Toth, P.P.; Ruscica, M.; Corsini, A.; Cicero, A.F.G. Efficacy and Safety of Mipomersen: A Systematic Review and Meta-Analysis of Randomized Clinical Trials. *Drugs* **2019**, *79*, 751–766. [CrossRef] [PubMed]
103. Gencer, B.; Mach, F. Potential of Lipoprotein (a)-Lowering Strategies in Treating Coronary Artery Disease. *Drugs* **2020**, *80*, 229–239. [CrossRef] [PubMed]
104. Zhou, J.; Zhang, Q.; Wang, Y.; Gao, P.; Chen, D. The effect and safety of anacetrapib in the treatment of dyslipidemia: A sys-tematic review and meta-analysis. *Postgrad. Med.* **2018**, *130*, 129–136. [CrossRef] [PubMed]
105. Nicholls, S.J.; Ruotolo, G.; Brewer, H.B.; Wang, M.D.; Liu, L.; Willey, M.B.; Deeg, M.A.; Krueger, K.A.; Nissen, S.E. Evacetrapib alone or in combination with statins lowers lipoprotein (a) and total and small LDL particle concentrations in mildly hypercholesterolemic patients. *J. Clin. Lipidol.* **2016**, *10*, 519–527. [CrossRef]
106. Afanasieva, O.I.; Ezhov, M.V.; Razova, O.A.; Afanasieva, M.I.; Utkina, E.A.; Pokrovsky, S.N. Apolipoprotein (a) phenotype determines the correlations of lipoprotein (a) and proprotein convertase subtilisin/kexin type 9 levels in patients with potential familial hypercholesterolemia. *Atherosclerosis* **2018**, *277*, 477–482. [CrossRef]
107. Chan, D.C.; Watts, G.F. The Promise of PCSK9 and Lipoprotein (a) as Targets for Gene Silencing Therapies. *Clin. Ther.* **2023**, *45*, 1034–1046. [CrossRef]
108. Yu, Z.; Hu, L.; Sun, C.; Wang, Z.; Zhang, X.; Wu, M.; Liu, L. Effect of Different Types and Dosages of Proprotein Convertase Subtilisin/Kexin Type 9 Inhibitors on Lipoprotein (a) Levels: A Network Meta-analysis. *J. Cardiovasc. Pharmacol.* **2023**, *81*, 445–453. [CrossRef]
109. Fogacci, F.; Yerlitaş, S.İ.; Giovannini, M.; Zararsız, G.; Lido, P.; Borghi, C.; Cicero, A.F.G. Sex X Time Interactions in Lp(a) and LDL-C Response to Evolocumab. *Biomedicines* **2023**, *11*, 3271. [CrossRef]
110. Cicero, A.F.G.; Fogacci, F.; Zambon, A.; Toth, P.P.; Borghi, C. Efficacy and safety of inclisiran a newly approved FDA drug: A systematic review and pooled analysis of available clinical studies. *Am. Heart J.* **2022**, *13*, 100127. [CrossRef]
111. Qu, K.; Ma, X.F.; Li, G.H.; Zhang, H.; Liu, Y.M.; Zhang, K.; Zeng, J.F.; Lei, J.J.; Wei, D.H.; Wang, Z. Vitamin C down-regulate apo(a) expression via Tet2-dependent DNA demethylation in HepG2 cells. *Int. J. Biol. Macromol.* **2017**, *98*, 637–645. [CrossRef]
112. Jenner, J.L.; Jacques, P.F.; Seman, L.J.; Schaefer, E.J. Ascorbic acid supplementation does not lower plasma lipoprotein (a) concentrations. *Atherosclerosis* **2000**, *151*, 541–544. [CrossRef]

113. Bostom, A.G.; Hume, A.L.; Eaton, C.B.; Laurino, J.P.; Yanek, L.R.; Regan, M.S.; McQuade, W.H.; Craig, W.Y.; Perrone, G.; Jacques, P.F. The effect of high-dose ascorbate supplementation on plasma lipoprotein (a) levels in patients with premature coronary heart disease. *Pharmacotherapy* **1995**, *15*, 458–464. [CrossRef]
114. Zeman, M.; Vecka, M.; Perlík, F.; Staňková, B.; Hromádka, R.; Tvrzická, E.; Širc, J.; Hrib, J.; Žák, A. Pleiotropic effects of niacin: Current possibilities for its clinical use. *Acta Pharm.* **2016**, *66*, 449–469. [CrossRef] [PubMed]
115. Yari, Z.; Tabibi, H.; Najafi, I.; Hedayati, M.; Movahedian, M. Effects of soy isoflavones on serum lipids and lipoprotein (a) in peritoneal dialysis patients. *Nutr. Metab. Cardiovasc. Dis.* **2020**, *30*, 1382–1388. [CrossRef] [PubMed]
116. Simental-Mendía, L.E.; Gotto, A.M.; Jr Atkin, S.L.; Banach, M.; Pirro, M.; Sahebkar, A. Effect of soy isoflavone supplementation on plasma lipoprotein (a) concentrations: A meta-analysis. *J. Clin. Lipidol.* **2018**, *12*, 16–24. [CrossRef] [PubMed]
117. Surma, S.; Sahebkar, A.; Banach, M.; endorsed by the International Lipid Expert Panel (ILEP). Low carbohydrate/ketogenic diet in the optimization of lipoprotein (a) levels: Do we have sufficient evidence for any recommendation? *Eur. Heart J.* **2023**, *44*, ehad635. [CrossRef] [PubMed]
118. Brandt, E.J.; Brandt, D.J.; Desai, N.R.; Spatz, E.S.; Nasir, K.; Mani, A. Association of vitamins, minerals, and lead with lipoprotein (a) in a cross-sectional cohort of US adults. *Int. J. Vitam. Nutr. Res.* **2023**, *93*, 99–110. [CrossRef]

Journal of
Clinical Medicine

MDPI

Brief Report

Clinical Expression of Familial Hypercholesterolemia in Patients from France and French Canada Carrying Identical-by-Descent Pathogenic *LDLR* Gene Variants: A Proof-of-Concept Study

Miriam Larouche [1], Olivier Bluteau [2], Alain Carrié [2], Alex Lauzière [1], Etienne Khoury [1], Diane Brisson [1], Daniel Gaudet [1,*,†] and Antonio Gallo [2,†]

[1] Departement of Medicine, Université de Montréal and ECOGENE-21, Chicoutimi, QC G7H 7K9, Canada; miriam.larouche@ecogene21.org (M.L.); alex.lauziere@usherbrooke.ca (A.L.); etienne.khoury@umontreal.ca (E.K.); diane.brisson@ecogene21.org (D.B.)

[2] Sorbonne-Université, Assistance Publique—Hôpitaux de Paris (APHP), INSERM Unité de Recherche sur les Maladies Cardiovasculaires et Métaboliques (UMRS) 1166, Hôpital Pitié-Salpêtrière, 75013 Paris, France; olivier.bluteau@aphp.fr (O.B.); alain.carrie@aphp.fr (A.C.); antonio.gallo@aphp.fr (A.G.)

* Correspondence: daniel.gaudet@umontreal.ca

† These authors contributed equally to this work.

Abstract: Background: Studying patients carrying identical-by-descent (IBD) pathogenic gene variants allows us to control for the disease-causing genetic background and to more accurately document the impact of modifiers. Familial hypercholesterolemia (FH) is characterized by elevated low-density lipoprotein cholesterol (LDL-c) levels and premature atherosclerosis and is often caused by defects in the *LDLR* gene. There is a high prevalence of FH in French Canada as a result of a founder effect from France in the 17th century. Several FH patients currently living in French Canada (founder population) and in France (colonizing population) carry IBD FH-causing variants. The expression of FH is affected by environmental and genetic modifiers, and patients with IBD variants may present different characteristics. **Methods:** In this study, we compared FH clinical expression patients carrying IBD *LDLR* pathogenic variants living in France or Canada. Four IBD variants, namely c.259T>G p.(Trp87Gly), c.2000G>A p.(Cys667Tyr), c.682G>A p.(Glu228Lys), and c.1048C>T p.(Arg350*), were selected. Untreated plasma lipid profiles, the apolipoprotein E (APOE) genotype, cardiovascular risk factors, and the occurrence of symptomatic ASCVD were compared in 105 adult carriers (30 from France and 75 from French Canada). **Results:** All parameters were similar between the two populations, except for untreated total cholesterol (10.14 ± 1.89 mmol/L vs. 8.65 ± 1.84 mmol/L, $p = 0.0006$) and LDL-c concentrations (7.94 ± 1.86 mmol/L vs. 6.93 ± 1.78 mmol/L, $p = 0.016$), which were significantly higher in FH patients living in France, an observation that was revealed across all studied *LDLR* variants. **Conclusions:** This study illustrates that FH patients sharing IBD pathogenic *LDLR* variants that have evolved in different geographic, cultural, and socio-economic environments for hundreds of years differ in terms of cholesterol levels, highlighting the importance of better understanding the interplay between genetic and environmental modulators of FH expression.

Keywords: familial hypercholesterolemia; founder effect; identical-by-descent variant

1. Introduction

Familial hypercholesterolemia (FH) is characterized by the accumulation of low-density lipoprotein (LDL) particles and elevated LDL-cholesterol (LDL-c) levels due to the lack of functionality or availability of LDL receptors (LDLR). FH is most often caused by pathogenic LDLR gene variants or by variants in genes having deleterious effects on LDLR functions [1,2]. Patients affected by FH generally have elevated LDL-c levels from birth (above 5 mmol/L in adulthood) and are at risk of developing atherosclerosis early in life [3,4]. FH prevalence is estimated at 1:250 globally, although its prevalence is significantly higher in some isolates or founder populations [5].

FH expression is affected by multiple modifiers and varies from one individual to another, even among carriers of the same FH-causing pathogenic variant [4]. Environmental and genetic modifiers can directly affect LDL-c concentration, and an increasing amount of evidence shows that these modifiers can also impact the epigenome and modulate FH clinical expression [6,7]. Unlimited combinations of genes and environmental factors therefore contribute to each person's unique blend of traits, health, and identity, making it difficult to precisely predict the individual trajectory of FH expression and response to treatment.

Identical-by-descent (IBD) pathogenic gene variants have emerged as interesting candidates to study the genetic underpinnings of atherosclerotic cardiovascular disease (ASCVD) as they are shared by individuals via common ancestors. Studying patients with IBD gene variants allows us to control for the disease-causing genetic background and to more accurately document the impact of modifiers (genetic, clinical, environmental, or socio-economic). Many research efforts have indeed been supporting the idea that studying IBD segments consists of a powerful method for controlling genetic background, while providing a more nuanced understanding of the role of various modifiers in disease expression and susceptibility. Additionally, advances in IBD detection methods have been recently developed, such as the RaPID tool, which aims to improve the ability to identify segments with high accuracy and speed, despite having large biobank-scale databases. In addition to controlling the genetic background, these tools are helpful for investigating the impact of environmental and other modifiers on disease expression, while detecting population structure and familial relationships in specific therapeutic areas [8,9].

French-Canadians provide an interesting example of a founder population where documented IBD pathogenic LDLR variants are more prevalent and originate from a common ancestral source from France in the 17th century (Figure 1) [10]. Consequently, some French and French-Canadian patients, today living on different continents, carry the same IBD FH-causing gene variants that have evolved for 4 centuries in different environments. In this proof-of-concept (PoC) study, we compared LDL-c levels and other clinical characteristics in heterozygous FH (HeFH) patients from France and French Canada carrying IBD gene variants.

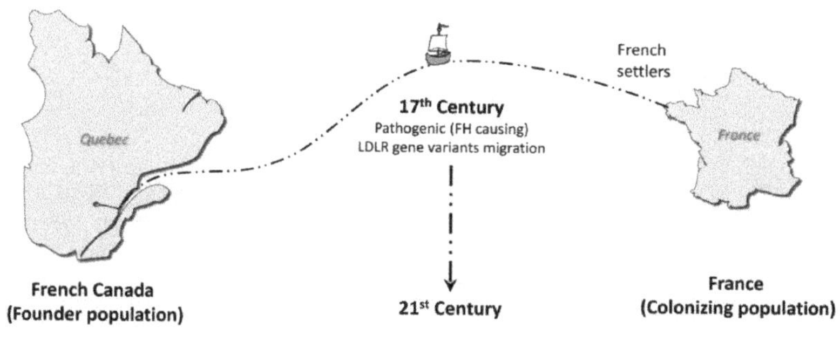

Baseline cholesterol levels in 105 FH carriers of identical by descent (IBD) LDLR gene variants from French Canada and France

Characteristics of FH patients (% or mean +/- SD)	Patients from French Canada (n=75)	Patients from France (n=30)	p-value
Men (%)	52	57	NS
Age (years) (median (IQR))	61.0 (44.0-74.0)	53.0 (35.8-70.5)	0.133
Baseline (highest untreated) total cholesterol (mmol/L) (mean +/- SD)	8.65 ± 1.84	10.14 ± 1.89	0.0006
Baseline (highest untreated) LDL-cholesterol (mmol/L) (mean +/- SD)	6.93 ± 1.78	7.94 ± 1.86	0.016

Figure 1. Baseline (untreated) total cholesterol and LDL-cholesterol levels in FH carriers of identical-by-descent (IBD) pathogenic *LDLR* gene variants in 75 FH patients from the French-Canadian founder population and 30 patients from France (colonizing population). Patients from both countries carried

either the c.259T>G p.(Trp87Gly) rs121908025, c.2000G>A p.(Cys667Tyr) rs28942083, c.682G>A p.(Glu228Lys) rs121908029, or c.1048C>T p.(Arg350*) rs769737896 *LDLR* gene variants, all pathogenic, having a proven French founder effect and having evolved in a different environment for 4 centuries. Both groups were comparable for ApoE genotype, smoking habits, anthropometric measurements, diabetes, and other cardiovascular risk factors. Patients were matched for age and sex ($\geq$3:1 for the p.(Trp87Gly) variant). Baseline cholesterol levels were significantly lower among French-Canadians in all genotypes (see text).

2. Methods

Four IBD FH-causing *LDLR* variants, namely c.259T>G p.(Trp87Gly) rs121908025, c.2000G>A p.(Cys667Tyr) rs28942083, c.682G>A p.(Glu228Lys) rs121908029, and c.1048C>T p.(Arg350*) rs769737896 originating from France with a proven French-Canadian founder effect were selected [10,11]. During their initial visit to the lipid clinics, FH patients were assessed by a multidisciplinary team. Data on lipid profiles, FH-related genotypes, treatment regimen, metabolic syndrome-associated parameters, and cardiovascular risks were collected from those who consented to participate in this study. Plasma lipid profiles at baseline (untreated), ApoE genotype, cardiovascular risk factors, and the occurrence of symptomatic ASCVD were compared in 105 adult carriers (30 from France and 75 from French Canada). For the most frequent variant, p.(Trp87Gly), patients in both groups were matched for age ($\pm$1 year) and sex in a $\geq$3:1 ratio. For the other variants, matching was dependent on the number of subjects. Data comparisons were made using Chi-square, Fisher's exact test, Student's *t*-tests and Wilcoxon–Mann–Whitney for independent samples. Statistical analyses were performed using SPSS package version 25 (IBM Corp., Armonk, NY, USA).

This research study (French National Agency for the Safety of Medicines and Health Products, protocol reference 2014-A01549–38 and its Canadian counterpart, protocol reference ECO HyperTG-Hyperchol) were conducted in accordance with the principles of the Declaration of Helsinki, consistent with the Good Clinical Practice guidelines of the International Conference on Harmonization. Ethical approval was obtained in France from the CCTIRS (Comité Consultatif sur le Traitement de l'Information en matière de Recherche dans le domaine de la Santé) and the CNIL (Commission National de l'Informatique et des libertés) in 2015 and in Canada from Advarra IRB in 2014. All subjects were screened at their respective lipid clinics and agreed to participate in this study. Informed consent was obtained from all participants, and a code that systematically de-identifies all clinical data was assigned to each subject [12]. Participants were included in this analysis based on the availability of lipid-associated parameter data.

3. Results

Subjects from both populations were comparable in terms of sex, age, smoking status (current or not), statin intolerance, diabetes, obesity, and hypertension (Table 1). Although not statistically significant, the prevalence of ApoE4 in this study was almost 2-fold more elevated among French-Canadians (29% vs. 17%). Mean baseline untreated total cholesterol (10.14 $\pm$ 1.89 mmol/L vs. 8.65 $\pm$ 1.84 mmol/L, p = 0.0006) and LDL-c concentrations (7.94 $\pm$ 1.86 mmol/L vs. 6.93 $\pm$ 1.78 mmol/L, p = 0.016) were significantly higher in the French cohort (Figure 1), and this was observed across all FH-causing variants (Table 2). The coronary artery anatomy of those who had a coronarography will be the subject of another publication.

Table 1. Characteristics of HeFH patients from France and French Canada.

Characteristics (% or Median (IQR))	France (n = 30)	French Canada (n = 75)	p-Value
Men (%)	57	52	NS
Age (years)	53.0 (35.8–70.5)	61.0 (44.0–74.0)	NS
ApoE2 carriers (%)	4	14	NS
ApoE4 carriers (%)	17	29	NS
Diabetes (%)	3	7	NS
Obesity (%)	11	19	NS
Hypertension (%)	17	22	NS
Current smokers (%)	31	22	NS
Statin intolerance (%)	4	19	NS
ASCVD (%)	33	33	NS
Age at first event (years)	49.0 (39.8–56.0)	45.0 (39.5–54.5)	NS

NS = $p > 0.05$. Continuous variables are median (IQR). ApoE: apolipoprotein E, ASCVD: atherosclerotic cardiovascular disease, IQR: interquartile range.

Table 2. Gene variant-specific differences in untreated LDL-cholesterol concentration in France versus French Canada.

IBD Pathogenic Variants	France n (%)	LDL-c (mmol/L) Mean ± SD	French Canada n (%)	LDL-c (mmol/L) Mean ± SD
All variants	30 (100)	7.94 ± 1.86	75 (100)	6.93 ± 1.78
p.(Trp87Gly)	10 (33.3)	7.15 ± 2.10	38 (50.7)	6.64 ±1.66
p.(Cys667Tyr)	2 (6.7)	8.34 ± 0.71	9 (12.0)	6.63 ± 1.28
p.(Glu228Lys)	11 (36.7)	7.72 ± 1.81	15 (20.0)	7.50 ± 2.14
p.(Arg350*)	7 (23.3)	8.49 ± 2.00	13 (17.3)	7.05 ± 2.04

p.(Trp87Gly): c.259T>G, rs121908025. p.(Cys667Tyr): c.2000G>A, rs28942083. p.(Glu228Lys): c.682G>A, rs121908029. p.(Arg350*): c.1048C>T, rs769737896.

4. Discussion

In this PoC study, we used LDL-cholesterol as a probe to highlight differences in HeFH expression between patients from two populations sharing IBD *LDLR* pathogenic variants. It illustrates that FH patients of similar age, sex, and risk profile, originating from France and French Canada, sharing well-documented IBD pathogenic LDLR variants having evolved in different geographic, cultural, and socio-economic environments for hundreds of years, may differ in terms of cholesterol levels (Figure 1), highlighting the importance of better understanding the interplay between genetic and environmental modulators of FH expression.

Higher plasma total cholesterol and LDL-c concentrations were observed in FH patients from France despite the fact that the ApoE4 allele (generally associated with higher cholesterol concentration) was 2-fold more prevalent among French-Canadians, who presented lower LDL-c than their French IBD FH counterparts.

Since the colonization of New France in the 17th century, the dissemination of FH-causing gene variants in French Canada was important due to large pedigrees (often > 12 children per nuclear family) and limited population migration movements due to the harshness of transport routes [11]. The combination of these factors led to a phenomenon called endogamy, resulting in the high prevalence of IBD FH in French Canada (1:80), which is much higher than in France and the rest of the world (1:250) [11]. In addition, most cases of FH in French Canada were mainly caused by a small number of IBD *LDLR* pathogenic variants [11]. The historical high prevalence of FH in French Canada is not a consequence of consanguinity but of endogamy [13]. Comparing the expression of IBD genetic diseases in a founder population and in the colonizing population offers a unique opportunity to explain differences in the clinical expression or the response to interventions, controlling for the effect of the disease-causing variant. Indeed, IBD pathogenic variants that have evolved for hundreds of years in different geographic environments allow us to control for the variance in FH clinical expression that is specifically due to the pathogenic variant, which is the case of LDL-c, the main feature of FH. One advantage of IBD pathogenic variants is that differences in the clinical expression of the disease are not determined by the pathogenic variant itself but rather by other modifying factors. This constitutes a real advantage in identifying key genetic, epigenetic, or environmental factors affecting FH expression, risk trajectory, or response to treatment. Specifically, when controlling for the genetic cause of FH, observed differences in LDL-c could contribute to the identification of genetic variants that increase susceptibility to LDL accumulation and atherogenicity beyond *LDLR*.

It is well documented that other genes, environmental factors, nutritional habits, physical activity, bacterial exposure, stress, and other factors affect the epigenome, gene expression, and the microbiota and could highly impact the lipid profile or ASCVD risk [14]. By controlling for the FH-causing gene variant (using IBD variants), the analysis of modifiers is simplified, potentially uncovering novel pathways that influence FH expression, risk trajectory, or response to current emerging therapies. In alignment with our study, Mszar et al. suggested that the investigation of patients carrying IBD pathogenic gene variants is pivotal for addressing the underdiagnosed rate of FH in specific geographical territories, while identifying CV risks in these genetically self-contained communities [15]. Similar findings were also described within the Indian population, showing the high prevalence of FH and unique genetic architecture caused by consanguineous marriage practices as well as multiple endogamous groups [16,17].

This PoC study has limitations. First, with a total of 105 participants, the sample size is small, although it offered sufficient power to highlight significant differences in lipid parameters. This said, it is worth mentioning that the pathogenic variants used in this PoC study were limited to those with a proven and published IBD origin. The establishment of a France–Canada transatlantic collaboration improves the identification of FH patients carrying proven IBD pathogenic variants in both countries, thus progressively contributing to the increase in the sample size. In addition, other FH-causing variants are currently being assessed for a common origin (founder effect). Such variants, if proven IBD, will be added in the next phases of the study, further increasing the patient pool. Second, this study specifically and only targets HeFH. We are currently integrating HoFH in order to maximize the advantages conferred by IBD pathogenic variants across various founder populations and multiple countries. Third, although available for several patients in secondary prevention, coronary anatomy data were not included in this PoC study. This will be the subject of a dedicated manuscript in a larger sample of age- and gender-matched FH patients with ASCVD.

In the next few years, planned analyses include exome sequencing, DNA methylation studies, as well as comprehensive endophenotypic, clinical, and environmental investigations in a larger sample of IBD patients. These efforts aim to better document modifiers of FH, uncover potential new targets for preventing ASCVD, and identify factors that modulate responses to emerging therapies. Integrating these diverse approaches within the clinical pathway will enhance our understanding of FH and help improve treatment strategies for affected populations on different continents. Populations from other countries, such as Lebanon, the USA, the UK, Turkey, India, and South Africa, will be involved in the next steps as these communities also share FH-causing IBD variants [18–20]. These populations importantly differ in terms of life habits and access to accurate diagnosis and treatment. Access issues and quality of life will also be assessed through this project as part of the SMASH initiative (System and Molecular Approaches of Severe Dyslipidemias) (accessed on 23 September 2024, www.smash-access.org).

Author Contributions: Conceptualization, M.L. and D.G.; methodology, M.L., O.B., A.C., D.G. and A.G.; validation, M.L., D.B., D.G. and A.G.; formal analysis, M.L. and D.B.; resources, D.G.; data curation, D.B. and A.G.; writing—original draft preparation, M.L. and D.G.; writing—review and editing, M.L., O.B., A.C., A.L., E.K., D.B., D.G. and A.G.; supervision, D.G. and A.G.; project administration, D.G. and A.G. All authors have read and agreed to the published version of the manuscript.

Funding: This project was supported by ECOGENE-21 dedicated funds for the SMASH program.

Institutional Review Board Statement: Ethical approval was obtained in France (protocol reference 2014-A01549–38) from the CCTIRS (Comité Consultatif sur le Traitement de l'Information en matière de Recherche dans le domaine de la Santé) and the CNIL (Commission National de l'Informatique et des libertés) in 2015 and in Canada (protocol reference ECO HyperTG-Hyperchol) from Advarra IRB in 2014 (last amendment approved on 17 December 2023).

Informed Consent Statement: Informed consent was obtained from all subjects involved in the study.

Data Availability Statement: The datasets presented in this article are not readily available because the data are part of an ongoing study. Genealogical data are not available due to privacy and ethical reasons. Requests concerning access to the datasets should be directed to the corresponding author.

Conflicts of Interest: The authors have no conflict of interest to disclose in this study.

References

1. Saadatagah, S.; Jose, M.; Dikilitas, O.; Alhalabi, L.; Miller, A.A.; Fan, X.; Olson, J.E.; Kochan, D.C.; Safarova, M.; Kullo, I.J. Genetic basis of hypercholesterolemia in adults. *NPJ Genom. Med.* **2021**, *6*, 28. [CrossRef] [PubMed]
2. Goldstein, J.L.; Hobbs, H.H.; Brown, M.S. Familial Hypercholesterolemia. In *The Online Metabolic and Molecular Bases of Inherited Disease*; Valle, D.L., Antonarakis, S., Ballabio, A., Beaudet, A.L., Mitchell, G.A., Eds.; McGraw-Hill Education: New York, NY, USA, 2019.
3. Cuchel, M.; Raal, F.J.; Hegele, R.A.; Al-Rasadi, K.; Arca, M.; Averna, M.; Bruckert, E.; Freiberger, T.; Gaudet, D.; Harada-Shiba, M.; et al. 2023 Update on European Atherosclerosis Society Consensus Statement on Homozygous Familial Hypercholesterolaemia: New treatments and clinical guidance. *Eur. Heart J.* **2023**, *44*, 2277–2291. [CrossRef] [PubMed]
4. Santos, R.D.; Gidding, S.S.; Hegele, R.A.; Cuchel, M.A.; Barter, P.J.; Watts, G.F.; Baum, S.J.; Catapano, A.L.; Chapman, M.J.; Defesche, J.C.; et al. Defining severe familial hypercholesterolaemia and the implications for clinical management: A consensus statement from the International Atherosclerosis Society Severe Familial Hypercholesterolemia Panel. *Lancet Diabetes Endocrinol.* **2016**, *4*, 850–861. [CrossRef] [PubMed]
5. Safarova, M.S.; Santos, R.D.; Moriarty, P.M. 34—Special Patient Populations: Familial Hypercholesterolemia and Other Severe Hypercholesterolemias. In *Clinical Lipidology*, 3rd ed.; Ballantyne, C.M., Ed.; Elsevier: New Delhi, India, 2024; pp. 320–335.e2. [CrossRef]
6. Block, T.; El-Osta, A. Epigenetic programming, early life nutrition and the risk of metabolic disease. *Atherosclerosis* **2017**, *266*, 31–40. [CrossRef] [PubMed]
7. Reeskamp, L.F.; Venema, A.; Pereira, J.P.B.; Levin, E.; Nieuwdorp, M.; Groen, A.K.; Defesche, J.C.; Grefhorst, A.; Henneman, P.; Hovingh, G.K. Differential DNA methylation in familial hypercholesterolemia. *EBioMedicine* **2020**, *61*, 103079. [CrossRef] [PubMed]
8. Tang, K.; Naseri, A.; Wei, Y.; Zhang, S.; Zhi, D. Open-source benchmarking of IBD segment detection methods for biobank-scale cohorts. *GigaScience* **2022**, *11*, giac111. [CrossRef] [PubMed]
9. Naseri, A.; Liu, X.; Tang, K.; Zhang, S.; Zhi, D. RaPID: Ultra-fast, powerful, and accurate detection of segments identical by descent (IBD) in biobank-scale cohorts. *Genome Biol.* **2019**, *20*, 143. [CrossRef] [PubMed]
10. Couture, P.; Morissette, J.; Gaudet, D.; Vohl, M.C.; Gagne, C.; Bergeron, J.; Despres, J.P.; Simard, J. Fine mapping of low-density lipoprotein receptor gene by genetic linkage on chromosome 19p13.1-p13.3 and study of the founder effect of four French Canadian low-density lipoprotein receptor gene mutations. *Atherosclerosis* **1999**, *143*, 145–151. [CrossRef] [PubMed]
11. Gaudet, D.; Tremblay, G.; Perron, P.; Gagne, C.; Ouadahi, Y.; Moorjani, S. Familial hypercholesterolemia in eastern Quebec: A public health problem? The experience of the hyperlipidemia clinic of Chicoutimi. *Union Med. Can.* **1995**, *124*, 54–60. [PubMed]
12. Gaudet, D.; Arsenault, S.; Belanger, C.; Hudson, T.; Perron, P.; Bernard, M.; Hamet, P. Procedure to protect confidentiality of familial data in community genetics and genomic research. *Clin. Genet.* **1999**, *55*, 259–264. [CrossRef]
13. Davignon, J.; Roy, M. Familial hypercholesterolemia in French-Canadians: Taking advantage of the presence of a "founder effect". *Am. J. Cardiol.* **1993**, *72*, 6D–10D. [CrossRef] [PubMed]
14. Zhang, M.; Hu, T.; Ma, T.; Huang, W.; Wang, Y. Epigenetics and environmental health. *Front. Med.* **2024**, *18*, 571–596. [CrossRef] [PubMed]
15. Mszar, R.; Buscher, S.; Taylor, H.L.; Rice-DeFosse, M.T.; McCann, D. Familial Hypercholesterolemia and the Founder Effect Among Franco-Americans: A Brief History and Call to Action. *CJC Open* **2020**, *2*, 161–167. [CrossRef]

16. Imran, M.; Bhoyar, R.C.; Jain, A.; Sahana, S.; Rophina, M.; Arvinden, V.R.; Senthivel, V.; Divakar, M.K.; Mishra, A.; Jolly, B.; et al. Genetic epidemiology of monogenic dyslipidemia and statin-associated adverse drug phenotypes in Indian population from whole-genomes of 1029 self-declared healthy individuals. *Hum. Gene* **2024**, *39*, 201252. [CrossRef]
17. Sharma, S.; Gaur, K.; Gupta, R. Trends in epidemiology of dyslipidemias in India. *Indian Heart J.* **2024**, *76*, S20–S28. [CrossRef]
18. Abifadel, M.; Rabes, J.P.; Jambart, S.; Halaby, G.; Gannage-Yared, M.H.; Sarkis, A.; Beaino, G.; Varret, M.; Salem, N.; Corbani, S.; et al. The molecular basis of familial hypercholesterolemia in Lebanon: Spectrum of *LDLR* mutations and role of *PCSK9* as a modifier gene. *Hum. Mutat.* **2009**, *30*, E682–E691. [CrossRef]
19. Leitersdorf, E.; Tobin, E.J.; Davignon, J.; Hobbs, H.H. Common low-density lipoprotein receptor mutations in the French Canadian population. *J. Clin. Investig.* **1990**, *85*, 1014–1023. [CrossRef] [PubMed]
20. Ashavaid, T.F.; Altaf, A.K.; Nair, K.G. Molecular basis of familial hypercholesterolemia: An Indian experience. *Indian J. Clin. Biochem.* **2000**, *15* (Suppl. S1), 11–19. [CrossRef] [PubMed]

Journal of
Clinical Medicine

MDPI

Article

Statin Use and Major Adverse Cardiovascular Events Among Patients with Ischemic Heart Diseases: A Multi-Center Retrospective Study

Awatif Hafiz [1,†], Sarah Aljohani [2,†], Hussam Kutbi [1], Nayyra Fatani [1], Lama Alkhathran [3], Majd Alyaqub [3], Meshal S. Alhamed [4], Abdulrhaman O. Alhaqbani [4], Abdulrahman A. Alhadlaq [4], Mohammed A. Alsalman [4], Majed S. Al Yami [3,5,6,*] and Omar A. Almohammed [7,8]

1 Department of Pharmacy Practice, Faculty of Pharmacy, King Abdulaziz University, Jeddah 22252, Saudi Arabia; whafidh@kau.edu.sa (A.H.); hkutbi1@kau.edu.sa (H.K.); nsfatani@kau.edu.sa (N.F.)
2 Department of Clinical Pharmacy, King Fahd Armed Forces Hospital, Jeddah 23311, Saudi Arabia; sarah_aljuhani@hotmail.com
3 Department of Pharmacy Practice, College of Pharmacy, King Saud bin Abdulaziz University for Health Sciences, Riyadh 11481, Saudi Arabia; alkhathran286@gmail.com (L.A.); majdalyaqub@gmail.com (M.A.)
4 College of Medicine, King Saud University, Riyadh 11451, Saudi Arabia; 439100663@student.ksu.edu.sa (A.O.A.); 439106386@student.ksu.edu.sa (A.A.A.); 439100704@student.ksu.edu.sa (M.A.A.)
5 King Abdullah International Medical Research Center, Riyadh 11481, Saudi Arabia
6 Pharmaceutical Care Department, King Abdulaziz Medical City, Riyadh 11481, Saudi Arabia
7 Department of Clinical Pharmacy, College of Pharmacy, King Saud University, Riyadh 11451, Saudi Arabia; oalmohammed@ksu.edu.sa
8 Pharmacoeconomics Research Unit, College of Pharmacy, King Saud University, Riyadh 11451, Saudi Arabia
* Correspondence: yamim@ksau-hs.edu.sa
† These authors contributed equally to this work.

Abstract: Objective: The objective of this study was to evaluate the effects of adherence to the ACC/AHA 2018 dyslipidemia guidelines on patient management of lipid-lowering therapy in patients with ischemic heart diseases (IHD) and its correlation with major adverse cardiovascular events (MACEs), including non-fatal MI, stroke, death, hospitalization for revascularization, and peripheral arterial disease. **Methods**: A multi-center retrospective observational study was conducted in patients with IHD between January 2019 and December 2020, who were followed for two years. The primary objective was to assess statin utilization and adherence to the 2018 ACC/AHA guidelines and the associated influence on MACE outcomes. Inferential statistical analyses, including chi-square tests and the Mann–Whitney test, were conducted to assess the associations between adherence to the guidelines, MACE rates, and LDL-C goal achievement. **Results**: The study included 1011 patients with ischemic heart disease (IHD), predominantly male (78.2%), with a mean age of 59 ± 10.9 years. Non-adherent patients had higher baseline LDL-C levels (3.0 ± 1.1 mmol/L vs. 2.7 ± 1.2 mmol/L; $p = 0.0005$), while adherent patients were more likely to be on cardiovascular medications, including statins (78.4% vs. 57.4%), aspirin (74.2% vs. 56.3%), and P2Y12 inhibitors (69.5% vs. 48.4%), compared to non-adherent patients. Adherence was associated with lower non-fatal MI rates (9.3% vs. 21.1%, $p < 0.0001$) and fewer revascularizations (9.3% vs. 16.8%; $p = 0.0024$). Additionally, 49.2% of adherent patients achieved target LDL-C goals, compared to 30.5% of the non-adherent patients ($p < 0.0001$). Notably, there were no significant differences in stroke, peripheral arterial disease, or mortality rates. **Conclusions**: The achievement of target LDL-C goals and reduced MACEs was observed with adherence to the 2018 ACC/AHA dyslipidemia guidelines. However, lipid management in IHD patients remains sub-optimal, highlighting opportunities for further enhancement.

Keywords: ischemic heart diseases; dyslipidemia; guideline; lipid management

1. Introduction

According to the American College of Cardiology/American Heart Association (ACC/AHA) guidelines, all patients with ischemic heart disease (IHD) and other atherosclerotic cardiovascular diseases (ASCVDs)—in the absence of contraindications—should receive a high-intensity statin indefinitely. There is strong evidence supporting the use of high-intensity statins as the first-line choice for lipid management in secondary prevention to prevent the recurrence of ASCVD or cardiovascular death [1,2]. Statins are extremely effective lipid-lowering agents, which work by reducing cholesterol biosynthesis and modulating lipid metabolism in the liver [3]. In patients who have experienced an ACS episode, initiating lipid-lowering agents (especially high-intensity statins) has been shown to improve cardiovascular outcomes, regardless of previous statin exposure. Therefore, introducing a high-intensity statin (e.g., atorvastatin or rosuvastatin) as early as possible after an ACS event is recommended [4–6]. In addition to the ability of statins to lower circulating LDL-C, they have also been shown to be effective in stabilizing or regressing plaque through multiple mechanisms, including the reduction of necrotic lipid cores, anti-inflammatory effects, and improving endothelial function. These mechanisms give statins the ability to lower morbidity and mortality related to cardiovascular events [4,7,8]. However, low adherence to guideline recommendations for the secondary prevention of IHD is a critical issue that hinders the effectiveness of cardiovascular disease (CVD) management. Despite the well-established benefits of statin therapy in reducing the risk of IHD, studies have consistently revealed sub-optimal adherence rates among eligible patients. This non-adherence can be attributed to various factors, including patient-related factors such as a lack of awareness, concerns about side effects, and medication costs, as well as healthcare system-related barriers such as inadequate physician–patient communication and gaps in guideline implementation [9–11]. Improving adherence to statin therapy could significantly reduce the incidence and burden of IHD, leading to improved patient outcomes and reduced healthcare costs. Therefore, it is imperative to identify and implement targeted interventions that address the barriers to adherence and promote the appropriate use of statins, in line with evidence-based guidelines for IHD prevention.

A strong inverse relationship exists between LDL-C levels and cardiovascular outcomes, leading to the concept "the lower the LDL, the better". This principle suggests a continuous relationship between LDL-C reduction and improved prognostic outcomes, without a specific lower limit posing risks [12]. The 2023 ESC ACS guidelines conferred values to be followed for secondary treatment; in particular, lowering LDL-C to less than 1.4 mmol/L (<55 mg/dL) and obtaining at least a 50% LDL-C reduction compared to the baseline. In another scenario, in patients experiencing a second cardiovascular event within 2 years (not necessarily of the same type as the first event), an LDL-C goal of <1.0 mmol/L (<40 mg/dL) as a treatment goal implied a greater benefit [13]. However, achieving these guideline-recommended LDL-C targets remains challenging in patients with acute coronary syndrome (ACS) [14].

This study aims to explore the relationship between statin utilization and major adverse cardiovascular events (MACEs), examining adherence to the 2018 ACC/AHA guidelines for high-intensity statin therapy in patients with IHD in Saudi Arabia. The findings of this study could inform clinical decision making, support policy development, and contribute to the overall improvement of cardiovascular disease management, potentially enhancing patient outcomes and reducing healthcare costs.

2. Materials and Methods

2.1. Study Design and Outcomes

This was a retrospective study, conducted to investigate the relationship between statin utilization according to the 2018 ACC/AHA guideline recommendations and MACEs among patients diagnosed with IHD. Adult patients (≥18 years old), who were admitted to King Abdulaziz University Hospital (KAUH) in Jeddah and King Abdulaziz Medical City (KAMC) and King Saud University Medical City (KSUMC) in Riyadh between January 2019 and December 2020, with a confirmed diagnosis of IHD at the time of enrollment, were included. The included patients were followed for two years. Patients with incomplete demographics and those prescribed high-intensity statins for other reasons than IHD were excluded. Patients were categorized into two groups: patients who were adherent to the guideline recommendations and those who were not. The data for this study were retrospectively collected from electronic medical records, including demographics, medical history, medication history, laboratory results, and MACE outcomes. The Biomedical Research Ethics Committee at all three sites approved the study, with the following reference numbers: KAUH (protocol number: 234-22), KAMC (SP22R/254/12), and KSUMC (protocol number: E-22-7285).

2.2. Definitions

Patients with IHD were operationally defined as patients presenting with either of the following at the time of enrollment: stable ischemic heart disease (SIHD), unstable angina (UA), non-ST elevation myocardial infarction (NSTEMI), and ST elevation myocardial infarction (STEMI). High-intensity statin was defined as receiving either rosuvastatin 20 or 40 mg or atorvastatin 40 or 80 mg. Patients who were classified as high-risk for ASCVD were those who had either multiple major ASCVDs or one major ASCVD with multiple high-risk conditions (Table 1). Adherence to the 2018 ACC/AHA guidelines was defined as meeting all three of the following criteria: (1) prescribing high-intensity or maximally tolerated statin, (2) obtaining an LDL level 4–6 weeks after statin initiation, and (3) utilization of non-statin therapy when the target LDL level was considered not to be achieved with statin alone, or if a trial with maximally tolerated statin did not achieve an LDL goal of less than 70 mg/dL. Major adverse cardiac events (MACEs) were defined as the occurrence of any of the following during the two-year follow-up period: non-fatal MI, stroke, death, hospitalization for revascularization or any cardiac cause, or peripheral arterial disease (PAD).

2.3. Statistical Analysis

Descriptive statistics were employed to summarize the demographic characteristics of the study population, including age, gender distribution, medical history, and medication history. The association between statin utilization and MACEs, as well as sub-group analyses based on the agent used and the doses for the adherent group, were assessed using appropriate inferential statistical analyses, including chi-square tests and the Mann–Whitney test, while adjusting for potential confounding variables.

Table 1. Very high risk for future ASCVD events [1].

Major ASCVD Events	High-Risk Conditions
• Recent ACS (within 12 month) • History of MI (other than the recent ACS) • History of ischemic stroke • Symptomatic PAD (history of claudication with ABI < 0.85 or previous revascularization or amputation)	• Age ≥ 65 y • Heterozygous familial hypercholesterolemia • History of prior CABG or PCI outside of the major ASCVD event(s) • Diabetes mellitus • Hypertension • Chronic kidney disease (eGFR 15–59 mL/min/1.73 m^2) • Smoking • Persistently elevated LDL-C (LDL-C ≥ 100 mg/dL) despite maximally tolerated statin therapy and ezetimibe • History of congestive heart failure

ACS: acute coronary syndrome, MI: myocardial infarction, PAD: peripheral arterial disease, ABI: ankle brachial index, CABG: coronary artery bypass grafting, PCI: percutaneous coronary intervention, eGFR: glomerular filtration rate, LDL-C: low-density lipoprotein.

3. Results

The study included a random sample of 1011 patients with IHD. The patients were predominantly male (78.2%), with an average age of 59.0 ± 10.9 years, with comparable age between the adherent and non-adherent groups (with respect to the 2018 ACC/AHA guidelines). The main comorbidities in the study population were diabetes (70.1%), hypertension (65.9%), and dyslipidemia (56.1%). These conditions were more prevalent in the non-adherent group, particularly hypertension (p = 0.001) and dyslipidemia (p = 0.0002). Additionally, heart failure was more frequent among non-adherent patients (25.8% vs. 17.1%; p = 0.0053). Both groups were obese on average, with a slightly higher mean body mass index (BMI) in the adherent group (30.7 ± 18.4 vs. 28.7 ± 5.1; p = 0.33). The medication history indicated significant differences in the use of guideline-recommended therapies between groups. Adherent patients had higher rates of using all recommended cardiovascular medications. Statin therapy was notably more frequent in the adherent group (78.4% vs. 57.4%), as were the uses of aspirin (74.2% vs. 56.3%) and P2Y12 inhibitors (69.5% vs. 48.4%). Beta-blockers and ACE inhibitors/ARBs were also more frequently prescribed to those adhering to the guidelines, underscoring a comprehensive approach to managing IHD (Table 2).

Table 2. Baseline demographics and clinical characteristics of patients based on adherence to the guideline's recommendations.

Characteristics	All Patients N = 1011	Adherence to Guideline Recommendations		p-Value †
		No N = 190 (18.8%)	**Yes N = 821 (81.2%)**	
Age	59.0 ± 10.9	59.5 ± 11.0	58.9 ± 10.9	0.4206
Male	791 (78.2)	137 (72.1)	654 (79.7)	**0.0230**
Body mass index (BMI)	30.3 ± 16.7	28.7 ± 5.1	30.7 ± 18.4	0.3328
Active smokers	306 (30.3)	53 (27.9)	253 (30.8)	0.5783
Comorbidities				
Diabetes mellitus	709 (70.1)	141 (74.2)	568 (69.2)	0.3909
Hypertension	666 (65.9)	146 (76.8)	520 (63.3)	**0.0013**
Dyslipidemia	567 (56.1)	132 (69.5)	435 (53.0)	**0.0002**

Table 2. *Cont.*

Characteristics	All Patients N = 1011	Adherence to Guideline Recommendations No N = 190 (18.8%)	Adherence to Guideline Recommendations Yes N = 821 (81.2%)	p-Value †
Heart failure	189 (18.6)	49 (25.8)	140 (17.1)	**0.0053**
HFrEF	161 (15.9)	44 (23.2)	117 (14.3)	**0.0098**
HFpEF	28 (2.8)	5 (2.6)	23 (2.8)	0.9458
Chronic kidney disease	84 (8.3)	23 (12.1)	61 (7.4)	0.0713
Ischemic stroke or TIA	46 (4.5)	7 (3.7)	39 (4.8)	0.4341
Hemorrhagic stroke	5 (0.5)	0 (0.0)	5 (0.6)	0.4502
Atrial fibrillation	37 (3.7)	10 (5.3)	27 (3.3)	0.3405
Peripheral arterial disease	16 (1.6)	1 (0.5)	15 (1.8)	0.4319
History of carotid stenosis	6 (0.6)	0 (0.0)	6 (0.7)	0.3108
Medication History				
Lipid-lowering agents	753 (74.5)	109 (57.4)	644 (78.4)	**<0.0001**
Aspirin	716 (70.8)	107 (56.3)	609 (74.2)	**<0.0001**
P2Y12 inhibitors	663 (65.6)	92 (48.4)	571 (69.5)	**<0.0001**
Beta Blockers	663 (65.6)	92 (48.4)	571 (69.5)	**<0.0001**
ACEI/ARB	563 (55.7)	80 (42.1)	483 (58.8)	**<0.0001**
Spironolactone	83 (8.2)	6 (3.2)	77 (9.4)	**<0.0001**

Numbers are presented as mean ± SD or frequency (%). † *p*-values are from the Mann–Whitney test for continuous not normally distributed data or chi-square test for categorical data; values in bold are statistically significant. Abbreviations: SD: standard deviation; BMI: body mass index; HFrEF: heart failure with reduced ejection fraction; HFpEF: heart failure with preserved ejection fraction; TIA: transient ischemic attack; ACEI: angiotensin-converting enzyme inhibitors; ARB: angiotensin receptor blocker.

Baseline LDL-C levels were notably higher in the non-adherent group (3.0 ± 1.1 mmol/L vs. 2.7 ± 1.2 mmol/L; $p = 0.0005$), with no significant differences in other lipid profiles (Table 3). Most patients were diagnosed with their first IHD event, more frequently in the adherent group (77.8% vs. 61.1%, $p < 0.0001$). NSTEMI was the predominant initial diagnosis, affecting 50.6% of the cohort, with stent placement via percutaneous coronary intervention (PCI) being more common among non-adherent patients (41.6% vs. 30.9%; $p = 0.0049$). Following the initial IHD event, patients were predominantly classified as "high risk" (38.9%) or "very high risk" (58.7%) for future cardiovascular events, underscoring the importance of guideline adherence in this high-risk population (Table 4).

In the context of medication adherence, 809 out of the 821 adherent patients (98.5%) were on high-intensity statin therapy, primarily involving atorvastatin (40 or 80 mg) and rosuvastatin (20 or 40 mg). In contrast, only 134 of the 190 non-adherent patients (70.5%) received high-intensity statins. Although the patients had comparable rates of utilizing ezetimibe or PCSK9 inhibitors (Table 5), the use of non-statin therapies during the study period was limited to ezetimibe and PCSK9 inhibitors, with therapy escalation occurring in a subset of patients.

Clinical outcomes demonstrated significant benefits associated with adherence to guideline recommendations. Patients adhering to the guidelines showed a lower rate of non-fatal MI, with incidents occurring in 9.3% compared to 21.1% in the non-adherent group ($p < 0.0001$). Revascularization rates were also lower among adherent patients, observed at 9.3% versus 16.8% for the non-adherent group ($p = 0.0024$). Additionally, a higher percentage of adherent patients achieved target LDL-C levels at the first or second follow-up, with 49.2% meeting these targets compared to 30.5% in the non-adherent group. Moreover, the LDL-C levels were significantly lower in adherent patients after both the first and second follow-up visits. However, there were no significant differences between the groups in terms of stroke, PAD, or mortality rates (Table 6).

Table 3. Laboratory values at baseline based on adherence to the guideline's recommendations.

Laboratory Test	All Patients	Adherence to Guideline Recommendations		p-Value †
		No	Yes	
HbA1C, %	8.0 ± 2.2	8.3 ± 2.3	7.9 ± 2.2	**0.0481**
Total cholesterol, mmol/L	4.4 ± 1.3	4.6 ± 1.3	4.4 ± 1.3	0.0747
LDL-C, mmol/L	2.8 ± 1.2	3.0 ± 1.1	2.7 ± 1.2	**0.0005**
HDL-C, mmol/L	1.0 ± 0.3	1.0 ± 0.2	1.0 ± 0.3	0.3386
Triglyceride, mmol/L	1.8 ± 1.1	1.9 ± 1.3	1.8 ± 1.1	0.4192
Serum creatinine, mg/dL	1.2 ± 0.9	1.1 ± 0.7	1.2 ± 1.0	0.3629
Creatinine clearance, mL/min	90.8 ± 38.9	88.0 ± 36.2	91.4 ± 39.5	0.4051

Numbers are presented as mean ±SD. † p-values are from the Mann–Whitney test for continuous not normally distributed data; values in bold are statistically significant. Abbreviations: SD: standard deviation.

Table 4. Classification of the index IHD event based on adherence to the guideline's recommendations.

Baseline Incident and Procedure	All Patients N = 1011	Adherence to Guideline Recommendations		p-Value †
		No N = 190 (18.8%)	Yes N = 821 (81.2%)	
Classification of the new IHD				**0.0172**
NSTEMI	512 (50.6)	105 (55.3%)	407 (49.6%)	
STEMI	241 (23.8)	28 (14.7%)	213 (25.9%)	
UA	108 (10.7)	26 (13.7%)	82 (10.0%)	
Stable IHD	15 (1.5)	2 (1.1%)	13 (1.6%)	
Number of diseased vessels				0.2038
One	306 (30.3)	46 (24.2)	260 (31.7)	
Two	181 (17.9)	37 (19.5)	144 (17.5)	
Three	208 (20.6)	37 (19.5)	171 (20.8)	
Four	91 (9.0)	21 (11.1)	70 (8.5)	
New or recurrent event				**<0.0001**
New	755 (74.7)	116 (61.1)	639 (77.8)	
Recurrent	230 (22.7)	65 (34.2)	165 (20.1)	**0.0215**
2nd	177 (17.5)	44 (23.2)	133 (16.2)	
3rd	36 (3.6)	14 (7.4)	22 (2.7)	
4th	12 (1.2)	3 (1.6)	9 (1.1)	
5th or more	5 (0.5)	4 (2.1)	1 (0.1)	
Not documented	26 (2.6)	9 (4.7)	17 (2.1)	
Procedure performed				
Stent PCI	333 (32.9)	79 (41.6)	254 (30.9)	**0.0049**
CABG	208 (20.6)	36 (18.9)	172 (21.0)	0.5383
Unspecified PCI	199 (19.7)	15 (7.9)	184 (22.4)	**<0.0001**
Medical therapy only	167 (16.5)	44 (23.2)	123 (15.0)	**0.0062**
Balloon PCI	47 (4.6)	7 (3.7)	40 (4.9)	0.4834
Not documented	94 (9.3)	17 (8.9)	77 (9.4)	0.8536
Risk category (after event)				0.2504
High risk	393 (38.9)	84 (44.2)	309 (37.6)	
Very high risk	593 (58.7)	102 (53.7)	491 (59.8)	

Numbers are presented as frequency (%). † p-values are from the chi-square test; values in bold are statistically significant. Abbreviations: IHD: ischemic heart disease; STEMI: ST-elevation myocardial infarction; NSTEMI: non-ST-elevation myocardial infarction; UA: unstable angina; PCI: percutaneous coronary intervention; CABG: coronary artery bypass grafting.

A sub-group analysis was performed in patients who were grouped to be adherent in order to examine the differences in outcomes with regard to the agent prescribed. When comparing rosuvastatin and atorvastatin, atorvastatin had statistically significantly lower non-fatal MI (7.1% vs. 20% $p \leq 0.0001$), revascularization (7.7% vs. 17.3% $p = 0.0010$), and stroke (1.8% vs. 4.3%; $p = 0.0397$) levels (Table S1), and no statistical differences in outcomes were observed when the doses of these agents were further sub-analyzed (Table S2).

Table 5. Lipid-lowering agents used after the index event and its distribution based on adherence to the guideline's recommendations.

Outcomes	All Patients N = 1011	Adherence to Guideline Recommendations		*p*-Value †
		No N = 190 (18.8%)	Yes N = 821 (81.2%)	
Statin agent used				**<0.0001**
Atorvastatin	780 (77.1)	100 (52.6)	680 (82.7)	
10 mg	4 (0.4)	3 (1.6)	1 (0.1)	
20 mg	29 (2.9)	27 (14.2)	2 (0.2)	
40 mg	417 (41.2)	44 (23.2)	373 (45.4)	
80 mg	330 (32.6)	26 (13.7)	304 (37.0)	
Rosuvastatin	220 (21.8)	80 (42.1)	140 (17.1)	
10 mg	24 (2.4)	16 (8.4)	8 (1.0)	
20 mg	158 (15.6)	52 (27.4)	106 (12.9)	
40 mg	38 (3.8)	12 (6.3)	26 (3.2)	
Simvastatin	11 (1.1)	10 (5.3)	1 (0.1)	
10 mg	7 (0.7)	7 (3.7)	0 (0.0)	
20 mg	4 (0.4)	3 (1.6)	1 (0.1)	
Additional drug used				
Ezetimibe	229 (22.7)	37 (19.5)	192 (23.4)	0.5095
PCSK9 inhibitors	19 (1.9)	2 (1.1)	17 (2.1)	0.6470

Numbers are presented as frequency (%). † *p*-values are from the chi-square test; values in bold are statistically significant. Abbreviation: PCSK9: Proprotein convertase subtilisin/kexin type 9.

Table 6. Patients' outcomes based on adherence to the guideline's recommendations.

Outcomes	All Patients N = 1011	Adherence to Guideline Recommendations		*p*-Value †
		No N = 190 (18.8%)	Yes N = 821 (81.2%)	
Patient was at LDL-C goal at 1st or 2nd follow-up	462 (45.7)	58 (30.5)	404 (49.2)	**<0.0001**
LDL-C at first follow-up	2.1 ± 1.0	2.4 ± 1.1	2.0 ± 1.0	**0.0009**
LDL-C at second follow-up	1.9 ± 0.9	2.2 ± 0.8	1.9 ± 0.9	**0.0257**
Non-fatal MI	116 (11.5)	40 (21.1)	76 (9.3)	**<0.0001**
Revascularization	108 (10.7)	32 (16.8)	76 (9.3)	**0.0024**
Stroke	25 (2.5)	7 (3.7)	18 (2.2)	0.2328
Peripheral arterial disease	2 (0.2)	1 (0.5)	1 (0.1)	0.2621
Death from CVD	21 (2.1)	7 (3.7)	14 (1.7)	0.0848
Death due to any cause	19 (1.9)	4 (2.1)	15 (1.8)	0.7991

Numbers are presented as frequency (%). † *p*-values are from the chi-square test; values in bold are statistically significant. Abbreviations: MI: myocardial infarction; CVD: cardiovascular disease.

4. Discussion

In this observational study, we evaluated adherence to the 2018 ACC/AHA guideline recommendations for statin therapy in the treatment of patients with clinical ASCVD, particularly those with IHD. Our findings revealed that more than half of the study population was classified as being at very high risk, and 81.2% were adherent to guideline recommendations. More than one-third of our patients had their first episode of IHD at the time of enrollment, with 50% of these episodes being NSTEMI. Those who were adherent to the utilization patterns recommended by the guidelines had a lower incidence of non-fatal MI and hospitalization for revascularization. They were also observed to have their LDL-C at the target level during their first or second follow-up.

Maddox et al. have utilized the National Cardiovascular Data Registry's (PINNACLE: Practice Innovation and Clinical Excellence) database to assess the effects of the 2013 ACC/AHA cholesterol guidelines on current cardiovascular practice in the United States. Their results revealed that only 50% of the patients were on statin therapy alone, while the proportion of patients on non-statin therapy was about 3%. Furthermore, statin utilization was found to be less than 80% in low- and middle-income countries [15]. We found higher rates of high-intensity statin (81%) and non-statin (24%) utilization when compared to those in the study of Maddox et al. (50% and 3%, respectively). We postulate several reasons for such findings. Unlike the study conducted by Maddox et al., in which adherence to guidelines was examined in four statin benefit groups, our study mainly focused on IHD patients, in which 50% of the cases were NSTEMI and 24% were STEMI patients, and the majority of the population was considered to be at very high risk. Thus, the prescription patterns of clinicians tend to be more aggressive for these patients. Second, all three hospitals participating in this study were teaching hospitals, and, therefore, clinicians are updated regularly. Finally, all three centers require a clinical pharmacist as part of the care team [16]. On the other hand, non-adherence to guideline recommendations was about 18%. The retrospective nature of the study limited our ability to assess the barriers to guideline adherence. Reasons for non-adherence to guidelines based on practical experience include the patient's age (particularly age above 75), tolerability, cost, socio-economic status, and accessibility to healthcare services. All these factors warrant further exploration in subsequent studies in order to provide actionable insights and improve adherence to clinical guidelines.

It should be noted that we are still under-prescribing non-statin therapy to eligible patients. We propose several explanations for this finding. First, about 60% of our population presented with their first IHD episode, and such patients are usually not yet on a maximally tolerated statin dose. Second, the mean LDL-C at baseline was 2.8 mmol—close to the target of <2.6 mmol/L (100 mg/dL)—in which case the use of a statin alone can be expected to reduce it to target levels. Third, only 59 patients (6%) missed LDL-C monitoring at 4–6 weeks following statin initiation; thus, therapy was (in most cases) intensified as needed. It is important to note that non-statin therapies play a crucial role in helping patients to achieve target LDL-C levels, particularly in those who are unable to tolerate high-intensity statins or fail to reach target LDL-C levels despite maximal statin therapy. In our study, the overall utilization of ezetimibe was 22.7%, while PCSK9 inhibitors were used in 1.9% of patients. These therapies, when used in combination with statins, promote additional LDL-C reduction through complementary mechanisms, as supported by previous studies, in which ezetimibe has been shown to reduce LDL-C by about 30% [17], whilst PCSK9 inhibitors can cut cholesterol levels by an average of 50–60% [18]. Nevertheless, there remains a significant gap in their adoption, particularly in non-adherent patients. Potential barriers include cost considerations, limited access to PCSK9 inhibitors, and variations in the prescribing practices of clinicians.

The 2013 ACC/AHA guidelines did not specify LDL-C targets or monitoring recommendations, whereas the 2018 guidelines reintroduced these. In our study, 50% of guideline-adherent patients achieved LDL-C targets at follow-up, compared to 31% of non-adherent patients ($p < 0.0001$); meanwhile, 59 patients (6%) did not have an LDL-C value measured after statin initiation. However, this was a lower proportion of missed

LDL-C lab values post-statin initiation when compared to available studies. For instance, the ACS EuroPath IV project assessed the effect of the ESC/EAS 2019 guidelines on lipid management in 2650 patients with ACS between March and June of 2022, in comparison with data collected from 2650 patients who participated in the ACS EuroPath I survey in 2018. In this study, 10% of the patients did not have lipid panel testing in 2022 [14]. Sarak et al. examined lipid testing performed in the hospital or within 90 days of discharge in patients with at least one-year survival after an ACS event between 2012 and 2018. The study included 27,979 patients, among whom 3750 patients (13.4%) did not have lipid testing [19]. It is worth noting that atherosclerotic plaque stabilization is a key mechanism through which lipid-lowering therapy (LLT) exerts its clinical benefits. High-intensity statins, in particular, play a critical role through reducing necrotic lipid cores, suppressing inflammation, and improving endothelial function, ultimately leading to more stable plaques that are less prone to rupture. Achieving LDL-C targets amplifies these effects, promoting not only the stabilization of plaque but also its regression. A recent review has emphasized that these mechanisms translate into significant reductions in major adverse cardiovascular events, including myocardial infarction and stroke [20]. In our study, patients adhering to guideline-directed LLT demonstrated higher LDL-C target attainment, which may have contributed to the observed reductions in non-fatal MI and revascularization rates. This highlights the importance of achieving LDL-C goals as a means to enhance plaque stability and improve clinical outcomes in high-risk populations.

Real-world data examining the effects of statin therapy on mortality and morbidity outcomes remain limited. In a study conducted between January 2003 and January 2011, 1528 patients who underwent PCI for ACS were followed for three months to assess all-cause mortality. About 60% of the patients were on high-intensity statins, while 40% were either on a low-dose statin or not on statins at all. A statistically significant reduction in all-cause mortality during the 3-month follow-up was observed in those receiving high-intensity statins. All-cause mortality occurred in 8 patients (0.9%) receiving high-intensity statin therapy and 21 patients (3.5%) taking low-intensity statins or no statin therapy at discharge (hazard ratio 0.244, 95% confidence interval [CI] 0.108–0.551; p = 0.001) [21]. Although not statistically significant, our study observed a numerically lower incidence of mortality due to cardiovascular disease (1.7% vs. 3.7%) or death from any cause (1.8% vs. 2.1%) among patients who were adherent to guideline recommendations, mostly receiving high-intensity statins (98.5% of these patients). However, this numerically lower incidence can be explained by the statistically significant difference in utilization rates of recommended therapies for secondary prevention of ACS, such as aspirin, $P2Y_{12}$ inhibitors, beta-blockers, ACEI/ARBs, and spironolactone.

To shed light on morbidity-related outcomes such as non-fatal MI, hospitalization, and/or revascularization, Timothy et al. conducted a meta-analysis of RCTs or systematic reviews on coronary heart disease to determine the effectiveness of statins. In particular, RCTs or systematic reviews published between January 1966 and December 2002 were included, for a total of 25 studies enrolling 69,511 individuals. Statin therapy reduced non-fatal MI by 25% (relative risk 0.75; 95%CI, 0.71–0.79) [22]. Our study revealed a statistically significant lower incidence of non-fatal MI between the group who were adherent to the guidelines and those who were not (9.3% vs. 21.1%; $p < 0.0001$). Additionally, hospitalization for revascularization was also statistically significant between the two groups (9.3% vs. 16.8%; $p < 0.0024$). Notably, it was observed that when a lower LDL-C level was achieved, a greater benefit in terms of ASCVD reduction was obtained. As mentioned above, about 50% of the patients in the group who were adherent to the guidelines had their LDL-C at target (<70 mg/dL), compared to 31% of those patients who were not in alignment with guidelines.

Although our study was a multi-center study, it had some limitations. The retrospective nature of the study might introduce some documentation bias due to the complexity of the chart review process. This might have also led to the difficulty of assessing adverse events that highly impact statin adherence. Compared to other real-world data studies, we had a small sample size. In addition, a reduced amount of data collection occurred during the COVID-19 pandemic period, which may have affected access to and availability of laboratory testing. Furthermore, in the middle of the study period, the 2022 ACC Expert Consensus Report further reduced the threshold for consideration of non-statin therapy to 55 mg/dL for patients with clinical ASCVD who are at very high risk. However, we doubt that this alteration impacted our results, as it was published in November of 2022, while our patients were followed to the end of 2022 only.

5. Conclusions

In conclusion, this study is among the first to evaluate adherence to the 2018 ACC/AHA guidelines for lipid management in a real-world, multi-center setting within a Saudi Arabian population. Our findings highlighted the substantial benefits of adherence, including improved LDL-C goal attainment and reductions in non-fatal MI and revascularization rates. The novelty of this study lies in its focus on a diverse, multi-racial population living in Saudi Arabia, where limited data regarding the applicability of international guidelines are available at present. By demonstrating that the benefits of guideline-directed therapies extend to this population, we provide a foundation for assessing current prescribing practices and identifying actionable strategies to optimize care and outcomes in this unique context. To further enhance adherence, we conclude that including a pharmacist in the care team, who can update the team via teaching once relevant guidelines are updated, could potentially help to bring prescribing patterns in line with the recommendations of such guidelines. Several postulated theories should be further examined for their capacity to enhance LDL testing and further target level achievement, including reminding patients about their upcoming lab tests, as well as monitoring the tolerability and utilization of non-statin therapy when effective levels of statins are deemed intolerable.

Supplementary Materials: The following supporting information can be downloaded at: https://www.mdpi.com/article/10.3390/jcm14030908/s1, Table S1: Adherant patients' outcomes based on agents used; Table S2: Adherant patients' outcomes based on agents' doses used.

Author Contributions: Conceptualization, A.H., S.A., H.K., M.S.A.Y. and O.A.A.; methodology, A.H., S.A., H.K., M.S.A.Y. and O.A.A.; software and data analysis, O.A.A.; validation, A.H., S.A., H.K., M.S.A.Y. and O.A.A.; investigation, A.H., S.A., N.F., L.A., M.A., M.S.A., A.O.A., A.A.A. and M.A.A.; resources, A.H., S.A., L.A., M.S.A., M.S.A.Y. and O.A.A.; data curation, A.H., S.A., N.F., L.A., M.A., M.S.A., A.O.A., A.A.A. and M.A.A.; writing—original draft preparation, A.H., S.A., N.F. and M.S.A.Y.; writing—review and editing, A.H., S.A., H.K., N.F., L.A., M.A., M.S.A., A.O.A., A.A.A., M.A.A., M.S.A.Y. and O.A.A.; supervision, A.H., M.S.A.Y. and O.A.A.; project administration, A.H., M.S.A.Y. and O.A.A.; funding acquisition, O.A.A. All authors have read and agreed to the published version of the manuscript.

Funding: The author (OAA) received funding from the Research Supporting Project (RSP2025R77), King Saud University, Riyadh, Saudi Arabia to support the publication of this article. The funding agency played no role in designing the study, analyzing and interpreting the data, or writing the manuscript.

Institutional Review Board Statement: The study was approved by the supervising institutional review boards (IRBs) at the three study sites: KAUH on April 2022 (ref. no. 234-22, KAMC on 26 December 2022 (ref. no. SP22R/254/12), and KSUMC on 8 November 2022 (Ref. no. E-22-7285).

Informed Consent Statement: The need for written consent was waived by the ethics committee because of the retrospective nature of the study.

Data Availability Statement: The datasets used and/or analyzed during the current study are available from the corresponding author upon reasonable request.

Acknowledgments: The authors would like to extend their appreciation to King Saud University for funding this work through the Researcher Supporting Project (RSP2025R77), King Saud University, Riyadh, Saudi Arabia.

Conflicts of Interest: The authors declare that they have no competing interests.

References

1. Grundy, S.M.; Stone, N.J.; Bailey, A.L.; Beam, C.; Birtcher, K.K.; Blumenthal, R.S.; Braun, L.T.; de Ferranti, S.; Faiella-Tommasino, J.; Forman, D.E.; et al. 2018 AHA/ACC/AACVPR/AAPA/ABC/ACPM/ADA/AGS/APhA/ASPC/NLA/PCNA Guideline on the Management of Blood Cholesterol: Executive Summary: A Report of the American College of Cardiology/American Heart Association Task Force on Clinical Practice Guidelines. *J. Am. Coll. Cardiol.* **2019**, *73*, 3168–3209. [CrossRef] [PubMed]
2. Smith, S.C., Jr.; Benjamin, E.J.; Bonow, R.O.; Braun, L.T.; Creager, M.A.; Franklin, B.A.; Gibbons, R.J.; Grundy, S.M.; Hiratzka, L.F.; Jones, D.W.; et al. AHA/ACCF Secondary Prevention and Risk Reduction Therapy for Patients with Coronary and other Atherosclerotic Vascular Disease: 2011 update: A guideline from the American Heart Association and American College of Cardiology Foundation. *Circulation* **2011**, *124*, 2458–2473. [CrossRef] [PubMed]
3. Stancu, C.; Sima, A. Statins: Mechanism of action and effects. *J. Cell Mol. Med.* **2001**, *5*, 378–387. [CrossRef]
4. Rosa, G.M.; Carbone, F.; Parodi, A.; Massimelli, E.A.; Brunelli, C.; Mach, F.; Vuilleumier, N.; Montecucco, F. Update on the efficacy of statin treatment in acute coronary syndromes. *Eur. J. Clin. Investig.* **2014**, *44*, 501–515. [CrossRef] [PubMed]
5. Ference, B.A.; Ginsberg, H.N.; Graham, I.; Ray, K.K.; Packard, C.J.; Bruckert, E.; Hegele, R.A.; Krauss, R.M.; Raal, F.J.; Schunkert, H.; et al. Low-density lipoproteins cause atherosclerotic cardiovascular disease. 1. Evidence from genetic, epidemiologic, and clinical studies. A consensus statement from the European Atherosclerosis Society Consensus Panel. *Eur. Heart J.* **2017**, *38*, 2459–2472. [CrossRef]
6. Navarese, E.P.; Kowalewski, M.; Andreotti, F.; van Wely, M.; Camaro, C.; Kolodziejczak, M.; Gorny, B.; Wirianta, J.; Kubica, J.; Kelm, M.; et al. Meta-analysis of time-related benefits of statin therapy in patients with acute coronary syndrome undergoing percutaneous coronary intervention. *Am. J. Cardiol.* **2014**, *113*, 1753–1764. [CrossRef]
7. Baigent, C.; Keech, A.; Kearney, P.M.; Blackwell, L.; Buck, G.; Pollicino, C.; Kirby, A.; Sourjina, T.; Peto, R.; Collins, R.; et al. Efficacy and safety of cholesterol-lowering treatment: Prospective meta-analysis of data from 90,056 participants in 14 randomised trials of statins. *Lancet* **2005**, *366*, 1267–1278. [CrossRef]
8. Ward, N.C.; Watts, G.F.; Eckel, R.H. Statin Toxicity. *Circ. Res.* **2019**, *124*, 328–350. [CrossRef]
9. Arnold, S.V.; Spertus, J.A.; Tang, F.; Krumholz, H.M.; Borden, W.B.; Farmer, S.A.; Ting, H.H.; Chan, P.S. Statin use in outpatients with obstructive coronary artery disease. *Circulation* **2011**, *124*, 2405–2410. [CrossRef]
10. Cassagnol, M.; Hai, O.; Sherali, S.A.; D'Angelo, K.; Bass, D.; Zeltser, R.; Makaryus, A.N. Impact of cardiologist intervention on guideline-directed use of statin therapy. *World J. Cardiol.* **2020**, *12*, 419–426. [CrossRef]
11. Schoen, M.W.; Salas, J.; Scherrer, J.F.; Buckhold, F.R. Cholesterol treatment and changes in guidelines in an academic medical practice. *Am. J. Med.* **2015**, *128*, 403–409. [CrossRef] [PubMed]
12. Pedro-Botet, J.; Pintó, X. Colesterol LDL, cuanto más bajo mejor. *Clínica Investig. Arterioscler.* **2019**, *31*, 16–27. [CrossRef] [PubMed]
13. Byrne, R.A.; Rossello, X.; Coughlan, J.J.; Barbato, E.; Berry, C.; Chieffo, A.; Claeys, M.J.; Dan, G.A.; Dweck, M.R.; Galbraith, M.; et al. 2023 ESC Guidelines for the management of acute coronary syndromes. *Eur. Heart J.* **2023**, *44*, 3720–3826. [CrossRef] [PubMed]
14. Laufs, U.; Catapano, A.L.; de Caterina, R.; Schiele, F.; Sionis, A.; Zaman, A.; Jukema, J.W. The effect of the 2019 ESC/EAS dyslipidaemia guidelines on low-density lipoprotein cholesterol goal achievement in patients with acute coronary syndromes: The ACS EuroPath IV project. *Vasc. Pharmacol.* **2023**, *148*, 107141. [CrossRef]
15. Maddox, T.M.; Borden, W.B.; Tang, F.; Virani, S.S.; Oetgen, W.J.; Mullen, J.B.; Chan, P.S.; Casale, P.N.; Douglas, P.S.; Masoudi, F.A.; et al. Implications of the 2013 ACC/AHA cholesterol guidelines for adults in contemporary cardiovascular practice: Insights from the NCDR PINNACLE registry. *J. Am. Coll. Cardiol.* **2014**, *64*, 2183–2192. [CrossRef]

16. Cornelison, P.; Marrs, J.C.; Anderson, S.L. Clinical Pharmacist Outreach to Increase Statin Use for Patients with Cardiovascular Disease in a Safety-Net Healthcare System. *Am. Health Drug Benefits* **2021**, *14*, 63–69. [PubMed] [PubMed Central]
17. Cannon, C.P.; Blazing, M.A.; Giugliano, R.P.; McCagg, A.; White, J.A.; Theroux, P.; Darius, H.; Lewis, B.S.; Ophuis, T.O.; Jukema, J.W.; et al. Ezetimibe Added to Statin Therapy after Acute Coronary Syndromes. *N. Engl. J. Med.* **2015**, *372*, 2387–2397. [CrossRef]
18. Sabatine, M.S.; Giugliano, R.P.; Keech, A.C.; Honarpour, N.; Wiviott, S.D.; Murphy, S.A.; Kuder, J.F.; Wang, H.; Liu, T.; Wasserman, S.M.; et al. Evolocumab and Clinical Outcomes in Patients with Cardiovascular Disease. *N. Engl. J. Med.* **2017**, *376*, 1713–1722. [CrossRef]
19. Sarak, B.; Savu, A.; Kaul, P.; McAlister, F.A.; Welsh, R.C.; Yan, A.T.; Goodman, S.G. Lipid Testing, Lipid-Modifying Therapy, and PCSK9 (Proprotein Convertase Subtilisin-Kexin Type 9) Inhibitor Eligibility in 27 979 Patients With Incident Acute Coronary Syndrome. *Circ. Cardiovasc. Qual. Outcomes* **2021**, *14*, e006646. [CrossRef]
20. Cesaro, A.; Acerbo, V.; Indolfi, C.; Filardi, P.P.; Calabrò, P. The Clinical Relevance of the Reversal of Coronary Atherosclerotic Plaque. *Eur. J. Intern. Med.* **2024**, *129*, 16–24. [CrossRef]
21. Tentzeris, I.; Rohla, M.; Jarai, R.; Farhan, S.; Freynhofer, M.K.; Unger, G.; Nürnberg, M.; Geppert, A.; Wessely, E.; Wojta, J.; et al. Influence of High-Dose Highly Efficient Statins on Short-Term Mortality in Patients Undergoing Percutaneous Coronary Intervention With Stenting for Acute Coronary Syndromes. *Am. J. Cardiol.* **2014**, *113*, 1099–1104. [CrossRef] [PubMed]
22. Wilt, T.J.; Bloomfield, H.E.; MacDonald, R.; Nelson, D.; Rutks, I.; Ho, M.; Larsen, G.; McCall, A.; Pineros, S.; Sales, A. Effectiveness of statin therapy in adults with coronary heart disease. *Arch. Intern. Med.* **2004**, *164*, 1427–1436. [CrossRef] [PubMed]

Journal of
Clinical Medicine

MDPI

Article

Efficacy and Safety of Statin Treatment in Children with Familial Hypercholesterolemia: Outcomes of 20 Years of Experience

Radosław Motkowski [1,*], Paweł Abramowicz [1], Jolanta Kubalska [2], Bożena Mikołuć [1] and Jerzy Konstantynowicz [1]

1 Department of Pediatrics, Rheumatology, Immunology and Metabolic Bone Diseases, Medical University of Bialystok, 15-274 Bialystok, Poland; pawel.abramowicz@umb.edu.pl (P.A.); bozena.mikoluc@umb.edu.pl (B.M.); jurekonstant@o2.pl (J.K.)
2 Department of Genetics, Institute of Psychiatry and Neurology, 02-957 Warsaw, Poland
* Correspondence: radek@umb.edu.pl; Tel.: +48-85-7450-622

Abstract: Background: The objective of this retrospective cohort study was to present the experience of 20-year-long comprehensive care of pediatric patients with familial hypercholesterolemia (FH) in a single academic center. Methods and Results: The study included 84 children aged 1–18 years with FH. For the whole study group, 535 medical visits were recorded. The mean follow-up period was 33.6 months. Molecular testing performed in 55 children (65%) provided genetic confirmation of the diagnosis in 36 children (43%). Twenty-seven children (32%) were treated pharmacologically with statins. Follow-up during the treatment averaged 29 months. Treatment with statins was associated with a mean reduction in total cholesterol and LDL-cholesterol levels of 24 and 33% from the baseline. Symptoms of statin intolerance occurred incidentally and did not require amendment in the treatment protocol. Significantly higher values of body weight, height, and BMI were found only among girls older than 10 years who were treated with statins. Conclusions: These data confirm a high efficacy and a good safety profile of statin treatment in children with FH, demonstrating no harm to physical development. However, there is a need for further cause-and-effect research regarding associations between long-term treatment with low-cholesterol, low-fat diets, statin therapy, and excessive weight gain.

Keywords: atherosclerosis; statins; children; familial hypercholesterolemia; safety

1. Introduction

Familial hypercholesterolemia (FH) is a congenital metabolic disorder (OMIM #143890, #144010, #107703, #607786), which is connected to increased serum low-density lipoprotein cholesterol (LDL-C), leading to premature atherosclerosis and diseases of the cardiovascular system [1]. The average age of the first hospitalization due to cardiovascular disease in this group of patients is 45 years, i.e., approximately 20 years earlier than in the general population [2]. The incidence of familial hypercholesterolemia in Europe has been estimated at 1:217 according to recent studies [3]. In contrast, the mortality due to circulatory system diseases in these patients is 100 times higher compared with the general population [4,5]. Lipid-lowering treatments initiated early significantly reduce the risk later in life [6,7].

According to current clinical practice, the most common hypolipemic therapeutic management used among FH children is statins [8]. The safety and efficacy of statin treatment in children were evaluated a couple of years ago in several meta-analyses [9], including those incorporated in the Cochrane Reviews Evidence [10]. Unfortunately, these reports concerned only studies with a maximum follow-up duration of 2 years, thereby suggesting a necessity for longer and well-designed observations in this specific group. In an analysis for the Cochrane Library, the importance of the careful monitoring of lipid parameters, the incidence of adverse effects, other risk factors of atherosclerosis, and child growth and development during statin treatment [10].

Existing evidence on the efficacy of statin therapy renders it ethically impossible to design a long-term randomized trial. Further, it is all the more essential to monitor and follow-up on children already undergoing hypolipemic treatment concerning treatment tolerance, several aspects of statin safety, and the children's development [11].

The recent literature encompassing longer follow-ups have usually reported aggregated data originating from many centers, including a 5-year follow-up of the efficacy and safety of the treatment in a UK cohort of 232 children [12], Norwegian data covering 302 children [13] and also combined data from Canada and the United States covering 289 pediatric patients [14].

Specific evidence for the effectiveness of statin treatment was provided by a 20-year follow-up from The Netherlands [15]. This report did not compare children treated vs. not treated with statins, but children with FH treated with statins and their healthy siblings and affected parents. The researchers showed that the risk of cardiovascular disease before the age of 39 for untreated parents was 26% (7% died during that time), whereas for their children treated from the age of 13, it was 1%. Moreover, the early initiation of statins in children with FH alleviated the progression of carotid intima-media thickness [15].

A parameter called Cumulative LDL-C burden is used to determine the risk of developing ischemic heart disease. The level of 160, associated with the development of ischemic heart disease, is reached by a person without FH at the age of 55. In contrast, a patient with heterozygous FH reaches it at the age of 35 years. If lipid-lowering therapy in an individual with FH is initiated at 18 years, the cumulative LDL cholesterol burden of 160 will be achieved at the age of 48. If the treatment with statins is initiated at the 10th year of life, a similar cumulative LDL cholesterol burden will be reached around the age of 53 years. [7].

This retrospective cohort study aimed to present the experience of 20 years of care in pediatric patients with familial hypercholesterolemia in a single specialist academic center. The efficacy and safety of the hypolipemic treatment with statins were reviewed in detail, especially in the context of growth and physical development measured with basic anthropometric parameters.

2. Materials and Methods

2.1. Study Participants

The study included 84 children (42 girls) aged 1 to 18 years who were consulted at least twice between 2001 and 2021 at the Metabolic Outpatient Clinic of the University Children's Hospital in Bialystok, Northeastern Poland, for familial hypercholesterolemia diagnosed using the Simon Broome Criteria [16]. For the whole study group, 535 medical visits were recorded, with an average of 6 for each patient (range: 2–27). The mean follow-up time was 33.63 months (SD 37.3), the shortest 2 months, and the longest 173 months (14.5 years). All children in this study had a family history of hypercholesterolemia and/or premature cardiovascular disease. Molecular testing was performed in 55 children (65%). The tests revealed the presence of a known gene mutation underlying the diagnosis of FH in 36 children (43%). In 19 children, molecular testing failed to identify a known mutation in the LDL receptor or apolipoprotein B genes.

A low-cholesterol diet, with restrictions on saturated and trans fats, was recommended to all studied children, and the rules were consistently reminded to the children and caregivers at each follow-up visit. Cholestyramine treatment was attempted in five children between 2005 and 2010 and was discontinued due to intolerance of the form and taste of the preparation. Twenty-seven children (32%) were treated pharmacologically with statins. Treatment was usually implemented at the 4th visit, after an average follow-up of 34 months (SD 29.26; min. 3 months, max. 100 months), with a mean age of 13 years (SD 2.47; range: 8.5–17 years). The first follow-up visit was held after two months (1–3 months) and the follow-up time during treatment averaged 29 months (SD 24.27; the most extended observation was 75 months). A total of 18 participants (66%) were treated with simvastatin at the time of the last visit (twelve subjects with a dose of 10 mg, six subjects with 20 mg), and 9 participants were receiving rosuvastatin (6 with a dose of 5 mg, 2 with 10 mg, and 1 with 20 mg).

The remaining 57 children (68%) did not receive pharmacological treatment due to age limitations associated with the registration and product characteristics for hypolipidemic drugs (8 years for rosuvastatin and 10 years for simvastatin) or because of a lack of parental consent. Detailed characteristics of children treated with the diet and statins and those treated with the diet alone are shown in Table 1.

Table 1. Characteristics of hypercholesterolemic groups. Data are presented as means and standard deviations, where applicable.

	Treated with Statins (n = 27)	Without Statins (n = 57)	p
Age at baseline [y] during the first visit	10.03 (3.57)	8.09 (3.60)	0.009
Sex	16 girls, 11 boys	26 girls, 31 boys	0.243
Family history of hypercholesterolemia:			
Siblings	17 (63%)	25 (44%)	0.102
Parents	27 (100%)	52 (91%)	0.113
Grandparents	19 (70%)	47 (82%)	0.491
Mutation status:			
- LDL-R	15 (56%)	12 (21%)	0.001
- APO-B	7 (26%)	2 (4%)	
- neither LDL nor APO-B	2 (7%)	17 (30%)	
- not performed or under testing	3 (11%)	26 (46%)	
Time of observation [months]	64.44 (42.61)	29.75 (28.76)	0.001
Number of visits	11.67 (5.21)	3.88 (2.77)	0.001
Age [y] during the last visit	15.63 (2.36)	10.55 (3.68)	0.001

2.2. Methods

The study was based on a retrospective review of medical records. Anthropometric data and clinical features (body weight, body height, heart rate, and blood pressure values), as well as available biochemical test results (lipid profile, glucose level, creatinine kinase, and aminotransferase activity), were included in the study. Data on body weight, height, and a standard formula for BMI were also cross-referenced with reference values for age- and sex-matched normative values (growth charts, Z-score).

We also analyzed recorded information on chronic complaints, concomitant diseases, co-morbidities, and, in the group of children treated with statins, treatment tolerance (i.e., occurrence of adverse reactions and side effects). The protocol was approved by the Bioethics Committee at the Medical University of Bialystok. The study was supported by the Medical University of Bialystok No. SUB/1/DN/19/001/1126.

Blood for testing was collected in the morning after 12 h of fasting. Glucose was determined using the enzymatic hexokinase/glucose 6-phosphate dehydrogenase method (COBAS 6000 C501, Roche, Mannheim, Germany). Lipids (i.e., total cholesterol, LDL- and HDL-cholesterol, and triglycerides), alanine and aspartate aminotransferase activities, and creatinine kinase were measured with the colorimetric enzymatic method (COBAS 6000 C501, Roche, Mannheim, Germany).

Molecular tests were performed using the PCR RFLP method and MLPA sequencing, and in some patients, the next-generation sequencing method (NGS) on the MiSeq platform (Illumina Inc., San Diego, CA, USA) using the ADH MASTR (Multiplicom, Niel, Belgium) kit. The tests were performed at the Institute of Psychiatry and Neurology in Warsaw and the University Clinical Center of the Medical University of Gdańsk.

Statistical analysis was performed using the arithmetic mean and standard deviation (SD) for quantitative variables. The Chi^2 test assessed the significance of differences in qualitative variables. The examined continuous variable distribution was evaluated with the Kolmogorov–Smirnov test. For the analysis of the variables distributed normally, the Student's t-test was used, and for the variables inconsistent with the normal distribution, the Mann–Whitney U test was used. Stepwise multiple regression analysis was conducted to determine relationships between the selected variables included in the models.

The anthropometric parameters converted to Z-scores were calculated separately for subgroups stratified by age and sex (with a 1-year range precision) based on population data published elsewhere [17]. The following standard formula was used to determine the Z-score: Z-score = (parameter—SD for corresponding age and sex)/median for corresponding age and sex.

In the calculations, the level of $p < 0.05$ was accepted as statistically significant, authorizing the rejection of individual null hypotheses. The data were processed using the Polish version of Statistica 13.0 statistical software for Windows PCs. Raw data used in the publication are available in Supplementary Materials.

3. Results

3.1. Lipid Profile

In the study group, the mean total cholesterol at the first visit was 258 mg/dL (SD 42.23), and LDL-C was 185 mg/dL (SD 43.93). Total cholesterol and LDL-C levels found at the beginning of the follow-up in the FH children who later received statin treatment were higher compared with peers who did not receive such treatment later (Table 2, Figure 1). After treatment with the dietary regimen alone, a similar decrease in total cholesterol was observed in both groups, with a mean reduction of 5.27% in the group subsequently treated with statins and 4.68% in the untreated group, and a decrease in LDL-C by 4.45% and 13.7%, respectively. Only in the group of children who had never been treated with statins were these differences significant ($p < 0.001$).

Table 2. Lipid profile in study groups during follow-up. Data are presented as means and standard deviations in parentheses. The letters in the superscript indicate statistically significant differences from $p < 0.001$. The symbols in the superscript indicate significant differences from $p < 0.01$.

	Treated with Statins (n = 27)				Without Statins (n = 57)	
	First Visit	Start of Treatment	Control Visit	Last Visit	First Visit	Last Visit
Total cholesterol [mg/dL]	284.00 ^{a,e} (35.97)	279.23 ^{k} (30.36)	213.11 ^{k} (36.65)	204.26 ^{c,e} (26.30)	245.37 $^{a,\#}$ (39.43)	232,96 $^{c,\#}$ (46.56)
HDL cholesterol [mg/dL]	58.29 (23.88)	59.88 (18.64)	60.56 $^{\$}$ (14.42)	55.54 $^{\$}$ (13.57)	56.93 (13.37)	55.37 (11.49)
LDL cholesterol [mg/dL]	211.53 ^{b,f} (37.56)	204.50 ^{m} (27.14)	138.63 ^{m} (32.78)	134.27 ^{d,f} (23.78)	171.80 $^{b,\%}$ (41.03)	160.06 $^{d,\%}$ (46.72)
Triglycerides [mg/dL]	86.42 (52.59)	81.20 (35.57)	73.78 (29.80)	71.84 (26.26)	94.66 (63.88)	87.15 (38.88)

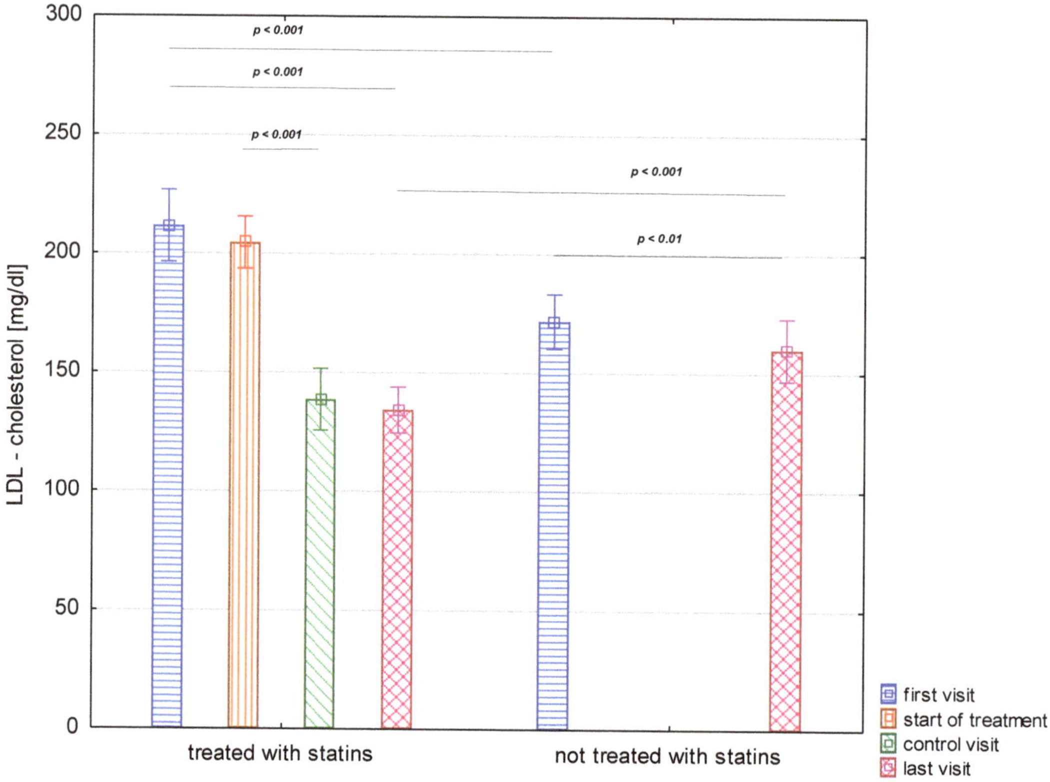

Figure 1. LDL lipoprotein cholesterol levels in the study group stratified by statin treatment.

Treatment with statins was associated with a mean reduction of 24 and 33% from the baseline in total cholesterol and LDL-C levels after just two months (control visit) (Table 2, Figure 1). Subsequent months of treatment resulted in further reductions in total cholesterol and LDL-C, and during the entire follow-up, the values were lower by 27% and 36% than the baseline, respectively.

Based on records from the most recent available visits, total cholesterol and LDL-C concentrations in the children treated concurrently with the diet and statins for a mean follow-up of 29 ± 24.26 months were significantly lower than for children treated with diet alone after 29 ± 28.76 months of follow-up (Table 2, Figure 1). At the last recorded visit, 14 (52%) of the statin-treated children still had LDL-C levels above 130 mg/dL, but only 2 (7%) had levels above 160 mg/dL. In the group of children not treated with statins, LDL-C levels above 130 mg/dL were observed in 38 (66%) children, and those above 160 mg/dL were found in almost 1 in 3 children (20 of 57–35%).

There were no differences in HDL lipoprotein cholesterol and triglyceride levels, except for a slight decrease in HDL lipoprotein cholesterol during statin treatment (Table 1). The decline in HDL lipoprotein cholesterol levels during the entire follow-up averaged 7.7% in this group and averaged 10% in the diet-only treatment group. Triglyceride levels in the diet-only children decreased by 4%, whereas, in the statin-treated group, the TG levels eventually reduced by an average of 3%.

3.2. Comorbidities and Tolerability of Statin Treatment

During each of the 535 analyzed medical consultations, caregivers of children with hypercholesterolemia were asked questions about comorbidities and the tolerance of treatment. Two patients dropped out of further treatment and lipid care after attempting oral cholestyramine. Coexisting celiac disease and hypothyroidism were found in two patients.

The 27 children treated with statins were consulted 315 times. Two boys were diagnosed with scoliosis during puberty, and one boy developed avascular necrosis of the hip. One patient was diagnosed with an ovarian cyst and obesity; another female patient showed overweight, hypertension, and menstrual disorders. One boy was diagnosed with congenital macular dystrophy, another one had psoriasis, and one girl was diagnosed with epilepsy during follow-up.

One patient experienced a transient increase in total cholesterol after being introduced to retinoids for severe acne lesions. Another patient was switched to rosuvastatin due to intolerance to simvastatin (headache, weakness, fatigue). In one boy, due to lack of parental consent, the treatment was discontinued for 6 months because of exacerbated psoriatic lesions that coincided with the introduction of simvastatin treatment. No progression of skin lesions was then observed after restarting treatment.

Nine children had fasting blood glucose values > 100 mg/dL in single measurements, but only one boy had a fasting blood glucose greater than 120 mg/dL. Three children had single glycemic values < 60 mg/dL. No child was diagnosed with diabetes.

Only one boy with hepatic steatosis of unknown etiology, diagnosed prior to treatment, had elevated aminotransferase activity. After achieving target LDL-cholesterol values with normal aminotransferase activities, the patient discontinued treatment and care at the Metabolic Clinic.

Four patients had increased creatinine kinase activity, all of which was due to the test being performed the day after excessive exercise. The values exceeded five times the upper limit in only two of them. The parents of one of these patients, whose molecular testing did not reveal the presence of a pathogenic mutation, waived further drug treatment. Another patient with a strong family history and a confirmed mutation in the LDL receptor gene returned to treatment with the previously used dose of rosuvastatin. With the rule of one day's rest from sports, before the test was performed, he was never again found to have increased creatinine kinase activity afterward.

Nine children showed heart rates higher than 90/min two or more times, and one boy showed bradycardia below 60/min. Blood pressure values were recorded during 176 visits and averaged 116.7 mmHg and 71.3 mmHg systolic and diastolic, respectively (75–95 centile according to standard reference). Two or more abnormal systolic blood pressure measurements (>120 mmHg) were found in 10 children. Five children also demonstrated elevated diastolic blood pressure values (>80 mmHg). Two of them were not treated with statins due to being too young at the time of the study. In all of these children, further diagnostics confirmed the diagnosis of so-called white coat hypertension.

3.3. Anthropometric Measurements

The distribution of body weight, height, and BMI of the male and female participants in relation to the standard reference is shown in Figure 2 (3rd and 97th centile according to OLAF) [17]. The body height remained within normal limits. There were no deficiencies in body weight throughout the follow-up period. The summary data presented in the graph revealed a higher prevalence of weight above the age standard (97th centile) in older children, more prevalent among girls, and more frequent among children treated with statins. The prevalence of obesity, defined as a BMI above the 97th percentile, was found less frequently but still more often among older, mainly female children and those treated with statins.

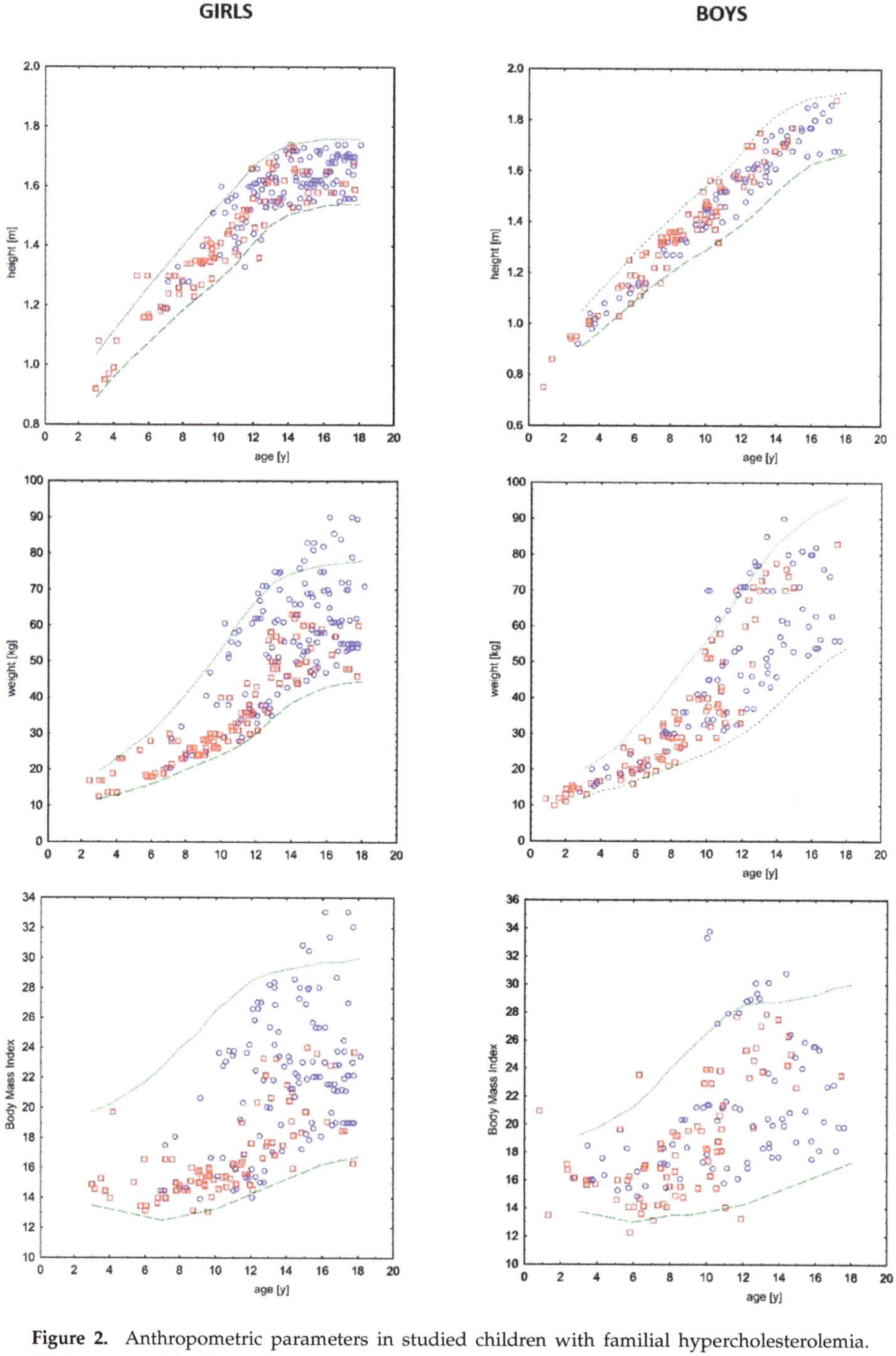

Figure 2. Anthropometric parameters in studied children with familial hypercholesterolemia. Circles—treated finally with statins; squares—never treated with statins; dashed line—3rd centile; dotted line—97th centile according to the standard reference from OLAF study [17].

The Z-score values for body weight in participants treated with statins were statistically significantly higher than in the children treated with diet alone, averaging 1.13 (SD 1.49) vs. 0.49 (SD 1.15). A similar relationship was found by assessing the Z-score values for BMI, with an average of 0.98 (SD 1.38) vs. 0.25 (SD 1.15). Differences in the body height Z-score were not significant.

A multiple regression analysis was performed to determine the significance of the differences regarding anthropometry (height, weight, and BMI) as dependent variables, and age, sex, total cholesterol, and statin treatment as independent variables. There was an association of body height only with age (R 0.93) and sex (R 0.1), as well as body weight with age (R 0.86), sex (R 0.15), TC levels (R −0.08), and statin treatment (R −0.12). The BMI values depended less on age (R 0.55), sex (R 0.19), and total cholesterol (R −0.07) but more distinctly on the statin treatment (R −0.22) in this model.

Based on the above results, the differences in the anthropometric parameters between children treated with statins and those treated with diet alone were stratified by age and sex subgroups (children younger or older than 10 years). The age threshold we adopted was arbitrarily determined based on two rationales—the only existing comparable report [12], which also adopted the age of 10 years as a criterion for stratification, and the registration restrictions of simvastatin (the most commonly used statin), which has been approved for pediatric treatment in individuals aged over 10 years.

There were no significant differences among boys except for a slightly greater height in older boys treated with statins. There were no significant differences between the younger girls either. In contrast, significantly higher values of body weight, height, and BMI were found among girls older than 10 years who were treated with statins compared to those who were treated with the diet alone. The analysis of anthropometric measurements related to sex and age (Z-scores) did not confirm differences in body height but again showed higher Z-scores for body weight and BMI in the group of statin-treated girls over 10 years of age (Table 3).

Table 3. Anthropometric parameters in study groups divided according to sex and age. Data is presented as means and standard deviations in brackets. The quantity n denotes the number of available measurements.

			Treated with Statins n = 232	**Without Statins n = 195**	p
Boys					
<10 years	Weight n = 86	[kg]	27.46 (11.41)	24.39 (9.45)	0.19
		Z-score	1.05 (1.31)	0.66 (1.14)	0.21
	Height n = 75	[m]	1.21 (0.15)	1.22 (0.17)	0.62
		Z-score	0.56 (0.81)	0.89 (1.11)	0.11
	BMI n = 75	[kg/m^2]	17.96 (3.48)	16.83 (2.69)	0.07
		Z-score	0.92 (1.27)	0.41 (1.29)	0.06
≥10 years	Weight n = 98	[kg]	59.40 (15.43)	54.28 (17.05)	0.14
		Z-score	1.14 (1.57)	1.41 (1.24)	0.24
	Height n = 88	[m]	1.63 (0.12)	1.57 (0.13)	0.04
		Z-score	0.75 (0.84)	1.06 (0.96)	0.12
	BMI n = 88	[kg/m^2]	22.3 (4.44)	22.87 (4.16)	0.81
		Z-score	1.15 (1.56)	1.29 (1.22)	0.29

Table 3. *Cont.*

			Treated with Statins $n = 232$	Without Statins $n = 195$	p
Girls					
<10 years	Weight $n = 60$	[kg]	29.38 (8.89)	23.59 (5.49)	0.08
		Z-score	0.62 (1.17)	0.26 (1.09)	0.41
	Height $n = 48$	[m]	1.31 (0.10)	1.25 (0.13)	0.45
		Z-score	0.69 (1.02)	0.64 (1.27)	0.92
	BMI $n = 48$	[kg/m^2]	16.12 (2.27)	14.93 (1.23)	0.29
		Z-score	0.23 (1.05)	−0.39 (0.70)	0.16
≥10 years	Weight $n = 183$	[kg]	58.26 (14.09)	44.83 (10.47)	0.01
		Z-score	1.19 (1.53)	0.02 (0.81)	0.01
	Height $n = 161$	[m]	1.61 (0.09)	1.56 (0.10)	0.01
		Z-score	0.34 (1.1)	0.19 (1.12)	0.39
	BMI $n = 161$	[kg/m^2]	22.33 (4.34)	18.31 (2.82)	0.01
		Z-score	0.97 (1.32)	−0.05 (0.69)	0.01

4. Discussion

This study summarizing a 20-year-long follow-up of a pediatric population with FH showed that statin therapy, when introduced reasonably early, is safe, provides benefits, and does not cause health hazards during growth. Importantly, there is still a limited number of published data on statin use in children and adolescents and related associations.

The mean age of children who had been treated later with statins was higher at the time of their first visit to our center than the mean age of children in whom treatment was not initiated. A similar relationship and almost identical values were observed in the Norwegian cohort [13]. There is no such direct data in the UK report, and the mean duration of treatment in the North American study was 2.7 years [14]. The time to introduce statins into treatment was later than recommended (10 years of age) in all populations: 11 years in the UK, 12.5 years in Norway and North America, and 13 years in our center. As reported elsewhere, this is due to a delayed diagnosis associated with cascade screening in these countries and a lack of population-based screening [18].

In a study conducted in Norway, children treated with statins demonstrated a 38% reduction in LDL-C between the first and last visits, whereas children not treated with statins had 4% [13]. In a similar study from the UK, this difference was 35% [12]. A recent report encompassing data from eight European countries described reductions in LDL-C of 28% to 57%. However, when data from Greece, where population-based screening was conducted between the 1st and 3rd years of age, were excluded from the analysis, the mean reduction in LDL-C during statin treatment was much greater, i.e., 33.5% [18]. Another study from Poland showed a 34.4% decrease in LDL-C following one-year treatment with rosuvastatin, although at different doses [19].

In our study, we observed a similar efficacy in children treated with statins. We reported a 33% reduction in LDL-C levels after just two months and 36% during the entire follow-up. We found a concomitant more significant (13.7%) decrease in LDL lipoprotein cholesterol levels in the group on long-term diet and lifestyle modification than in the Norwegian (4.5%) or the UK (5.4%) studies. This may be similar to an option of dietary correction of lipid disorders in children, as described in the literature, ranging from 10 to 15% [20,21]. We hypothesized that such an outcome may have resulted from regular consultations on low-fat, hypolipemic diet rules and also the involvement of both parents and children. Other studies have no data on the frequency of dietary counseling.

In the above-mentioned Norwegian study, a higher proportion of statin-treated children achieved target LDL-C levels than in our study (71% vs. 48%). In the study by Ramaswami et al., the percentage of children whose LDL-C levels fell below 130 mg/dL was 54% after excluding data from Greece, where up to 99% of children achieved the therapeutic goal [18]. In the study from North America, 51% of studied children failed to reach this strategic goal [14]. Notably, our results (like those in other studies on pediatric populations) were much better compared with some published studies among adults, where only 2.7% reached the target concentration [22]. In an interesting Norwegian paper, 22% of young adults reached the treatment goal, and 30% of children and young adults experienced treatment adherence problems [23]. We found more significant differences in children who did not receive pharmacological treatment. In the Norwegian study, 41% of such children did not reach the therapeutic goal, while in our study, 66% did. Unfortunately, significantly higher LDL-C levels than the target (>160 mg/dL) were present in up to 35% of our participants. No such data are available from other studies.

To date, there are no evidence-based recommendations addressing the degree of LDL-C reduction in children with FH that would effectively prevent the development of atherosclerosis and cardiovascular disease. However, the 32% reduction in LDL-C described in a Dutch longitudinal observational study is comparable to the effect obtained in most studies described above, so it reduced the risk of early cardiovascular disease from 26 to 1% [15]. This reduction in LDL-C was possible in our studied children after statins were used in monotherapy, at the lowest available doses, and in a short time—following approximately two months of intervention.

Regarding our patients with FH, we included data on comorbidities found in a number of these subjects during a longstanding follow-up, up to 15 years in some cases. Associations between coexisting conditions and events with the treatment cannot be ruled out, nor can they be confirmed. Available data do not report such diseases occurring in association with statin treatment in children or even in extensively studied adult populations. The most common reports of adverse effects attributable to statin treatment involve abnormal muscle and liver enzymes and the occurrence of diabetes. A Cochrane Library meta-analysis of nine studies involving 1177 children treated with statins for 4 to 24 months found incident adverse events only. The incidence was not different between children treated with statins and those receiving placebo [10].

In the Norwegian report, 5% of the children had adverse effects but were not associated with biochemical abnormalities. We found increased, though unrelated to treatment, aminotransferase activity in one patient, whereas none of the Norwegian studies showed such an abnormality. In both studies, an increase in creatinine kinase activity associated with increased exercise was observed in several children. Of importance, no one experienced symptoms of myopathy or rhabdomyolysis [13]. In the UK study, none of the participants showed increased creatinine kinase or aminotransferase activities [12]. In a report from Canada and the US, 5% ($n = 15$) of the children had increased creatinine kinase activity, but none had clinical symptoms, thus, no treatment modification was required. Increased aminotransferase activity was observed in 4%, which was normalized after the discontinuation of therapy and did not increase when treatment was restarted. Twenty patients (7%) experienced muscular pain, fatigue, rash, and abdominal pain but did not require a change in treatment [14]. In the Dutch cohort, there were no statistically significant differences in liver enzymes and creatinine kinase activity between statin-treated children with FH and their healthy siblings [15].

In our study, as reported elsewhere, symptoms of statin intolerance occurred incidentally and usually did not require amendment in the treatment protocol. In the adult population, such symptoms are equally rare (5 to 10%) but more often require treatment modification of the dosage, change of the active agent, or introduction of polytherapy to the treatment [24]. A recent meta-analysis of 62 studies involving more than 120,000 adults found that treatment with statins was associated with a small but significant risk of muscle complaints or liver dysfunction. These manifestations were mostly transient, depended on the type and dose of statin used, and also occurred in the placebo group [25]. Muscle damage occurs in less than 0.1% of adults, and the risk of liver damage occurs in 0.001%. When assessing the potential risk of adverse effects, the absolute benefits of statin therapy in preventing cardiovascular disease should be kept in mind, e.g., a 10% reduction in mortality with each 39 mg% reduction in LDL-cholesterol [21].

We also evaluated other atherosclerosis risk factors to determine target LDL-C levels while monitoring treatment for lipid disorders. None of the children in our study were diagnosed with hypertension or diabetes. No patient admitted to smoking cigarettes either. Nevertheless, more attention was needed to monitor the prevalence of overweight and obesity.

To our knowledge, only aggregate data on mean weight and height, or BMI, of children with hypercholesterolemia treated with statins are available in the current literature. None of our studied children were malnourished or short-statured during treatment. Obesity, defined as body weight or BMI > 97th centile for sex and age, was also less frequent in the entire group than in the general population. However, a detailed analysis of available data from 535 follow-up visits and their reference to reference charts showed a higher prevalence of obesity among children treated with statins (Figure 2). A multiple regression analysis confirmed that body weight and BMI were related to statin treatment, and a subgroup analysis showed that obesity was significantly more common in statin-treated girls older than ten years.

In the British report, children did not differ in weight or height at diagnosis. The anthropometric parameters assessed at the last follow-up visit were higher in those who started treatment before the age of 10 years compared with those not treated. No such differences were found in the group of children who began treatment after the age of 10 years [12]. In the North American study, the mean body weight centile before treatment implementation was 84 (ranging from 51 to 96), and it was 86 (53–97) at the last follow-up visit, but this difference was not significant. The mean BMI centile before treatment initiation was 89 (62–98), and it was 87 (54–97) after treatment [14]. The Dutch cohort showed a marked change in BMI from 19.6 to 25.4 after several years of treatment, but these results were unrelated to centile charts or Z-scores [15]. Medeiros et al. found that 14.1% of patients with FH had a BMI above the 95th percentile compared to 33.8% of patients with hypercholesterolemia of other etiologies [26].

The interpretation of the relationship found in our study is hampered by the lack of comparable reports that would have included multiple assessments of anthropometric parameters over a more extended follow-up period. Based on clinical experience in pediatric patients with FH, an explanation is that patients and their families often discontinue a low-cholesterol diet after the introduction of pharmacotherapy has been initiated. Every patient at our center was reminded during follow-up visits of the low-cholesterol diet, with a restriction of saturated fats, and was advised to maintain appropriate physical activity. Unfortunately, in many cases, numerous errors were reported by parents. What is challenging and questionable is the lack of a significant increase in body weight among boys who were more likely to make dietary mistakes than adolescent girls. Perhaps this may be related to boys' greater physical activity during puberty. However, it is noteworthy that obesity is an independent risk factor for atherosclerosis and the development of cardiovascular disease. Studies among adults have not found a higher incidence of obesity in people treated with statins, but this may be related to the age at which treatment began [27].

Some recommendations have indicated only the supportive nature of dietary treatment in these patients [4,5]. A lack of evidence for the advisability of low-fat and low-cholesterol diets in patients with FH has also been raised, however, at the same time, low-carbohydrate diets' potential benefits have been pointed out [28]. The explanation of the phenomenon described above requires further well-designed prospective studies. However, regardless of the reasons for the observed tendency to increase body weight during drug therapy, dietary monitoring should remain an essential part of care in children with FH [1]. Consistent dietary counseling can be critical in preventing overweight and obesity [27].

A limitation of our study is its observational and retrospective nature. In addition, the number of patients enrolled was relatively small compared to the expected prevalence since FH remains underdiagnosed and undertreated in children. Notably, the average age of diagnosis for FH is 44 years, and only 2.1% of those affected are diagnosed in their teens [22]. Another limitation is that only a limited proportion of all participants had a molecular diagnosis. However, the initiation of treatment was not restrictively determined by the result of a genetic test. Furthermore, the availability of the method was very limited at those times, i.e., during the first years of our follow-up. All children included in the study were diagnosed with FH using recognized clinical criteria.

We had no control over the disruptions that were associated with some children remaining in care for extended periods and some children dropping out of care early. Further research is also needed to assess the reasons why some parents opt for drug treatment for their children, whereas others do not. On the other hand, the strength of our study is the long follow-up duration and the large number of follow-up visits analyzed. Furthermore, the unified management of a child and the parents for a child with hypercholesterolemia within a single center, as well as the amount of routinely collected data, including anthropometric data, are noteworthy.

Atherosclerotic cardiovascular disease occurs worldwide and is regarded as the most common cause of death in adults. Many of these conditions could be prevented by diagnosing FH early enough. Unfortunately, although the disease is the most common monogenic condition, it is undoubtedly underestimated and diagnosed only in a small proportion of affected individuals and usually only after the onset of clinically apparent atherosclerosis [29]. The hypolipemic treatment used in secondary prevention would always be more complicated than that in primary prevention. An effective treatment initiated in childhood can significantly extend the healthy life span of patients with FH.

The results of our study presenting 20 years of experience from only one center confirm a high efficacy, good safety profile, and overall benefits of statin treatment in children with familial hypercholesterolemia. These data support the view of the necessity of the early implementation of statin therapy for pediatric patients with FH. There is a need for further cause-and-effect research regarding associations between long-term treatment with low-cholesterol and low-fat diets and excessive weight gain during pharmacotherapy.

Supplementary Materials: The following supporting information can be downloaded at: https://www.mdpi.com/article/10.3390/jcm12237197/s1.

Author Contributions: R.M. conceived and planned the study; R.M., J.K. (Jolanta Kubalska) and B.M. designed the work and study protocol; R.M. and P.A. acquired and analyzed the data; R.M., P.A. and J.K. (Jerzy Konstantynowicz) interpreted the results; R.M. obtained funding and wrote the first draft of the manuscript; R.M., P.A. and J.K. (Jerzy Konstantynowicz) were responsible for writing and editing the final version of the report. All authors have read and agreed to the published version of the manuscript.

Funding: The study was supported with a grant of the Medical University of Bialystok No. SUB/1/DN/19/001/1126.

Institutional Review Board Statement: The protocol was approved by the Bioethics Committee at the Medical University of Bialystok.

Informed Consent Statement: Informed consent was obtained from all subjects involved in the study.

Data Availability Statement: Raw data used in the publication are available in Supplementary Materials.

Conflicts of Interest: The authors declare no conflict of interest.

References

1. Wiegman, A. Lipid Screening, Action, and Follow-up in Children and Adolescents. *Curr. Cardiol. Rep.* **2018**, *20*, 80. [CrossRef] [PubMed]

2. Mundal, L.; Igland, J.; Ose, L.; Holven, K.B.; Veierød, M.B.; Leren, T.P.; Retterstøl, K. Cardiovascular Disease Mortality in Patient with Genetically Verified Familial Hypercholesterolemia in Norway during 1992–2013. *Eur. J. Prev. Cardiol.* **2016**, *24*, 137–14 [CrossRef] [PubMed]
3. Nordestgaard, B.G.; Benn, M. Genetic Testing for Familial Hypercholesterolaemia Is Essential in Individuals with High LDL Cholesterol: Who Does It in the World? *Eur. Heart J.* **2017**, *38*, 1580–1583. [CrossRef] [PubMed]
4. Goldberg, A.C.; Hopkins, P.N.; Toth, P.P.; Ballantyne, C.M.; Rader, D.J.; Robinson, J.G.; Daniels, S.R.; Gidding, S.S.; de Ferrant S.D.; Ito, M.K.; et al. Familial Hypercholesterolemia: Screening, Diagnosis and Management of Pediatric and Adult Patient Clinical Guidance from the National Lipid Association Expert Panel on Familial Hypercholesterolemia. *J. Clin. Lipidol.* **2011**, *5* S1–S8. [CrossRef] [PubMed]
5. Myśliwiec, M.; Walczak, M.; Małecka-Tendera, E.; Dobrzańska, A.; Cybulska, B.; Filipiak, K.J.; Mazur, A.; Jarosz-Chobot, P. Szadkowska, A.; Rynkiewicz, A.; et al. Management in Familial Hypercholesterolaemia in Children and Adolescents. Position o the Lipid Expert Forum. *Kardiol. Pol.* **2013**, *71*, 1099–1105. [CrossRef]
6. Narverud, I.; Retterstøl, K.; Iversen, P.O.; Halvorsen, B.; Ueland, T.; Ulven, S.M.; Ose, L.; Aukrust, P.; Veierød, M.B.; Holven, K.B Markers of Atherosclerotic Development in Children with Familial Hypercholesterolemia: A Literature Review. *Atherosclerosis* **2014**, *235*, 299–309. [CrossRef]
7. Nordestgaard, B.G.; Chapman, M.J.; Humphries, S.E.; Ginsberg, H.N.; Masana, L.; Descamps, O.S.; Wiklund, O.; Hegele, R.A. Raal, F.J.; Defesche, J.C.; et al. Familial Hypercholesterolaemia Is Underdiagnosed and Undertreated in the General Population Guidance for Clinicians to Prevent Coronary Heart Disease. *Eur. Heart J.* **2013**, *34*, 3478–3490. [CrossRef]
8. Cohen, H.; Stefanutti, C.; Giacomo, S.D.; Morozzi, C.; Widhalm, K.; Bjelakovic, B.B.; Berni, A.; Martino, F.; Bosco, G. Current Approach to the Diagnosis and Treatment of Heterozygote and Homozygous FH Children and Adolescents. *Curr. Atheroscler Rep.* **2021**, *23*, 30. [CrossRef]
9. Dombalis, S.; Nash, A. The Effect of Statins in Children and Adolescents With Familial Hypercholesterolemia: A Systematic Review. *J. Pediatr. Health Care* **2020**, *35*, 292–303. [CrossRef]
10. Vuorio, A.; Kuoppala, J.; Kovanen, P.T.; Humphries, S.E.; Tonstad, S.; Wiegman, A.; Drogari, E.; Ramaswami, U. Statins for Children with Familial Hypercholesterolemia. *Cochrane Database Syst. Rev.* **2019**, *2019*, CD006401. [CrossRef]
11. Martin, A.C.; Gidding, S.S.; Wiegman, A.; Watts, G.F. Knowns and Unknowns in the Care of Pediatric Familial Hypercholesterolemia. *J. Lipid Res.* **2017**, *58*, 1765–1776. [CrossRef] [PubMed]
12. Ramaswami, U.; Cooper, J.; Humphries, S.E.; Group, F.P.R.S. The UK Paediatric Familial Hypercholesterolaemia Register Preliminary Data. *Arch. Dis. Child.* **2017**, *102*, 255–260. [CrossRef] [PubMed]
13. Bogsrud, M.P.; Langslet, G.; Wium, C.; Johansen, D.; Svilaas, A.; Holven, K.B. Treatment Goal Attainment in Children with Familial Hypercholesterolemia: A Cohort Study of 302 Children in Norway. *J. Clin. Lipidol.* **2018**, *12*, 375–382. [CrossRef] [PubMed]
14. Kavey, R.-E.W.; Manlhiot, C.; Runeckles, K.; Collins, T.; Gidding, S.S.; Demczko, M.; Clauss, S.; Harahsheh, A.S.; Mietus-Syder, M.; Khoury, M.; et al. Effectiveness and Safety of Statin Therapy in Children: A Real-World Clinical Practice Experience. *CJC Open* **2020**, *2*, 473–482. [CrossRef]
15. Luirink, I.K.; Wiegman, A.; Kusters, D.M.; Hof, M.H.; Groothoff, J.W.; de Groot, E.; Kastelein, J.J.P.; Hutten, B.A. 20-Year Follow-up of Statins in Children with Familial Hypercholesterolemia. *N. Engl. J. Med.* **2019**, *381*, 1547–1556. [CrossRef]
16. Wiegman, A.; Gidding, S.S.; Watts, G.F.; Chapman, M.J.; Ginsberg, H.N.; Cuchel, M.; Ose, L.; Averna, M.; Boileau, C.; Borén, J.; et al. Familial Hypercholesterolaemia in Children and Adolescents: Gaining Decades of Life by Optimizing Detection and Treatment. *Eur. Heart J.* **2015**, *36*, 2425–2437. [CrossRef]
17. Kułaga, Z.; Różdżyńska-Świątkowska, A.; Grajda, A.; Gurzkowska, B.; Wojtyło, M.; Góźdź, M.; Świąder-Leśniak, A.; Litwin, M. Percentile charts for growth and nutritional status assessment in Polish children and adolescents from birth to 18 year of age. *Stand. Med. Pediatr.* **2015**, *12*, 119–135.
18. Ramaswami, U.; Futema, M.; Bogsrud, M.P.; Holven, K.B.; van Lennep, J.R.; Wiegman, A.; Descamps, O.S.; Vrablik, M.; Freiberger, T.; Dieplinger, H.; et al. Comparison of the Characteristics at Diagnosis and Treatment of Children with Heterozygous Familial Hypercholesterolaemia (FH) from Eight European Countries. *Atherosclerosis* **2020**, *292*, 178–187. [CrossRef]
19. Hennig, M.; Brandt-Varma, A.; Wołoszyn-Durkiewicz, A.; Bautembach-Minkowska, J.; Buraczewska, M.; Świętoń, D.; Mickiewicz, A.; Rynkiewicz, A.; Gruchała, M.; Limon, J.; et al. Monitoring the Effects of Hypolipidemic Treatment in Children with Familial Hypercholesterolemia in Poland. *Life* **2020**, *10*, 270. [CrossRef]
20. Lehtovirta, M.; Matthews, L.A.; Laitinen, T.T.; Nuotio, J.; Niinikoski, H.; Rovio, S.P.; Lagström, H.; Viikari, J.S.A.; Rönnemaa, T.; Jula, A.; et al. Achievement of the Targets of the 20-Year Infancy-Onset Dietary Intervention—Association with Metabolic Profile from Childhood to Adulthood. *Nutrients* **2021**, *13*, 533. [CrossRef]
21. Michos, E.D.; McEvoy, J.W.; Blumenthal, R.S. Lipid Management for the Prevention of Atherosclerotic Cardiovascular Disease. *N. Engl. J. Med.* **2019**, *381*, 1557–1567. [CrossRef] [PubMed]
22. Cuchel, M.; McGowan, M.P. Familial Hypercholesterolaemia: Too Many Lost Opportunities. *Lancet* **2021**, *398*, 1667–1668. [CrossRef] [PubMed]
23. Langslet, G.; Johansen, A.K.; Bogsrud, M.P.; Narverud, I.; Risstad, H.; Retterstøl, K.; Holven, K.B. Thirty Percent of Children and Young Adults with Familial Hypercholesterolemia Treated with Statins Have Adherence Issues. *Am. J. Prev. Cardiol.* **2021**, *6*, 100180. [CrossRef]

24. Stroes, E.S.; Thompson, P.D.; Corsini, A.; Vladutiu, G.D.; Raal, F.J.; Ray, K.K.; Roden, M.; Stein, E.; Tokgözoğlu, L.; Nordestgaard, B.G.; et al. Statin-Associated Muscle Symptoms: Impact on Statin Therapy—European Atherosclerosis Society Consensus Panel Statement on Assessment, Aetiology and Management. *Eur. Heart J.* **2015**, *36*, 1012–1022. [CrossRef] [PubMed]
25. Cai, T.; Abel, L.; Langford, O.; Monaghan, G.; Aronson, J.K.; Stevens, R.J.; Lay-Flurrie, S.; Koshiaris, C.; McManus, R.J.; Hobbs, F.D.R.; et al. Associations between Statins and Adverse Events in Primary Prevention of Cardiovascular Disease: Systematic Review with Pairwise, Network, and Dose-Response Meta-Analyses. *BMJ* **2021**, *374*, n1537. [CrossRef] [PubMed]
26. Medeiros, A.M.; Alves, A.C.; Aguiar, P.; Bourbon, M.; on behalf of the Pediatric Investigators of the Portuguese Familial Hypercholesterolemia Study. Cardiovascular Risk Assessment of Dyslipidemic Children: Analysis of Biomarkers to Identify Monogenic Dyslipidemia. *J. Lipid Res.* **2014**, *55*, 947–955. [CrossRef]
27. Vallejo-Vaz, A.J.; Stevens, C.A.T.; Lyons, A.R.M.; Dharmayat, K.I.; Freiberger, T.; Hovingh, G.K.; Mata, P.; Raal, F.J.; Santos, R.D. Global Perspective of Familial Hypercholesterolaemia: A Cross-Sectional Study from the EAS Familial Hypercholesterolaemia Studies Collaboration (FHSC). *Lancet* **2021**, *398*, 1713–1725. [CrossRef]
28. Diamond, D.M.; Alabdulgader, A.A.; de Lorgeril, M.; Harcombe, Z.; Kendrick, M.; Malhotra, A.; O'Neill, B.; Ravnskov, U.; Sultan, S.; Volek, J.S. Dietary Recommendations for Familial Hypercholesterolaemia: An Evidence-Free Zone. *BMJ Evid. Based Med.* **2020**, *26*, 295–301. [CrossRef]
29. Groselj, U.; Wiegman, A.; Gidding, S.S. Screening in Children for Familial Hypercholesterolaemia: Start Now. *Eur. Heart J.* **2022**, *43*, 3209–3212. [CrossRef]

Journal of
Clinical Medicine

MDPI

Article

Lipid-Lowering Therapy in PURE Poland Cohort Study

Paweł Lubieniecki [1,*], Maria Wołyniec [2], Katarzyna Połtyn-Zaradna [2], Katarzyna Zatońska [2] and Andrzej Szuba [3]

[1] Clinical Department of Diabetology and Internal Disease, Wroclaw Medical University, Borowska Street 213, 50-556 Wroclaw, Poland
[2] Department of Social Medicine, Wroclaw Medical University, 50-345 Wrocław, Poland; maria.wolyniec@umw.edu.pl (M.W.); katarzyna.poltyn-zaradna@umw.edu.pl (K.P.-Z.); katarzyna.zatonska@umw.edu.pl (K.Z.)
[3] Clinical Department of Angiology and Internal Disease, Wroclaw Medical University, Borowska Street 213, 50-556 Wroclaw, Poland; andrzej.szuba@umw.edu.pl
* Correspondence: pawel.lubieniecki@usk.wroc.pl

Abstract: The aim of this study is to present data on the use of lipid-lowering therapy (LLT) in relation to calculated cardiovascular risk (CVR) and an additionally defined target LDL-C concentration. The cohort consisted of 1287 participants in the Polish edition of the Prospective Urban and Rural Epidemiological Study (PURE). CVR was calculated for each participant using the SCORE2 or SCORE2-OP scale, and for patients with diabetes mellitus (DM), chronic kidney disease (CKD) or atherosclerotic cardiovascular disease (ASCVD) according to the respective criteria. In the cohort analysed, 107 of 212 people (50.5%) in the low cardiovascular risk (CVR) group, 284 of 414 people (68.6%) in the moderate CVR group, 562 of 612 people (91.8%) in the high CVR group and 48 of 49 people (98%) in the very high CVR group did not meet the target LDL-c criterion. Of those in the low CVR group, 86% of participants were not receiving lipid-lowering therapy (LLT); in the moderate CVR group, the proportion was 77.8%; in the high CVR group, 68.1% and in the very high CVR group, 75%. In each cardiovascular risk group, participants who did not meet the target LDL-c concentration criterion and did not take LLT made up the larger group.

Keywords: systematic coronary risk evaluation 2; prospective urban and rural epidemiological study; cardiovascular risk; lipid-lowering therapy

1. Introduction

Cardiovascular disease (CVD) is the most common cause of death both worldwide and in Poland. In 2021, 180,760 people in Poland died from this cause, accounting for 34.8% of all such events [1]. The basis for estimating the probability of morbidity or death from this cause is the calculation of cardiovascular risk (CVR). This is a rough, estimated predictive value that determines the possibility of CVD or death from CVD over a 10-year period. Calculating an individual's CVR is the basis for appropriate primary prevention and further identification of optimal therapy.

Currently, the European Society of Cardiology recommends using the Systematic Coronary Risk Evaluation 2 (SCORE2) scale and the Systematic Coronary Risk Evaluation 2-Older Persons (SCORE2-OP) scale to assess cardiovascular risk. This is an update of the existing SCORE scale and is based on current data on the prevalence of cardiovascular disease and its possible consequences.

It takes into account age, sex, systolic blood pressure (SBP), non-HDL cholesterol (nHDL-C) and smoking status [2,3]. It is applied to a population excluding those with atherosclerotic cardiovascular disease (ASCVD), diabetes mellitus (DM) or chronic kidney disease (CKD) with a glomerular filtration rate (eGFR) below 60 min/1.73 m^2. Such individuals are immediately assigned to high- or very-high-risk groups for future cardiovascular incidents.

The risk calculation provides a baseline for adopting an appropriate individual strategy for each patient. The basis should be the improvement of modifiable factors, such as weight reduction, increased physical activity, smoking cessation, conservative or pharmacological treatment of hypertension or hyperlipidemia [4,5]. The basis of protective measures should be adequate patient education, including public awareness of the basics of healthy eating or proper physical activity.

In cases of dyslipidemia, lipid-lowering therapy (LLT) is used for secondary prevention. There are a number of studies showing a significant effect of statins and other hypolipemic drugs in reducing cardiovascular events [6–8].

We analysed a group of participants in the Polish cohort of the Prospective Urban and Rural Epidemiologic Study (PURE), which looked at CVD risk factors in residents of Wroclaw and the surrounding countryside. An individual CVR was determined for each participant, and it was determined whether they should be taking LLT according to current guidelines and whether they were actually doing so. Adequate risk identification at each stage of patient care can improve quality of life and prevent premature cardiac deaths as well as the higher expenses associated with treating CVD complications. The results are presented below.

2. Materials and Methods

Baseline data were collected between 2019 and 2022 and were part of the Global Prospective Urban and Rural Epidemiological Study (PURE), which has been ongoing since 2007, with data collected at 3-year intervals. All participants were screened according to the PURE study protocol [9,10], which included a questionnaire survey (individual health, household, family, food frequency questionnaire and International Physical Activity Questionnaire (IPAQ)), anthropometric measurements, blood pressure measurement, blood draw, ECG and spirometry. The baseline cohort consisted of 2035 adult participants (1281 women and 754 men) aged 30–85 years (mean: 55 years, SD $\pm$ 10). The study group included participants from urban areas (the city of Wroclaw) and rural areas (the villages surrounding Wroclaw) in Lower Silesia.

Diabetes was determined by self-reported diabetes and/or self-reported use of antidiabetic medications and/or measurement of fasting blood glucose $\geq$ 126 mg/dL [11]. Hypertension was determined by self-reported hypertension and/or self-reported antihypertensive medications and/or the mean of two blood pressure measurements $\geq$ 140/90 mmHg [12]. The presence of cardiovascular disease (CVD) and respiratory disease was reported by participants. The CVD category included participants who reported heart failure, coronary artery disease and other heart diseases. Attitudes toward tobacco smoking were self-reported by the participants. In the case of tobacco smoking, participants could have chosen one of three possible answers: "formerly used tobacco products", "currently use tobacco products", or "never used tobacco products".

Lipid disorders and use of LLT were self-reported by participants. The individual health questionnaire had four questions directly related to this:

(1) Do you have high cholesterol?
(2) Are you taking medications regularly to lower your cholesterol?
(3) In the last 12 months, were you taking medications for lowering cholesterol but then stopped?
(4) In the past month, how often did you take your cholesterol medications as the doctor prescribed?

As for question three, the participant could choose from the following reasons:

(1) Doctor advised me to stop because cholesterol was under control; Felt unwell from cholesterol medication(s) so was told to stop; Felt well, no need to take my medications.
(2) Self-decision to stop because cholesterol was under control; Felt unwell from cholesterol medications so decided to stop; Felt well, no need to take my medications; Cannot afford cholesterol medications; The pharmacy is too far away from me; I have to take too many medications; My cholesterol medication is often not available in my pharmacy.

The study was reviewed and approved by the Bioethics Committee of the Medical University of Wrocław on 6. October 2006 and was therefore conducted in accordance with the ethical standards set out in the relevant version of the 1964 Declaration of Helsinki (positive opinion of the Bioethics Committee of the Medical University of Wrocław No. KB-443/2006).

The SCORE2 and SCORE2-OP scales were calibrated against four country categories, which were determined from national CVD mortality rates published by WHO [13]. Poland was classified as a high-risk country. An individual CVR for each patient was then calculated based on age, sex, smoking status, nHDL-c concentration and SBP; the participant was then assigned to one of four age- and value-appropriate categories—low-, moderate-, high- or very-high-risk—according to the SCORE2 and SCORE2-OP tables applicable to high-risk countries [2,3].

This CVR assessment scheme is not applicable to patients with ASCVD, DM and CKD. These individuals fall into one of three risk categories—moderate, high or very high [14]—according to the following findings:

I Patients with CKD without DM or ASCVD:

- High for moderate CKD (eGFR 30–44 mL/min/1.73 m^2 and ACR (albumin-to-creatinine ratio) < 30 or eGFR 45–59 mL/min/1.73 m^2 and ACR 30–300 or eGFR > 60 mL/min/1.73 m^2 and ACR > 300).
- Very high for severe CKD (eGFR < 30 mL/min/1.73 m^2 or eGFR 30–44 mL/min/1.73 m^2 and ACR > 30).

II Patients with DM 2 and patients with DM 1 over 40 years of age [15]:

- Moderate for well-controlled, short-lived diabetes (<10 years) without data indicating TOD (target organ damage) and without additional ASCVD risk factors.
- High for patients with DM without ASCVD and/or severe TOD [16] and do not meet criteria for moderate risk.
- Very high for DM patients with ASCVD and/or severe TOD or eGFR < 45 mL/min/1.73 m^2 regardless of albuminuria or eGFR 45–59 mL/min/1.73 m^2 and microalbuminuria (ACR 30–300 mg/g) or proteinuria (ACR > 300 mg/g) or presence of microvascular disease in at least 3 locations.

III Patients with diagnosed ASCD:

- Very high for documented ASCVD, either clinically or unequivocally on imaging studies. Clinically documented ASCVD includes previous AMI (acute myocardial infarction), ACS (acute coronary syndrome), coronary revascularization and other arterial revascularization procedures, stroke, TIA (transient ischemic attack), aortic aneurysm and PAD (peripheral artery disease). ASCVD found unequivocally on imaging studies includes the presence of atherosclerotic plaque found on coronary angiography or ultrasound of the carotid arteries, or on CTA (computed tomography angiography).

Statistica 13.3 (TIBCO. Software Inc., Palo Alto, CA, USA) was used for statistical analysis. The work presents the results classified as the so-called industry statistics, using both descriptive statistics (age, sex) and mathematical statistics.

3. Results

3.1. Overall Results

The analysis included 1287 participants in the PURE study. Participants with ASCVD, CKD and DM who knew the duration of the last disease—a factor necessary to qualify the patient for the appropriate CVR group—were analysed. For participants without these diseases, all participants with the full set of data necessary to calculate SCORE2 or SCORE2-OP (age, sex, smoking status, SBP and nHDL-c) were analysed. The remaining participants were excluded from this analysis. The cohort consisted of 441 men (34.7%) and 846 women (65.3%). Based on place of residence, the number of urban residents amounted to 877 (68.1%), while the number of rural residents amounted to 410 (31.9%).

A total of 347 people (27%) reported using LLT. Of those, 30 participants had discontinued such treatment in the past 12 months, including 8 who discontinued treatment because of a physician's decision: 7 participants due to good lipid control and 1 participant due to poor health resulting from the use of the aforementioned medications. A total of 22 participants discontinued treatment on their own: 6 due to lack of effects, 7 due to poor health resulting from the use of LLT, 7 who did not feel the need to use LLT while feeling well, and 2 who discontinued treatment due to too much medication in daily use.

When calculating CVR using the SCORE-2 and SCORE-2-OP scales, 1064 people were included: 712 women and 352 men or, taking into account place of residence, 742 urban residents and 322 rural residents. The group with DM, CKD or ASCVD included 223 people: 134 women and 89 men or, considering place of residence, 135 urban residents and 88 rural residents. Overall results are shown in Table 1.

Table 1. Overall results.

Polish Cohort of the PURE Study	2035
participants analysed	1287
patients with DM, ASCVD, CKD	223
other patients	1064
urban residents/rural residents	877/410
men/women	441/846
patients with low CVR	212
patients with moderate CVR	414
patients with high CVR	612
patients with very high CVR	49

3.2. Outcomes in Specific Cardiovascular Risk Groups

3.2.1. Patients Classified in the Low CVR Group

Patients classified in the low CVR group comprised 212 participants (16.4%). Of these, 105 achieved the target LDL cholesterol concentration (LDL-c) (49.5%) and 107 participants did not (50.5%). A pooled analysis of the results without disaggregating patients by comorbidities is shown in Table 2. Among these 107 participants, 92 participants (86%) were not taking LLT. This group included 69 urban residents (75%) or 33 men (35.9%).

Table 2. Summary analysis of results without dividing patients by comorbidities.

	Low CVR	Moderate CVR	High CVR	Very High CVR
number of people	212	414	612	49
urban residents	155 (73.1%)	275 (66.4%)	416 (68%)	31 (67.2%)
men	63 (29.7%)	147 (35.5%)	205 (33.55%)	26 (53.1%)
have achieved the target LDL-c	105 (49.5%)	130 (31.4%)	50 (8.2%)	1 (2%)
were taking LLT	23 (21.9%)	31 (23.8%)	24 (48%)	0 (0%)
were not taking LLT	82 (78.1%)	99 (76.2%)	26 (52%)	1 (100%)
have not achieved the target LDL-c concentration	107 (50.5%)	284 (68.6%)	562 (91.8%)	48 (98%)
were taking LLT	15 (14%)	63 (22.2%)	179 (31.9%)	12 (25%)
were not taking LLT	92 (86%)	221 (77.8%)	383 (68.1%)	36 (75%)

Patients with ASCVD, DM and CKD did not qualify for the low CVR group.

The group of 107 individuals without ASCVD, DM and CKD represented those who did not meet the LDL-c target criterion in the low CVR group. Of these, 15 people (14% of the subgroup) were taking LLT. A total of 92 people (86% of the subgroup) refused treatment. In the group of people meeting the target LDL-c concentration criterion, 23 people (21.9% of the subgroup) were receiving appropriate drug treatment. In contrast, 82 people (the remaining 78.1% of the subgroup) were not receiving any treatment.

3.2.2. Patients with Moderate CVR

Among those with moderate CVR, of whom there were 414 (32.2%), 130 achieved the target LDL-c concentration (31.4%), while 284 did not reach the target concentration (68.6%). Of those 284 people, 221 people (77.8%) were not taking LLT. This group included 156 urban residents (70.6%) or, by sex, 85 men (38.4%).

The 111 participants with ASCVD, DM and CKD were assigned to the moderate CVR group. The target concentration was reached by 55 participants (49.5%).

The number of participants with ASCVD, DM and CKD with moderate CVR who did not reach the target LDL-c concentration amounted to 56 (50.5%). Of those, 16 patients (28.6% of the subgroup) were using pharmacological treatment for lipid disorders. In contrast, 40 participants in the study (71.4% of the subgroup not meeting LDL target criteria) refused such treatment.

A total of 303 participants without ASCVD, DM and CKD were allocated to the moderate CVR group. The target concentration was reached by 75 participants (24.8%).

The group without ASCVD, DM and CKD with moderate CVR who did not reach the target LDL concentration included 228 participants (75.2%). Of those, 47 participants (20.6% of the subgroup) were using pharmacological treatment for lipid disorders. In contrast, 181 participants (79.4% of the subgroup of those not meeting the target LDL-c concentration criteria) refused such treatment.

3.2.3. Patients Classified in the High CVR Group

There were 612 patients (47.6%) in the high CVR group. Only 50 patients reached the target LDL-c concentration (8.2%), while up to 562 patients (91.8%) had impaired lipid metabolism. Of the 562 people who did not reach the target LDL-c concentration for a given CVR, 383 were not taking LLT (68.1%). This group included 274 urban residents (71.5%) or, by sex, 125 men (32.6%).

A total of 63 individuals with ASCVD, DM, CKD were assigned to the high CVR group. The target concentration was reached by 12 participants (19%).

The group of those with ASCVD, DM, CKD with a high CVR who did not reach the target LDL-c concentration included 51 people (81%). Of those, 15 people (29.4% of the subgroup) were using pharmacological treatment for lipid disorders. In contrast, 36 study participants (70.6% of the subgroup of people not meeting the target LDL-c concentration criteria) refused such treatment.

A total of 549 participants were allocated to the group without ASCVD, DM and CKD with high CVR. Of those, 38 (6.9%) met the target LDL-c concentration criteria.

The group of 511 participants (93.1%) without ASCVD, DM and CKD represented those who did not meet the target LDL-c concentration criteria in the group with high CVR. Of those, 164 participants (32.1% of the subgroup) were taking LLT. In contrast, 347 people (67.9% of the subgroup) refused treatment.

3.2.4. Patients Classified as Having a Very High CVR

In the case of very high CVR, out of 49 people (3.8%), as many as 48 people (98%) did not reach the target LDL-c concentration. Among those individuals, 36 people (75%) were not taking LLT—22 urban residents (61.1%) or, by gender, 19 men (50%).

In the group of patients without comorbidities, such as ASCVD, DM and CKD, there were no patients meeting the criteria for very high CVR.

Outcomes by patients counted according to the SCORE2 scale and patients with DM, CKD and ASCVD are shown in Figure 1.

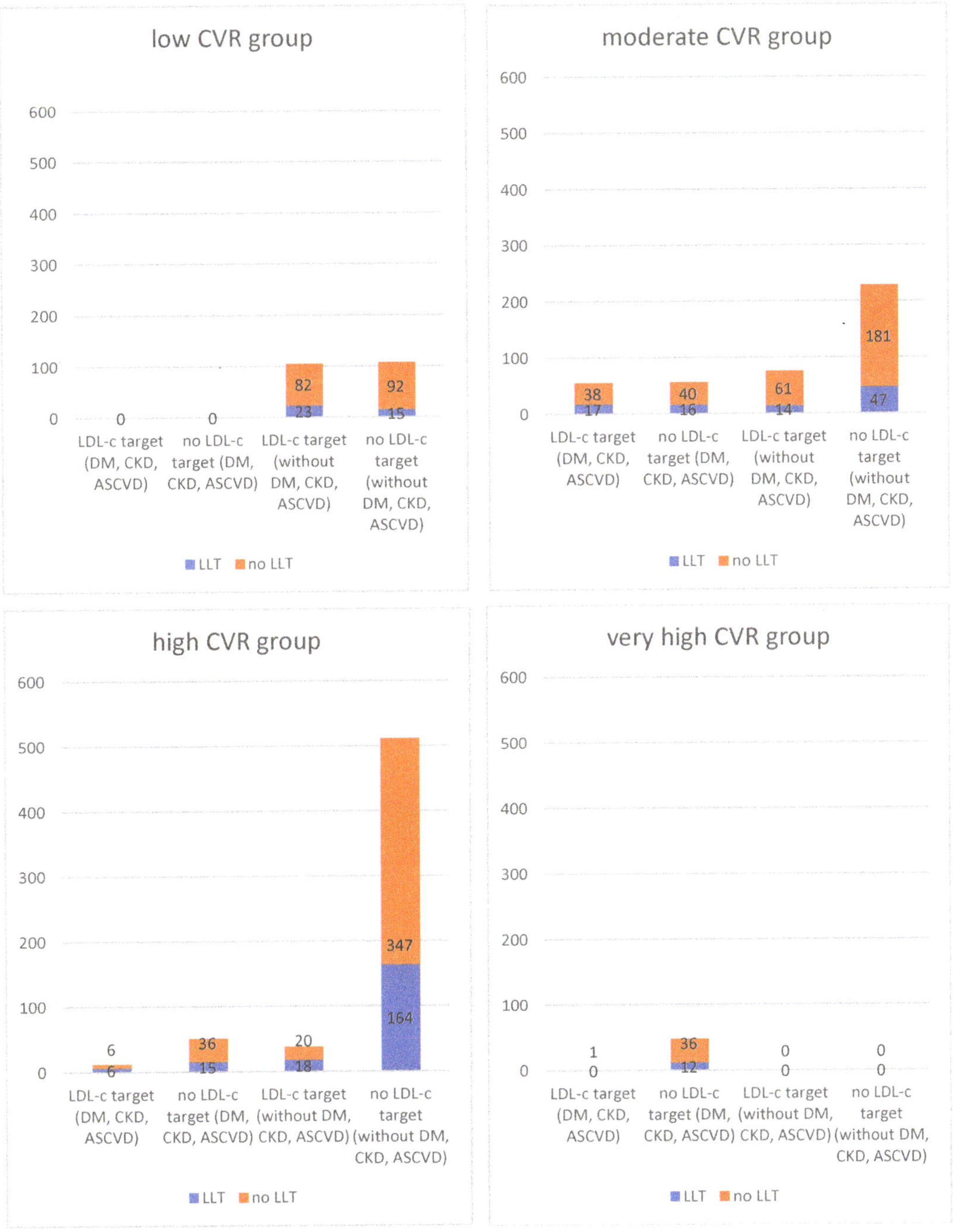

Figure 1. Outcomes by patients counted according to the SCORE2 scale and patients with DM, CKD and ASCVD.

4. Discussion

CVR assessment remains one of the primary tools for primary prevention. In August/September 2021, the European Society of Cardiology approved the SCORE2 and SCORE2-OP scales for use. They allow for estimation of an individual's risk of cardiovascular events over the next 10 years in apparently healthy individuals. Unlike their predecessor, the SCORE scale, they calculate the risk not only of fatal episodes due to cardiovascular disease, but also of non-fatal episodes such as strokes and heart attacks. Also updated from its predecessor is the consideration of nHDL-c concentration (the difference between total cholesterol and HDL-cholesterol (HDL-c) concentration) instead of total cholesterol concentration. Due to the proatherogenic effect of apoB-containing lipoproteins, thereby contributing to the formation and progression of atherosclerotic plaques, it is important to correctly estimate their amount. The concentration of LDL cholesterol can be influenced by the concentration of triglycerides; so, according to later studies and recent guidelines, the determination of n-HDL cholesterol is preferred for the determination of CVR [17,18].

Another novelty is the approach to people over 70 years of age. Included in this population are analyses that take into account competing risks; that is, deaths from causes other than CVD. The SCORE2-OP algorithm estimates the five-year and 10-year incidence of non-fatal and fatal cardiovascular events adjusted for competing risks in apparently healthy individuals over 70 years of age [3].

Calculating an individual's CVR is the first and most important step in primary prevention. Once the patient is classified into the appropriate group, we can adopt an individualized strategy. Starting with education, it is important to remember that a patient can be moved to a lower risk category by influencing modifiable risk factors through lifestyle changes. First and foremost, patients should be encouraged to quit smoking, as this element is one of the strongest modulators of cardiovascular disease [19]. Other aspects that can be improved include increased physical activity and proper nutrition, which reduces BMI (body mass index), which has a positive effect on CVR [20] and also has a positive effect on lipidogram profile. From a clinical point of view, one of the most important issues is the control and possible treatment of hypertension. This is a modifiable risk factor, an increase of which above established norms has a linear effect on increasing CVR [21].

Patients in the high and very high CVR groups should receive special attention and care. In our study, they accounted for more than half of all participants: 612 people (47.6%) in the high group and 49 people (3.8%) in the very high-risk group, respectively. For such individuals, pharmacological treatment of the modifiable CVD risk factors described above should be strongly considered for high and recommended for very high CVR [14]. In the absence of risk factor reduction by non-pharmacological methods, pharmacological methods, including LLT, should be considered.

In our study, 91.8% of those in the high CVR group and 98% of those in the very high CVR group did not meet the target LDL-c concentration criterion, a strong risk factor for cardiovascular disease [22,23]. Of those who did not meet the target LDL-c concentration, 68.1% of those in the high CVR group were not taking LLT. The percentage of such individuals in the high-risk group was 75%.

Pajak et al., in the WOBASZ II study, described that 60% of respondents with hypercholesterolemia were unaware of the condition, and only 6% of respondents were treated and achieved the recommended therapeutic goal. The WOBASZ II survey conducted in 2013–2014 was the second edition of the cross-sectional WOBASZ survey conducted on random samples of the Polish population in 2003–2005. One of the findings was that, relative to the first edition, the level of hypercholesterolemia remained stable and high [24].

One of the goals of the PURE study is to compare the risk factors for lifestyle diseases of urban and rural populations. Our results show that, in each risk group of people not meeting the target LDL-c concentration, urban residents were in the majority. This was 73.8% in the low CVR group, 67.6% in the moderate CVR group, 69.4% in the high CVR group and 62.5% in the very high group, respectively. One of the strongest inducers of lipid disorders is obesity. Anza-Ramirez et al. described, in their article, that residents of more densely populated cities are more likely to have increased BMI and obesity compared to those living in less urban areas [25]. Jungah et al. similarly showed a strong correlation between greater urbanization and obesity among the population in Seoul [26]. Carrillo-Larco et al. described a higher prevalence of obesity in people from urban areas and rural migrants compared to people from rural backgrounds [27].

Failure to meet the target LDL-c concentration criterion can have various causes. For those who do not require pharmacological intervention, the cause may be an abnormal lifestyle associated with an unhealthy diet. Such a group consists of people who are younger and without multimorbidity. In other cases, there is often a delay in the doctor's inclusion of appropriate treatment. Currently, LLT is included at too late a stage. This affects the patient as an individual, as well as the overall economics of the health care system. Ciaran et al. described the significant cost-effectiveness of prophylactic statin treatment for the health care system [28].

Among those who require pharmacological intervention, the reasons for the alarmingly low percentage of patients who do not achieve target LDL levels and do not adhere to LLT may include economic considerations, lack of access to healthcare or medications, overly complicated treatment regimens, the patient's general condition, and intentional nonadherence related to lack of faith in the effectiveness of prescribed medications or fear of their side effects. Choudry et al. described that, in a cohort of U.S. retired post-MI patients with significantly lower incomes, only 38.6% were receiving statins [29]. Nieuwerk et al. studied the effect of active counselling on adherence to statin use. Patients were randomly assigned to a standard care group and a group in which the intervention consisted of individualized, nurse-led counselling. At the end of the study, patient-reported adherence to LLT was significantly higher in the intervention group (100% vs. 95%; $p < 0.05$) [30].

Patient noncompliance is also influenced by the chronic nature of the disease and the need for long-term, largely indefinite treatment [31]. It is also necessary to take into account the diverse substrate of hyperlipidemia, the heterogeneity of this condition (including atherogenic hyperlipidemia), and thus the possible different treatment regimens [32]. Khan et al., in their article, highlighted the role of ezetimibe and PCSK9 inhibitors in reducing non-fatal myocardial infarctions and strokes [33]. Currently, these drug groups are rarely included by physicians and represent a negligible proportion of LLT.

5. Conclusions

In our study, we showed that 91.8% of patients in the high CVR group and 98% in the very high CVR group did not meet the target LDL-c criterion. Moreover, 68.1% of those in the first described group and 75% in the second group were not taking LLT. It is important to remember that even a small reduction in LDL-c levels in patients with high or very high CVR can improve prognosis and reduce the absolute number of vascular events in the future [34]. Greater awareness among practising physicians may lead to a greater focus on the problem and, as a result, a reduction in CVR in more people. Achieving target LDL levels while reducing CVR can be achieved by educating the patient on lifestyle changes, including diet, or, if ineffective, by incorporating LLT into treatment and then enforcing medical recommendations.

Author Contributions: Conceptualization, K.Z. and A.S.; methodology, P.L. and K.P.-Z.; software, P.L.; validation, M.W., P.L. and K.P.-Z.; formal analysis, P.L.; investigation, M.W., K.P.-Z. and P.L.; resources, K.Z., A.S., M.W., K.P.-Z. and P.L.; data curation, M.W. and P.L.; writing (original draft preparation), P.L.; writing (review and editing), A.S. and K.Z.; visualization, A.S.; supervision, K.Z. and A.S.; project administration, M.W., K.Z. and A.S.; funding acquisition, K.Z. and A.S. All authors have read and agreed to the published version of the manuscript.

Funding: This research received no external funding.

Institutional Review Board Statement: The study was conducted in accordance with the Declaration of Helsinki and approved by the Ethics Committee of Wroclaw Medical University (no. KB-443/2006).

Informed Consent Statement: Informed consent was obtained from all subjects involved in the study.

Data Availability Statement: The data are available upon request.

Conflicts of Interest: The authors declare no conflict of interest.

References

1. Raport: Sytuacja Zdrowotna Ludności Polski i Jej Uwarunkowania. Available online: https://www.pzh.gov.pl/raport-sytuacja-zdrowotna-ludnosci-polski-i-jej-uwarunkowania (accessed on 3 April 2023).
2. SCORE2 Working Group and ESC Cardiovascular risk Collaboration. SCORE2 risk prediction algorithms: New models to estimate 10-year risk of cardiovascular disease in Europe. *Eur. Heart J.* **2021**, *42*, 2439–2454. [CrossRef]
3. SCORE2-OP Working Group and ESC Cardiovascular Risk Collaboration. SCORE2-OP risk prediction algorithms: Estimating incident cardiovascular event risk in older persons in four geographical risk regions. *Eur. Heart J.* **2021**, *42*, 2455–2467. [CrossRef] [PubMed]
4. Dudina, A.; Cooney, M.T.; Bacquer, D.D.; Backer, G.D.; Ducimetière, P.; Jousilahti, P.; Keil, U.; Menotti, A.; Njølstad, I.; Oganov, R.; et al. Relationships between body mass index, cardiovascular mortality, and risk factors: A report from the SCORE investigators. *Eur. J. Cardiovasc. Prev. Rehabil.* **2011**, *18*, 731–742. [CrossRef] [PubMed]
5. Cornelius, M.E.; Wang, T.W.; Jamal, A.; Loretan, C.G.; Neff, L.J. Tobacco Product Use Among Adults—United States, 2019. *MMWR Morb. Mortal Wkly. Rep.* **2020**, *69*, 1736–1742. [CrossRef] [PubMed]
6. Ward, S.; Lloyd Jones, M.; Pandor, A.; Holmes, M.; Ara, R.; Ryan, A.; Yeo, W.; Payne, N. A systematic review and economic evaluation of statins for the prevention of coronary events. *Health Technol. Assess.* **2007**, *11*, 1–160. [CrossRef] [PubMed]
7. Aznaouridis, K.; Masoura, C.; Vlachopoulos, C.; Tousoulis, D. Statins in Stroke. *Curr. Med. Chem.* **2019**, *26*, 6174–6185. [CrossRef] [PubMed]
8. Almeida, S.O.; Budoff, M. Effect of statins on atherosclerotic plaque. *Trends Cardiovasc. Med.* **2019**, *29*, 451–455. [CrossRef] [PubMed]
9. Zatońska, K.; Zatoński, W.A.; Szuba, A. Prospective urban and rural epidemiology Poland—Study design. *J. Health Inequalities* **2016**, *2*, 136–141. [CrossRef]
10. Polskie Towarzystwo. Diabetologiczne. Zalecenia kliniczne dotyczące postępowania u chorych na cukrzycę 2019. *Diabetol. Prakt.* **2019**, *5*, 7–10.
11. Teo, K.; Chow, C.K.; Vaz, M.; Rangarajan, S.; Yusuf, S.; PURE Investigators-Writing Group. The Prospective Urban Rural Epidemiology (PURE) study: Examining the impact of societal influences on chronic noncommunicable diseases in low-, middle-, and high-income countries. *Am. Heart J.* **2009**, *158*, 1–7.e1. [CrossRef]
12. Szuba, A.; Martynowicz, H.; Zatońska, K.; Ilow, R.; Regulska-Ilow, B.; Różańska, D.; Wołyniec, M.; Połtyn-Zaradna, K.; Zatoński, W. Prevalence of hypertension in Polish population of PURE Poland study. *J. Health Inequalities* **2016**, *2*, 157–162. [CrossRef]
13. World Health Organization. Disease Burden and Mortality Estimates. Available online: https://www.who.int/data/gho/data/themes/mortality-and-global-health-estimates (accessed on 5 April 2023).
14. Visseren, F.L.; Mach, F.; Smulders, Y.M.; Carballo, D.; Koskinas, K.C.; Back, M.; Benetos, A.; Biffi, A.; Boavida, J.M.; Capodanno, D.; et al. 2021 ESC guidelines on cardiovascular disease prevention in clinical practice. *Eur. Heart J.* **2021**, *42*, 3227–3337. [CrossRef] [PubMed]
15. Livingstone, S.J.; Looker, H.C.; Hothersall, E.J.; Wild, S.H.; Lindsay, R.S.; Chalmers, J.; Cleland, S.; Leese, G.P.; McKnight, J.; Morris, A.D.; et al. Risk of cardiovascular disease and total mortality in adults with type 1 diabetes: Scottish registry linkage study. *PLoS Med.* **2012**, *9*, e1001321. [CrossRef] [PubMed]
16. Sattar, N.; Rawshani, A.; Franzén, S.; Rawshani, A.; Svensson, A.M.; Rosengren, A.; McGuire, D.K.; Eliasson, B.; Gudbjörnsdottir, S. Age at diagnosis of type 2 diabetes mellitus and associations with cardiovascular and mortality risks. *Circulation* **2019**, *139*, 2228–2237. [CrossRef] [PubMed]
17. Pischon, T.; Girman, C.J.; Sacks, F.M.; Rifai, N.; Stampfer, M.J.; Rimm, E.B. Non-high-density lipoprotein cholesterol and apolipoprotein B in the prediction of coronary heart disease in men. *Circulation* **2005**, *112*, 3375–3383. [CrossRef] [PubMed]
18. Ridker, P.M.; Rifai, N.; Cook, N.R.; Bradwin, G.; Buring, J.E. Non-HDL cholesterol, apolipoproteins A-I and B100, standard lipid measures, lipid ratios, and CRP as risk factors for cardiovascular disease in women. *JAMA* **2005**, *294*, 326–333. [CrossRef] [PubMed]
19. Larsson, S.C.; Burgess, S. Appraising the causal role of smoking in multiple diseases: A systematic review and meta-analysis of Mendelian randomization studies. *EBioMedicine* **2022**, *82*, 104154. [CrossRef]
20. Samson, R.; Ennezat, P.V.; Le Jemtel, T.H.; Oparil, S. Cardiovascular Disease Risk Reduction and Body Mass Index. *Curr. Hypertens. Rep.* **2022**, *24*, 535–546. [CrossRef]
21. Whelton, S.P.; McEvoy, J.W.; Shaw, L.; Psaty, B.M.; Lima, J.A.; Budoff, M.; Nasir, K.; Szklo, M.; Blumenthal, R.S.; Blaha, M.J. Association of normal systolic blood pressure level with cardiovascular disease in the absence of risk factors. *JAMA Cardiol.* **2020**, *5*, 1011–1018. [CrossRef]
22. Duarte Lau, F.; Giugliano, R.P. Lipoprotein(a) and its Significance in Cardiovascular Disease: A Review. *JAMA Cardiol.* **2022**, *7*, 760–769. [CrossRef]

23. Klop, B.; Elte, J.W.; Cabezas, M.C. Dyslipidemia in obesity: Mechanisms and potential targets. *Nutrients* **2013**, *5*, 1218–1240. [CrossRef] [PubMed]
24. Pająk, A.; Szafraniec, K.; Polak, M.; Polakowska, M.; Kozela, M.; Piotrowski, W.; Kwaśniewska, M.; Podolecka, E.; Kozakiewicz, K.; Tykarski, A.; et al. Changes in the prevalence, treatment, and control of hypercholesterolemia and other dyslipidemias over 10 years in Poland: The WOBASZ study. *Pol. Arch. Med. Wewn.* **2016**, *126*, 642–652. [CrossRef] [PubMed]
25. Anza-Ramirez, C.; Lazo, M.; Zafra-Tanaka, J.H.; Avila-Palencia, I.; Bilal, U.; Hernández-Vásquez, A.; Knoll, C.; Lopez-Olmedo, N.; Mazariegos, M.; Moore, K.; et al. The urban built environment and adult BMI, obesity, and diabetes in Latin American cities. *Nat. Commun.* **2022**, *13*, 7977. [CrossRef] [PubMed]
26. Kim, J.; Shon, C.; Yi, S. The Relationship between Obesity and Urban Environment in Seoul. *Int. J. Environ. Res. Public Health* **2017**, *14*, 898. [CrossRef] [PubMed]
27. Carrillo-Larco, R.M.; Bernabé-Ortiz, A.; Pillay, T.D.; Gilman, R.H.; Sanchez, J.F.; Poterico, J.A.; Quispe, R.; Smeeth, L.; Miranda, J.J. Obesity risk in rural, urban and rural-to-urban migrants: Prospective results of the PERU MIGRANT study. *Int. J. Obes.* **2016**, *40*, 181–185. [CrossRef] [PubMed]
28. Kohli-Lynch, C.N.; Lewsey, J.; Boyd, K.A.; French, D.D.; Jordan, N.; Moran, A.E.; Sattar, N.; Preiss, D.; Briggs, A.H. Beyond 10-Year Risk: A Cost-Effectiveness Analysis of Statins for the Primary Prevention of Cardiovascular Disease. *Circulation* **2022**, *145*, 1312–1323. [CrossRef]
29. Choudhry, N.K.; Setoguchi, S.; Levin, R.; Winkelmayer, W.C.; Shrank, W.H. Trends in adherence to secondary prevention medications in elderly post-myocardial infarction patients. *Pharmacoepidemiol. Drug Saf.* **2008**, *17*, 1189–1196. [CrossRef]
30. Nieuwkerk, P.T.; Nierman, M.C.; Vissers, M.N.; Locadia, M.; Greggers-Peusch, P.; Knape, L.P.; Kastelein, J.J.; Sprangers, M.A.; de Haes, H.C.; Stroes, E.S. Intervention to improve adherence to lipid-lowering medication and lipid-levels in patients with an increased cardiovascular risk. *Am. J. Cardiol.* **2012**, *110*, 666–672. [CrossRef]
31. Haynes, R.B.; McKibbon, K.A.; Kanani, R. Systematic review of randomised trials of interventions to assist patients to follow prescriptions for medications. *Lancet* **1996**, *348*, 383–386. [CrossRef]
32. Hagström, E.; Steg, P.G.; Szarek, M.; Bhatt, D.L.; Bittner, V.A.; Danchin, N.; Diaz, R.; Goodman, S.G.; Harrington, R.A.; Jukema, J.W.; et al. Apolipoprotein B, Residual Cardiovascular Risk After Acute Coronary Syndrome, and Effects of Alirocumab. *Circulation* **2022**, *146*, 657–672. [CrossRef]
33. Khan, S.U.; Yedlapati, S.H.; Lone, A.N.; Hao, Q.; Guyatt, G.; Delvaux, N.; Bekkering, G.E.T.; Vandvik, P.O.; Riaz, I.B.; Li, S.; et al. PCSK9 inhibitors and ezetimibe with or without statin therapy for cardiovascular risk reduction: A systematic review and network meta-analysis. *BMJ* **2022**, *377*, e069116. [CrossRef] [PubMed]
34. Mihaylova, B.; Emberson, J.; Blackwell, L.; Keech, A.; Simes, J.; Barnes, E.H.; Voysey, M.; Gray, A.; Collins, R.; Baigent, C. The effects of lowering LDL cholesterol with statin therapy in people at low risk of vascular disease: Meta-analysis of individual data from 27 randomised trials. *Lancet* **2012**, *380*, 581–590. [CrossRef] [PubMed]

Journal of
Clinical Medicine

MDPI

Article

The Dynamics of Cardiovascular Risk—An Analysis of the Prospective Urban Rural Epidemiology (PURE) Poland Cohort Study

Paweł Lubieniecki [1,*], Łukasz Lewandowski [2], Maria Wołyniec [3], Katarzyna Połtyn-Zaradna [3], Katarzyna Zatońska [3,4] and Andrzej Szuba [5]

[1] Clinical Department of Diabetology and Internal Disease, Wroclaw Medical University, Borowska Street 213, 50-556 Wroclaw, Poland
[2] Department of Medical Biochemistry, Wroclaw Medical University, Chalubinskiego 10, 50-368 Wroclaw, Poland; lukasz.lewandowski@umw.edu.pl
[3] Population Health Department, Wroclaw Medical University, 50-345 Wrocław, Poland; maria.wolyniec@umw.edu.pl (M.W.); katarzyna.poltyn-zaradna@umw.edu.pl (K.P.-Z.); katarzyna.zatonska@umw.edu.pl (K.Z.)
[4] Calisia University, 62-800 Kalisz, Poland
[5] Clinical Department of Angiology and Internal Disease, Wroclaw Medical University, Borowska Street 213, 50-556 Wroclaw, Poland; andrzej.szuba@umw.edu.pl
* Correspondence: pawel.lubieniecki@usk.wroc.pl

Abstract: Background: The purpose of this study was to analyze the major cardiovascular risk (CVR) factors and their trends in the study population. **Methods**: The results of subjects in the Polish Prospective Urban and Rural Epidemiological Study (PURE) study group were interpreted. CVR was calculated for each participant according to the Systematic Coronary Risk Evaluation (SCORE2) scale or the Systematic Coronary Risk Evaluation–Older Persons (SCORE2–OP) scale. Data from the beginning of the analysis (2013) and nine years later (2022) were included. In addition, the use of lipid–lowering therapy (LLT) and meeting the low–density lipoprotein cholesterol (LDL–c) target criterion at the beginning and end of the study were analyzed. **Results**: Patients in the high and very high CVR groups who had abnormal LDL–c results accounted for 64% and 91% of their group in 2013 and 70% and 92% in 2022, respectively. **Conclusions**: Regardless of age, patients using LLT at the start of the analysis had a greater increase in future CVR, especially if they had lipid abnormalities at the start of the study. This may be due to reverse causality and multimorbidity in these patients, highlighting the importance of appropriate treatment of lipid abnormalities.

Keywords: epidemiological study; cardiovascular risk; lipid–lowering therapy

1. Introduction

Data from the latest World Heart Federation (WHF) report show that the number of deaths worldwide from cardiovascular causes increased from 12.1 million in 1990 to 20.5 million in 2021. A total of 80% of the deaths occurred in low– and middle–income countries (LMICs) [1]. In Poland, classified as a high–income country, the Polish Society of Cardiology estimates that cardiovascular disease (CVD) accounts for 37% of all deaths. Given the constant progress and developments in various aspects of medicine, such as improvements in endovascular techniques, imaging, or the introduction of new drugs and the optimization of treatment regimens for CVD and comorbidities, these figures are particularly worrying.

In line with the Hippocratic maxim "prevention is better than cure", as a society, we should place greater emphasis on primary prevention, that is, by controlling potential risk factors, and preventing disease before it occurs. Such non–specific primary prevention of CVD includes education, which should be the cornerstone of any healthy society. Even the smallest lifestyle interventions can be fundamental to quality of life and reduction of major adverse cardiovascular events (MACE). These modifiable aspects include regular physical activity, a diet based on healthy eating principles and possible weight reduction, smoking cessation, and stress reduction.

Other modifiable risk factors are lipid disorders and abnormal blood pressure measurements. According to data from the National Health Fund, hypercholesterolemia is present in almost 60% of the adult Polish population and hypertension has been diagnosed in almost 10 million Poles [2]. The WOBASZ II study described a situation in which 60% of the study group with hypercholesterolemia were unaware of their current lipid disorders, and only 6% of participants had properly treated lipid management [3]. Similarly, lack of knowledge in the population characterizes the second modifiable risk factor, hypertension. Nowicki et al. described a situation in which only 55.33% of respondents identified hypertension as a cardiovascular risk factor (CVR) [4].

Two of the latest tools for predicting cardiovascular events are the SCORE2 (Systematic Coronary Risk Estimation2) scale and the SCORE2–OP (Systematic Coronary Risk Estimation2–Older Persons) scale for people without diagnosed atherosclerotic cardiovascular disease (ASCVD), chronic kidney disease (CKD), or diabetes mellitus (DM). The resulting score is a measure of the 10–year risk of CVD (heart attack, stroke) leading or not leading to death. The risk calculation takes into account smoking, gender, age, non–high–density lipoprotein–cholesterol fraction (nHDL–c), and systolic blood pressure (SBP). For people with CVD, DM, or CKD, the risk is determined according to current guidelines [5,6], taking into account the duration of the disease, laboratory parameters, or the presence of complications.

These models, and their results, can be used to inform patients about potential risks, the benefits of lifestyle modification, or the initiation of appropriate treatment. They can facilitate shared strategic decision–making between clinicians and patients regarding CVD risk management.

The aim of the study was to analyze trends in individual risk factors, achievement of lipid control goals and blood pressure measurements, and use of antihypertensive (AT) and lipid–lowering treatment (LLT) in the entire study cohort, as well as in individual CVR groups. The results are presented below.

2. Materials and Methods

2.1. Study Group

The analyzed group consisted of participants in the Polish part of the Prospective Urban and Rural Epidemiological (PURE) study residing in Wroclaw and surrounding rural areas. Each participant gave written consent to participate in long–term follow–up with periodic health monitoring. Data were collected during direct contact with each participant in cycles of every 3 years, starting in 2007. Information from 2013 and 2022 on patients without ASCVD, CKD, and DM was included in this study, as it was in these editions that all data necessary for the relevant analyses were available. The Bioethics Committee at the Medical University of Wroclaw gave a positive opinion on the conduct of the study in 2007 (No. KB–443/2006).

The survey instrument consisted of individual questionnaires on lifestyle, chronic diseases, or pharmacotherapy used, as well as home questionnaires. In addition, blood pressure was measured twice in each participant and anthropometric examinations including measurements of height, weight, and waist and hip circumference were performed. Venous blood was also collected, in which lipid profile and renal function parameters were determined. Participants over the age of 35 who gave informed verbal and written consent were included in the study, according to the guidelines of the PURE study. There was no exclusion criterion [7,8].

In this study, we used the SCORE2 and SCORE2–OP scales for a high–risk country. Poland was assigned to this category based on national CVD mortality rates published by WHO [9]. Then, based on age, sex, smoking, nHDL–c levels, and systolic blood pressure, an individual CVR was calculated for each patient, and the participant was assigned to one of four categories—low, moderate, high, or very high risk according to the SCORE2 and SCORE2–OP tables—appropriate for value and age [10,11].

The analysis in this study did not include individuals with significant cardiovascular disease, renal disease, or carbohydrate disorders. These individuals were assigned to the high or very high CVR category based on relevant guidelines [5].

2.2. Statistical Analyses

Data preprocessing, statistical modelling, and visualization were performed in STATISTICA 13.3 on the license of Wroclaw Medical University. Multi–way repeated measures ANOVA was performed to explore the multi–factor–adjusted (marginal) effect of factors (effects) taken into account in this study on the time–wise change (2013 vs. 2022, denoted as "TIME" in the manuscript) in CVR. This analysis was performed on the whole set of 2nd–degree interactions between "TIME" and each effect, in one model.

Subsequently, higher–degree effects were explored to analyze the influence of treatment– and demographical–related effects on treatment–wise changes in the time–related dynamics of the CVR. For this purpose, 3rd– or (eventually) 4th–order interactions were analyzed in the process of derivation of separate models and expanding them with new features. $p < 0.05$ was considered significant.

3. Results

3.1. Overall Outcomes of the Study Cohort and Lipid Disorder Scores in Each CVR Group

In 2013, the population sample counted 1153 participants. These were individuals who had a set of necessary data and a CVR group could be calculated for them. In 2022, 9 years later, the group represented 995 people. A total of 113 people refused to participate further in the study and 45 people died. The low CVR group in 2013 comprised 333 people. A total of 31% of this group had uncompensated lipid disorders, where 9 years later, in 2022, they already accounted for 57% of the total group (181 people). As for the group with moderate CVR, it included 459 people in 2013. Of this pool, 64% had abnormal LDL–c results; 9 years later, the group included 279 participants, and the percentage of those with lipid disorders had risen to 70%. In 2013, the group with high CVR included 361 participants. A total of 91% of participants in this group had elevated LDL–c levels. In 2022, the group size increased to 535 participants, and the percentage of those not meeting the target LDL–c criterion was 92%. There were no individuals in the cohort analyzed who fell into the very high CVR group. Detailed data are presented in Table 1.

Table 1. Distribution of participants by CVR group and meeting the target LDL–c concentration in 2013 and 2022.

	Low CVR	Moderate CVR	High CVR	Very High CVR
2013				
group size	333	459	361	0
have achieved the target LDL–c	229 (69%)	163 (36%)	32 (9%)	
have not achieved the target LDL–c concentration	104 (31%	296 (64%)	329 (91%)	
2022				
group size	181	279	535	0
have achieved the target LDL–c	78 (43%)	84 (30%)	56 (8%)	
have not achieved the target LDL–c concentration	103 (57%)	195 (70%)	(92%)	

3.2. *Time–Related Change in CVR and How the Selected Effects Modulated It in the Population Sample*

Based on the model (Table 2), the whole population showed a steep, approximately 59.94%, increase of the CVR (Figure 1A). Five variables in 2013 had an influence on these 9–year CVD risk dynamics, namely: age ($p < 0.001$), localization ($p \approx 0.026$), LLT ($p < 0.001$), hyperglycemia ($p \approx 0.033$), and whether the LDL–c target for the CVR was met ($p \approx 0.042$).

Table 2. Factorial analysis in context of changes of CVR over the studied time.

Hypothesis	SS	F	*p*
CVR did not change over the studied time...	290.20	41.28	<0.001
... and/or this trend was not affected by age	2149.78	305.83	<0.001
... and/or this trend was not affected by SBP	24.38	3.47	0.063
... and/or this trend was not affected by sex	3.10	0.44	0.507
... and/or this trend was not affected by localization	34.82	4.95	0.026
... and/or this trend was not affected by LLT	663.66	94.41	<0.001
... and/or this trend was not affected by AT	14.29	2.03	0.154
... and/or this trend was not affected by smoking status	10.45	1.49	0.223
... and/or this trend was not affected by hyperglycemic status	31.92	4.54	0.033
... and/or this trend was not affected by dyslipidemia (LDL–c > ref.)	29.23	4.16	0.042
... and/or this trend was not affected by obesity	6.99	0.99	0.319
–	7633.75		

Abbreviations: AT, anti–hypotensive treatment; LDL–c, low–density lipoprotein cholesterol; LLT, lipid–lowering therapy; SBP, systolic blood pressure; SS, sum of squares.

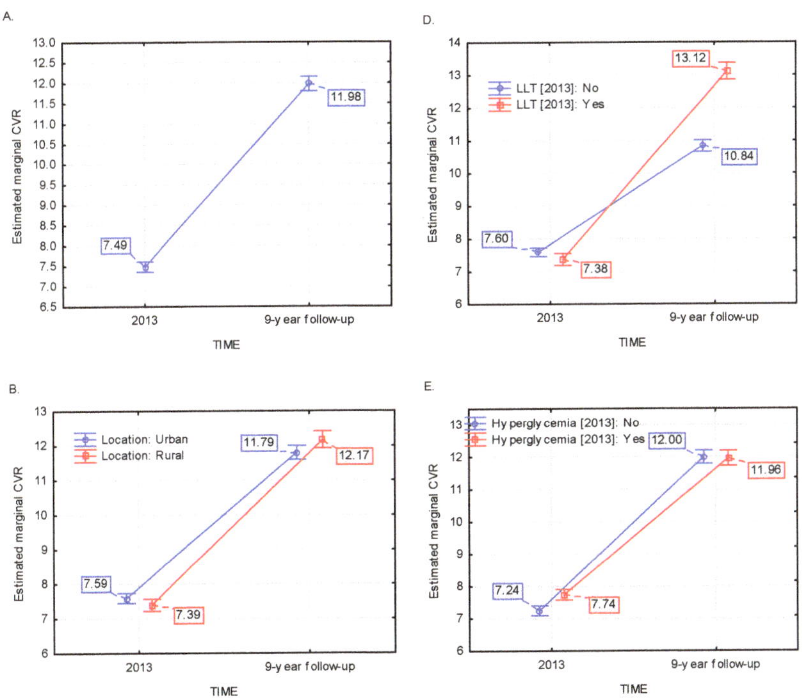

Figure 1. *Cont.*

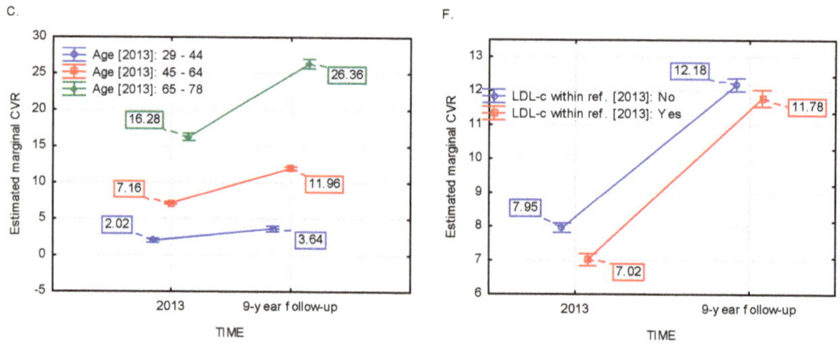

Figure 1. The dynamics of 9–year increase in CVR (**A**) and its change depending on effects (variables): localization (**B**), age (**C**), LLT (**D**), hyperglycemia (**E**) and meeting the LDL–c target for individual CVR (**F**).

Individuals living in rural areas were characterized by a 13.81% higher increase in CVR compared to those who lived in urban locations (Figure 1B). Moreover, the 9–year dynamics of CVR were positively associated with age (Figure 1C), reaching over 6.22–fold higher increase in individuals aged 65–78, compared to those aged 29–44. LLT in 2013 (Figure 1D), per se, was associated with approximately 77.16% higher increase of CVR compared to the stratum who was not subject to this treatment. Interestingly, hyperglycemia and meeting the LDL–c target level were associated with: 17.82% lower dynamics of CVR (Figure 1E) and 12.53% higher dynamics of CVR (Figure 1F), respectively.

3.3. Factors in 2013: Age, Localization, AT, and Meeting the CVR–Related LDL–c Target Value, Had a Significant Effect on How the LLT Was Associated with the Alteration of the 9–Year CVR Dynamics—Insights from the Analysis of 3rd– and 4th–Degree Interactions

Age more steeply influenced the 9–year dynamics of CVR among the individuals administered with LLT in 2013 ($p \approx 0.001$, Table A1). These individuals, compared to the subjects that did not receive such treatment, showed: 0.95, 2.74, and 3.76 percentage point higher 9–year increase of CVR at age strata: 29–44, 45–64, and 65–78, respectively (Figure 2).

The two different localizations (urban/rural) showed different dynamics in how the LLT in 2013 was associated with the 9–year dynamics of CVR ($p \approx 0.047$, Table A2). The inhabitants of rural areas who were admitted with LLT showed approximately 16.53% lower 9–year increase in CVR compared to individuals living in urban areas. However, among those under no LLT in 2013, the rural areas were associated with 12.15% higher increase in CVR, compared to urban (Figure 3).

The contrast in 9–year CVR dynamics in the context of LLT in 2013 (treatment vs. no treatment) was greater (2.01–fold vs. 1.63, Figure 4) among individuals who received AT in 2013 compared to those who did not receive it ($p \approx 0.007$, Table A3).

Interestingly, the association between LLT in 2013 and 9–year CVR dynamics was different depending on meeting the target LDL–c levels for CVR in individuals in 2013 ($p \approx 0.002$, Table A4). The LLT–wise contrast (treatment vs. no treatment) was lower among the individuals who met the target LDL–c level in 2013 compared to those who did not meet it (41.75% difference vs. 89.45% difference, Figure 5).

Since many factors influenced the association between 2013 with LLT and the 9–year dynamics in CVR, higher interactions (between more variables) were analyzed (Tables S1 and S2). Based on them, it could be stated that the association between age and the increase in 9–year CVR (Figure 3) was not affected by either the AT ($p \approx 0.885$, Table S1) or meeting the LDL–c target in 2013 ($p \approx 0.936$, Table S2). Moreover, the association between the LLT and the aforementioned risk (Figure 4) was not affected by the differences in localization ($p \approx 0.885$, Table S1). Interestingly, the simultaneous association between LLT and meeting the LDL–c target (in 2013) and the 9–year dynamics in CVR (Figure 5) was similar in urban and rural areas ($p \approx 0.936$, Table S2).

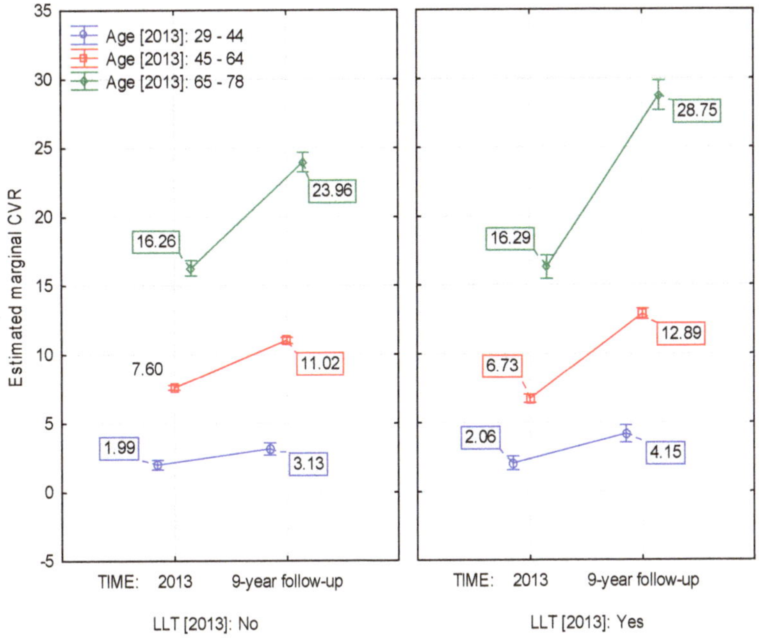

Figure 2. The influence of age in 2013 on the LLT–associated 9–year change in CVR.

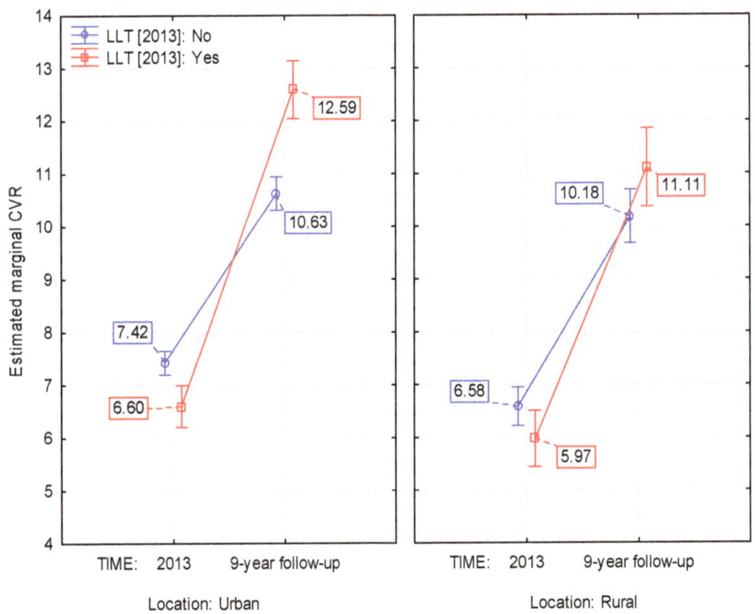

Figure 3. The influence of location in 2013 on the LLT–associated 9–year change in CVR.

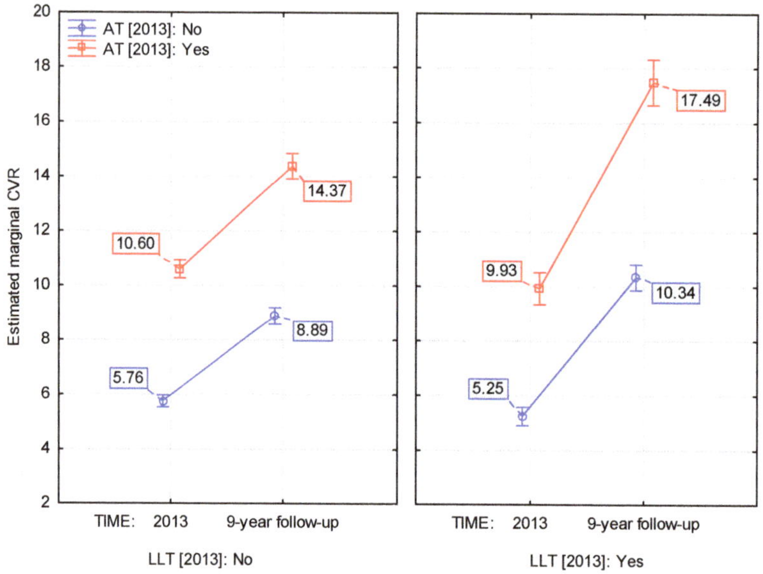

Figure 4. The association between AT in 2013 and the LLT–associated 9–year change in CVR.

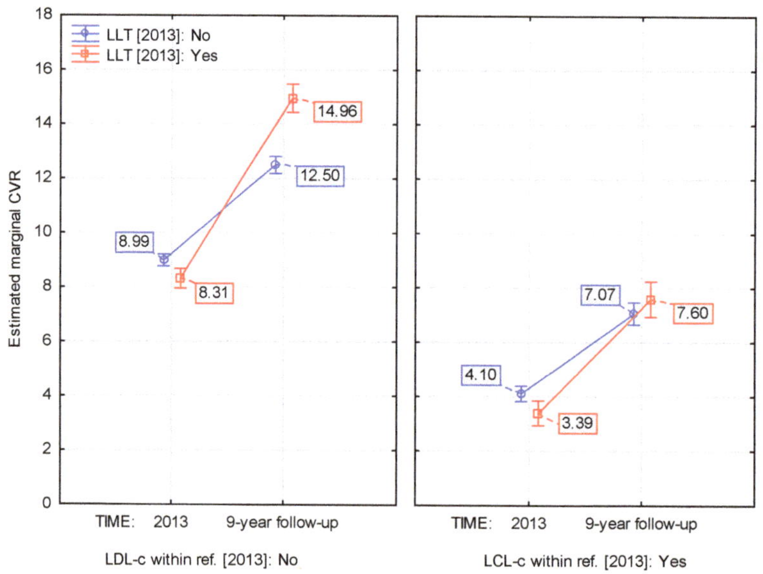

Figure 5. The influence of meeting the target LDL–c level in 2013 on the LLT–associated 9–year change in CVR.

4. Discussion

Nearly 20 million CVD–related deaths were reported in 2020, an increase of 18.7% from 2010 [12]. This shows the direction of challenges for modern medicine and how important it is to properly manage CVR. Both primary and secondary prevention have a place in the treatment of lipid disorders. In our study, we showed that people with abnormal lipid management results make up a larger proportion of each CVR group, and in subgroups with high CVR, they account for as much as 92%. Despite the passage of more years, greater public awareness, improvements in the diagnosis of hyperlipidemia, and improvements in LLT, the percentage of people with lipid problems has not decreased. Study after study shows how a very low percentage of people who qualify for LLT are actually treated. Mantel–Teeuwisse described the situation in the Dutch population, where only 3.2% of those eligible for LLT were both treated and controlled [13]. Hoerger et al. described in their study that 65% of those eligible for LLT receive no appropriate treatment [14]. Also, we, in our study related to the analysis of the Polish cohort of the PURE study, described that an overwhelming percentage of the group with high and very high CVR had abnormal LDL–c results (91.8% and 98%, respectively). Of these individuals, a significant proportion were not receiving LLT (68.1% and 75%, respectively) [15].

In our study, we showed that patients who used LLT during the initial analysis period had a higher risk of future CVD. This may be related to the phenomenon of reverse causality to which observational epidemiological studies are prone. It describes the relationship between two variables differently than one might expect. In a given situation, one of the variables is the cause, even though it appears to be the effect, and the other, by analogy, is the effect, despite the first impression that it might be the cause. Some refer to reverse causality as "cart–before–the–horse bias" to emphasize the unexpected nature of the correlation. In the study, this phenomenon was observed when the correlation between BMI (body mass index) and mortality was analyzed. Among the elderly, the highest risk was observed at low BMI levels. This was associated with unintentional weight loss with or without a diagnosed disease or a desire to improve health through proper nutrition [16,17].

Similarly, in our considerations, the outcome may have preceded its cause. LLT users, especially in the younger age categories, may have had poorer health, more disease compared to their peers, and thus a higher CVR. Physicians are more likely to start LLT in patients with this profile for secondary prevention than to implement the same treatment for primary prevention in a patient who is asymptomatic and without significant comorbidities. Therefore, it is important that all elements influencing CVR reduction are properly managed. One such component is the use of LLT and the reduction of lipid disorders. Numerous studies show that low adherence to LLT is associated with similar CVD mortality rates as placebo use. In contrast, adherence to LLT significantly reduces [18,19] the rate of cardiovascular events, such as coronary artery disease (CAD) without death, is significantly reduced when pharmacological recommendations are adhered to for a longer time [20]. An analogous situation exists for AT, where it has also been shown that each 20 mmHg reduction in SBP is associated with a twofold reduction in stroke mortality and a twofold difference in the rate of death from vascular causes such as ischemic heart disease [21].

Excessive LDL–c plays an important role in increasing CVR. There are several studies indicating its role in the initiation and progression of vascular disease [22,23]. In the above analysis, it was shown that abnormally elevated LDL–c levels at the beginning of the analysis period were associated with a significantly higher risk of future CVD. Similarly, the difference in future CVR increase between LLT users and non–users was higher in the group of individuals who did not achieve the target LDL–c concentration at the start of the analysis. This is supported by other analyses reporting that lowering LDL–c levels significantly reduces the incidence of myocardial infarction, revascularization or ischemic stroke [24]. Therefore, as Figorilli et al. emphasize, early identification of patients with LDL–c abnormalities and appropriate 10–year CVR stratification are the cornerstones of CVD prevention [25].

Recognition of lipid disorders and implementation of LLT is an essential component of secondary prevention of CVR reduction. The literature consistently shows results indicating a low percentage of patients adhering to recommendations and taking LLT [2–4]. Therefore, an important part of patient care is to promote appropriate health–promoting attitudes, including adherence to medical recommendations. To effectively promote the implementation of LLT, it is important to be aware of the limitations that contribute to such a high failure rate of implemented therapy.

Undoubtedly, socioeconomic status has a significant impact. A number of studies have shown the negative impact of rising drug fees on medication adherence [26,27]. LLT is often perceived by patients themselves as a low priority, and taking other medications, such as cardiovascular or antidiabetic drugs, is more important. The phenomenon of polypharmacy, or overuse of pills, also adversely affects the daily routine and every–time adherence. The solution is to use as many compounded preparations as possible. In addition to the excess of pills used daily, non–adherence is also influenced by the multiplicity of chronic diseases and their severity. Latry et al. showed that patients after a recent episode of myocardial infarction or with symptomatic heart disease had a higher rate of adherence to LLT use than those with chronic CAD and minimal symptoms or those using primary prevention [28].

Other reasons for poor adherence to LLT use include inadequate patient knowledge of the role and impact of cholesterol on CVR [29]. Insufficient education at the time of LLT inclusion can lead to a lack of acceptance of lipid disorder disease and skipping appropriate pharmacotherapy in daily life. In the Understanding Statin use in America and Gaps Education (USAGE) study, more than 10,000 respondents confirmed with their answers that adherence to statin use is affected by the manner and comprehensiveness of the physician's explanation at the time of statin inclusion about the role of cholesterol in CVR and the need to lower it [30]. Communicating potential side effects also has an impact on patient engagement. More extensive explanations of the advantages of statins over side effects, such as muscle symptoms, may contribute to less patient discouragement and more sustained adherence over time [31]. Inadequate information flow may also relate to communication between individual physicians. Kripalani et al. described that hospitalization summaries in the discharge chart are available in less than 34% of cases, and communication between the clinician and the primary care physician occurs in less than 20% of cases [32]. Poor communication can be an obstacle to compliance and discrepancies in medications prescribed in the hospital, which are not then monitored by the primary care physician.

Limitations on the part of the patient, as well as mistakes made by clinicians, affect non–adherence to medical recommendations for LLT. To improve treatment adherence rates, it is important not only to know why LLT is not being used on a daily basis, but also to provide active counseling. It has been shown that nurse–led interventions were associated with better lipid management than standard care. In a study where the intervention arm was a nurse, LDL cholesterol levels < 100 mg/dL were achieved in 97%, compared with 67% for standard care [33]. This shows how important and effective these smallest interventions are. Among these we can include a brief conversation, a reminder to use LLT at each visit. In considering the failure of the LLT used, we should also add the lack of escalation of the dose of the drug used, where low doses are repeatedly maintained.

Our analysis included the Polish cohort of the PURE study, which was designed to compare the lives of urban and rural residents in a number of ways. We showed that rural residents had a more dynamic increase in CVR overall and over time when they did not use LLT at the start of the analysis. In contrast, the increase in CVR over time was lower with hypolipemic treatment at the start of the analysis compared to urban residents. This may be influenced by poorer diagnosis of lipid disorders in rural residents and better treatment since diagnosis. The lifestyle of rural residents may determine higher mortality rates associated with chronic diseases such as cardiovascular disease, respiratory disease, kidney disease and diabetes. Such factors include smoking and obesity. Singh et al. describe that the prevalence of smoking was 16.9% in large metropolitan areas and 26.9% in non–metropolitan areas. Moreover, as recently as the 20th century, lung cancer mortality was significantly higher in metropolitan areas, while it is now higher in non–metropolitan areas [34]. The obesity problem also poses a greater challenge for rural residents. The prevalence of obesity in large metropolitan areas has increased 2.8–fold to 25.9% in recent years, while the prevalence of obesity in non–metropolitan areas has increased 3.5–fold to 33.2% [35]. In addition to individual lifestyle elements influencing the increase in CVR, systemic problems of rural areas must also be taken into account. These include disparities in access to health care. These can stem from cultural and financial constraints, which are often compounded by a shortage of qualified professionals and inadequate public transportation [36].

5. Conclusions

Treatment of lipid disorders is an important part of CVD prevention. Previous studies clearly show a low rate of LLT use, even if patients do not reach target LDL–c levels. In our study, we showed that this state of affairs has an impact on future CVR increases. Health–promoting education and raising awareness about the role of proper control and use of LLT is crucial to reducing CVD.

Supplementary Materials: The following supporting information can be downloaded at: https://www.mdpi.com/article/10.3390/jcm13133728/s1, Table S1: Three–way modulation of the change of CVR over time by: localization, LLT and AT—insights from logistic regression model with interactions. Table S2: Three–way modulation of the change of CVR over time by: localization, LLT and having LDL–c levels within the reference values in 2013—insights from logistic regression model with interactions.

Author Contributions: Conceptualization: A.S. and K.Z.; methodology: K.P.-Z., Ł.L. and P.L.; software: Ł.L. and P.L.; validation: K.P.-Z., P.L. and M.W.; formal analysis: P.L.; investigation: P.L., K.P.-Z. and M.W.; resources: M.W., K.P.-Z., P.L., A.S. and K.Z.; data curation: P.L., Ł.L. and M.W.; writing (original draft preparation): P.L.; writing (review and editing): K.Z. and A.S.; visualization: A.S.; supervision: A.S. and K.Z.; project administration: K.Z., A.S. and M.W.; funding acquisition: A.S. and K.Z. All authors have read and agreed to the published version of the manuscript.

Funding: The Polish Ministry of Science and Higher Education funded the Polish edition of the PURE study (grant number 290/W–PURE/2008/0). The study was also funded by the Medical University of Wroclaw, grant number SUBZ.E260.24.047.

Institutional Review Board Statement: The study was conducted in accordance with the Declaration of Helsinki and approved by the Ethics Committee of Wroclaw Medical University on 6 October 2006 (no. KB–443/2006).

Informed Consent Statement: Informed consent was obtained from all subjects involved in the study.

Data Availability Statement: The data are available upon request.

Conflicts of Interest: The authors declare no conflicts of interest.

Appendix A

Table A1. The influence of age in 2013 on the LLT–associated 9–year change in CVR—tabularized summary of the used logistic regression model.

Effect/Interaction	Hypothesis	SS	df	MS	F	*p*
TIME	CVR did not change over the studied time…	6251.61	1	6251.61	844.55	<0.001
(A) TIME × LLT [2013]	…and/or this trend was not affected by LLT	410.44	1	410.44	55.45	<0.001
(B) TIME × Age [2013]	…and/or this trend was not affected by age	1868.99	2	934.49	126.24	<0.001
TIME × LLT [2013] × Age [2013]	… and both above statements are not affected by differences in: age (A) or LLT (B)	103.52	2	51.76	6.99	0.001
Error		7898.24	1067	7.40		

SS—sums of squares; df—degrees of freedom; MS—mean square.

Table A2. The influence of location in 2013 on the LLT–associated 9–year change in CVR—tabularized summary of the used logistic regression model.

Effect/Interaction	Hypothesis	SS	df	MS	F	p
TIME	CVR did not change over the studied time...	7509.97	1	7509.97	820.27	<0.001
(A) TIME × Localization	... and/or this trend was not affected by localization	5.15	1	5.15	0.56	0.454
(B) TIME × LLT [2013]	... and/or this trend was not affected by LLT	437.21	1	437.21	47.75	<0.001
TIME × Localization ×LLT [2013]	... and both above statements were not affected by differences in: LLT (A) or localization (B)	36.37	1	36.37	3.97	0.047
Error		9787.17	1069	9.16		

SS—sums of squares; MS—mean square; df—degrees of freedom.

Table A3. The association between AT in 2013 and the LLT–associated 9–year change in CVR—tabularized summary of the used logistic regression model.

Effect/Interaction	Hypothesis	SS	df	MS	F	p
TIME	CVR did not change over the studied time...	7653.22	1	7653.22	849.73	<0.001
(A) TIME × LLT [2013]	... and/or this trend was not affected by LLT	663.04	1	663.04	73.62	<0.001
(B) TIME × AT [2013]	... and/or this trend was not affected by AT	194.08	1	194.08	21.55	<0.001
TIME × LLT [2013] × HT [2013]	... and both above statements were not affected by differences in: AT (A) or LLT (B)	65.59	1	65.59	7.28	0.007
Error		9628.09	1069	9.01		

df—degrees of freedom; MS—mean square; SS—sums of squares.

Table A4. The influence of meeting the target LDL–c level in 2013 on the LLT–associated 9–year change in CVR—tabularized summary of the used logistic regression model.

Effect/Interaction	Hypothesis	SS	df	MS	F	p
TIME	CVR did not change over the studied time...	7540.81	1	7540.81	840.51	<0.001
(A) TIME × LLT [2013]	... and/or this trend was not affected by LLT	479.22	1	479.22	53.42	<0.001
(B) TIME × LDL–c within reference value [2013]	... and/or this trend was not affected by dyslipidemia	223.45	1	223.45	24.91	<0.001
TIME × LLT [2013] × LDL–c within reference value [2013]	... and both above statements were not affected by differences in: dyslipidemic status (A) or LLT (B)	89.43	1	89.43	9.97	0.002
Error		9590.71	1069	8.97		

MS—mean square; df—degrees of freedom; SS—sums of squares.

References

1. Di Cesare, M.; Bixby, H.; Gaziano, T.; Hadeed, L.; Kabudula, C.; Vaca McGhie, D.; Mwangi, J.; Pervan, B.; Perel, P.; Piñeiro, D.; et al. *World Heart Report 2023: Confronting the World's Number One Killer*; World Heart Federation: Geneva, Switzerland, 2023.
2. National Health Fund of Poland. RAPORT NFZ: Nadciśnienie Tętnicze, Poland Government. 2022. Available online: https://www.nfz.gov.pl/aktualnosci/aktualnosci-centrali/raport-nfz-nadcisnienie-tetnicze,7352.html (accessed on 12 June 2024).
3. Pająk, A.; Szafraniec, K.; Polak, M.; Polakowska, M.; Kozela, M.; Piotrowski, W.; Kwaśniewska, M.; Podolecka, E.; Kozakiewicz, K.; Tykarski, A.; et al. Changes in the prevalence, treatment, and control of hypercholesterolemia and other dyslipidemias over 10 years in Poland: The WOBASZ study. *Pol. Arch. Med. Wewn.* **2016**, *126*, 642–652. [PubMed]
4. Nowicki, G.; Ślusarska, B.; Brzezicka, A. Analiza stanu wiedzy o czynnikach ryzyka chorób układu sercowo-naczyniowego wśród osób pracujących. *Nurs. Top.* **2009**, *17*, 321–327.
5. Visseren, F.L.J.; Mach, F.; Smulders, Y.M.; Carballo, D.; Koskinas, K.C.; Bäck, M.; Benetos, A.; Biffi, A.; Boavida, J.M.; Capodanno, D.; et al. 2021 ESC guidelines on cardiovascular disease prevention in clinical practice. *Eur. Heart J.* **2021**, *42*, 3227–3337. [CrossRef] [PubMed]
6. Livingstone, S.J.; Looker, H.C.; Hothersall, E.J.; Wild, S.H.; Lindsay, R.S.; Chalmers, J.; Cleland, S.; Leese, G.P.; McKnight, J.; Morris, A.D.; et al. Risk of cardiovascular disease and total mortality in adults with type 1 diabetes: Scottish registry linkage study. *PLoS Med.* **2012**, *9*, e1001321. [CrossRef] [PubMed]
7. Teo, K.; Chow, C.K.; Vaz, M.; Rangarajan, S.; Yusuf, S.; PURE Investigators-Writing Group. The Prospective Urban Rural Epidemiology (PURE) study: Examining the impact of societal influences on chronic noncommunicable diseases in low-, middle-, and high-income countries. *Am. Heart J.* **2009**, *158*, 1–7.e1. [CrossRef] [PubMed]
8. Zatońska, K.; Zatoński, W.A.; Szuba, A. Prospective urban and rural epidemiology Poland—Study design. *J. Health Inequal.* **2016**, *2*, 136–141. [CrossRef]
9. World Health Organization. Disease Burden and Mortality Estimates. Available online: https://www.who.int/data/gho/data/themes/mortality-and-global-health-estimates (accessed on 3 May 2024).
10. SCORE2 Working Group; ESC Cardiovascular Risk Collaboration. SCORE2 risk prediction algorithms: New models to estimate 10-year risk of cardiovascular disease in Europe. *Eur. Heart J.* **2021**, *42*, 2439–2454. [CrossRef]
11. SCORE2-OP Working Group; ESC Cardiovascular Risk Collaboration. SCORE2-OP risk prediction algorithms: Estimating incident cardiovascular event risk in older persons in four geographical risk regions. *Eur. Heart J.* **2021**, *42*, 2455–2467. [CrossRef] [PubMed]
12. Tsao, C.W.; Aday, A.W.; Almarzooq, Z.I.; Alonso, A.; Beaton, A.Z.; Bittencourt, M.S.; Boehme, A.K.; Buxton, A.E.; Carson, A.P.; Commodore-Mensah, Y.; et al. Heart Disease and Stroke Statistics-2022 Update: A Report From the American Heart Association. *Circulation* **2022**, *145*, e153–e639, Erratum in *Circulation* **2022**, *146*, e141. [CrossRef]
13. Mantel-Teeuwisse, A.K.; Verschuren, W.M.; Klungel, O.H.; Kromhout, D.; Lindemans, A.D.; Avorn, J.; Porsius, A.J.; de Boer, A. Undertreatment of hypercholesterolaemia: A population-based study. *Br. J. Clin. Pharmacol.* **2003**, *55*, 389–397. [CrossRef]
14. Hoerger, T.J.; Bala, M.V.; Bray, J.W.; Wilcosky, T.C.; LaRosa, J. Treatment patterns and distribution of low-density lipoprotein cholesterol levels in treatment-eligible United States adults. *Am. J. Cardiol.* **1998**, *82*, 61–65. [CrossRef] [PubMed]
15. Lubieniecki, P.; Wołyniec, M.; Połtyn-Zaradna, K.; Zatońska, K.; Szuba, A. Lipid-Lowering Therapy in PURE Poland Cohort Study. *J. Clin. Med.* **2024**, *13*, 60. [CrossRef] [PubMed]
16. Heiat, A.; Vaccarino, V.; Krumholz, H.M. An evidence-based assessment of federal guidelines for overweight and obesity as they apply to elderly persons. *Arch. Intern. Med.* **2001**, *161*, 1194–1203. [CrossRef] [PubMed]
17. Besser, L.M.; Brenowitz, W.D.; Meyer, O.L.; Hoermann, S.; Renne, J. Methods to Address Self-Selection and Reverse Causation in Studies of Neighborhood Environments and Brain Health. *Int. J. Environ. Res. Public Health* **2021**, *18*, 6484. [CrossRef] [PubMed]
18. Perreault, S.; Dragomir, A.; Blais, L.; Bérard, A.; Lalonde, L.; White, M.; Pilon, D. Impact of better adherence to statin agents in the primary prevention of coronary artery disease. *Eur. J. Clin. Pharmacol.* **2009**, *65*, 1013–1024. [CrossRef] [PubMed]
19. Ho, P.M.; Spertus, J.A.; Masoudi, F.A.; Reid, K.J.; Peterson, E.D.; Magid, D.J.; Krumholz, H.M.; Rumsfeld, J.S. Impact of medication therapy discontinuation on mortality after myocardial infarction. *Arch. Intern. Med.* **2006**, *166*, 1842–1847. [CrossRef] [PubMed]
20. Bouchard, M.H.; Dragomir, A.; Blais, L.; Bérard, A.; Pilon, D.; Perreault, S. Impact of adherence to statins on coronary artery disease in primary prevention. *Br. J. Clin. Pharmacol.* **2007**, *63*, 698–708. [CrossRef] [PubMed]
21. Lewington, S.; Clarke, R.; Qizilbash, N.; Peto, R.; Collins, R.; Prospective Studies Collaboration. Age-specific relevance of usual blood pressure to vascular mortality: A meta-analysis of individual data for one million adults in 61 prospective studies. *Lancet* **2002**, *360*, 1903–1913.
22. Tabas, I.; Williams, K.J.; Borén, J. Subendothelial lipoprotein retention as the initiating process in atherosclerosis: Update and therapeutic implications. *Circulation* **2007**, *116*, 1832–1844. [CrossRef]
23. Ference, B.A.; Ginsberg, H.N.; Graham, I.; Ray, K.K.; Packard, C.J.; Bruckert, E.; Hegele, R.A.; Krauss, R.M.; Raal, F.J.; Schunkert, H.; et al. Low-density lipoproteins cause atherosclerotic cardiovascular disease. 1. Evidence from genetic, epidemiologic, and clinical studies. A consensus statement from the European Atherosclerosis Society Consensus Panel. *Eur. Heart J.* **2017**, *38*, 2459–2472. [CrossRef]
24. Cholesterol Treatment Trialists' (CTT) Collaboration; Baigent, C.; Blackwell, L.; Emberson, J.; Holland, L.E.; Reith, C.; Bhala, N.; Peto, R.; Barnes, E.H.; Keech, A.; et al. Efficacy and safety of more intensive lowering of LDL cholesterol: A meta-analysis of data from 170,000 participants in 26 randomised trials. *Lancet* **2010**, *376*, 1670–1681. [PubMed]

25. Figorilli, F.; Mannarino, M.R.; Bianconi, V.; Pirro, M. Cholesterol-Lowering Therapy in Patients at Low-to-Moderate Cardiovascular Risk. *High Blood Press. Cardiovasc. Prev.* **2022**, *29*, 327–336. [CrossRef]
26. Simoens, S.; Sinnaeve, P.R. Patient co-payment and adherence to statins: A review and case studies. *Cardiovasc. Drugs Ther.* **2014**, *28*, 99–109. [CrossRef] [PubMed]
27. Choudhry, N.K.; Avorn, J.; Glynn, R.J.; Antman, E.M.; Schneeweiss, S.; Toscano, M.; Reisman, L.; Fernandes, J.; Spettell, C.; Lee, J.L.; et al. Full coverage for preventive medications after myocardial infarction. *N. Engl. J. Med.* **2011**, *365*, 2088–2097. [CrossRef] [PubMed]
28. Latry, P.; Molimard, M.; Dedieu, B.; Couffinhal, T.; Bégaud, B.; Martin-Latry, K. Adherence with statins in a real-life setting is better when associated cardiovascular risk factors increase: A cohort study. *BMC Cardiovasc. Disord.* **2011**, *11*, 46. [CrossRef] [PubMed]
29. Gazmararian, J.A.; Kripalani, S.; Miller, M.J.; Echt, K.V.; Ren, J.; Rask, K. Factors associated with medication refill adherence in cardiovascular-related diseases: A focus on health literacy. *J. Gen. Intern. Med.* **2006**, *21*, 1215–1221. [CrossRef] [PubMed]
30. Cohen, J.D.; Brinton, E.A.; Ito, M.K.; Jacobson, T.A. Understanding Statin Use in America and Gaps in Patient Education (USAGE): An internet-based survey of 10,138 current and former statin users. *J. Clin. Lipidol.* **2012**, *6*, 208–215. [CrossRef] [PubMed]
31. Wei, M.Y.; Ito, M.K.; Cohen, J.D.; Brinton, E.A.; Jacobson, T.A. Predictors of statin adherence, switching, and discontinuation in the USAGE survey: Understanding the use of statins in America and gaps in patient education. *J. Clin. Lipidol.* **2013**, *7*, 472–483. [CrossRef] [PubMed]
32. Kripalani, S.; LeFevre, F.; Phillips, C.O.; Williams, M.V.; Basaviah, P.; Baker, D.W. Deficits in communication and information transfer between hospital-based and primary care physicians: Implications for patient safety and continuity of care. *JAMA* **2007**, *297*, 831–841. [CrossRef]
33. Ruiz-Bustillo, S.; Ivern, C.; Badosa, N.; Farre, N.; Marco, E.; Bruguera, J.; Cladellas, M.; Enjuanes, C.; Cainzos-Achirica, M.; Marti-Almor, J.; et al. Efficacy of a nurse-led lipid-lowering secondary prevention intervention in patients hospitalized for ischemic heart disease: A pilot randomized controlled trial. *Eur. J. Cardiovasc. Nurs.* **2019**, *18*, 366–374. [CrossRef]
34. Singh, G.K.; Siahpush, M.; Williams, S.D. Changing urbanization patterns in US lung cancer mortality, 1950–2007. *J. Community Health* **2012**, *37*, 412–420. [CrossRef] [PubMed]
35. Schiller, J.S.; Lucas, J.W.; Ward, B.W.; Peregoy, J.A. Summary health statistics for U.S. adults: National Health Interview Survey, 2010. *Vital Health Stat.* **2012**, *252*, 1–20.
36. Douthit, N.; Kiv, S.; Dwolatzky, T.; Biswas, S. Exposing some important barriers to health care access in the rural USA. *Public Health* **2015**, *129*, 611–620. [CrossRef] [PubMed]

Journal of
Clinical Medicine

MDPI

Article

Is Insulin Resistance an Independent Predictor of Atherosclerosis?

Małgorzata Landowska [1,2], Bernadetta Kałuża [1,2,*], Cezary Watała [3], Emilia Babula [2], Aleksandra Żuk-Łapan [2], Kinga Woźniak [2], Aleksandra Kargul [2], Jonasz Jurek [2], Tomasz Korcz [4], Małgorzata Cicha-Brzezińska [4] and Edward Franek [1,2,5]

1 Department of Internal Medicine, Endocrinology and Diabetology, National Medical Institute of the Ministry of the Interior and Administration in Warsaw, 02-507 Warsaw, Poland; malgorzata.landowska97@wp.pl (M.L.); edward.franek@cskmswia.gov.pl (E.F.)
2 Students Scientific Group of the Medical University of Warsaw at the Department of Internal Medicine, Endocrinology and Diabetology, National Medical Institute of the Ministry of the Interior and Administration in Warsaw, 02-507 Warsaw, Poland; emilia.babula@wum.edu.pl (E.B.); aleksandrazuk11@gmail.com (A.Ż.-Ł.); kinga966@outlook.com (K.W.); aleksandra.k96@gmail.com (A.K.); jurekjonasz@gmail.com (J.J.)
3 Department of Haemostasis and Haemostatic Disorders, Medical University of Lodz, 92-215 Lodz, Poland; cezary.watala@umed.lodz.pl
4 Laboratory Diagnostics Unit, National Medical Institute of the Ministry of the Interior and Administration in Warsaw, 02-507 Warsaw, Poland; tomasz.korcz@cskmswia.gov.pl (T.K.); malgorzata.cicha@cskmswia.gov.pl (M.C.-B.)
5 Department of Human Epigenetics, Mossakowski Medical Research Centre Polish Academy of Sciences, 02-106 Warsaw, Poland
* Correspondence: bernadettta@o2.pl; Tel.: +47-722-14-05

Abstract: Background: Insulin resistance (IR) is a condition that precedes the onset of type 2 diabetes mellitus (T2DM), which is regarded as an established risk factor for atherosclerosis (AS). Considering that the same metabolic changes as those caused by IR are evidenced to promote the development of AS, we investigated whether IR estimated by the homeostasis model assessment of IR (HOMA-IR) could predict the occurrence of preclinical AS. **Methods:** The study participants were divided into two groups based on the presence of IR diagnosed during the baseline hospitalization and defined as a HOMA-IR value equal to or higher than 2.5. After a follow-up period of at least four years, a total of 79 (n = 79) were prospectively assessed in terms of the presence of preclinical AS, determined by either an abnormally low ankle–brachial index (ABI) (ABI < 0.9) or an increased carotid intima media thickness (CIMT) (CIMT > 1 mm). **Results:** Using the multivariate logistic regression analysis, it was demonstrated that the HOMA-IR was associated with an abnormally low ABI (odds ratio: 1.609, 95% confidence interval (CI): [1.041–2.487], p = 0.032). The Cox regression model revealed that the HOMA-IR was a predictor of both an abnormal ABI (hazard ratio: 1.435, CI: [1.076–1.913], p = 0.014) and increased CIMT (hazard ratio: 1.419, CI: [1.033–1.948], p = 0.031), independently of age, sex, dyslipidemia, smoking, triglycerides (TG), low-density lipoproteins (LDL), high-density lipoproteins (HDL), and total cholesterol levels. **Conclusions:** IR, as estimated by the HOMA-IR, may be considered as a predictor of preclinical AS, independently of cardiovascular risk factors.

Keywords: insulin resistance; atherosclerosis; carotid intima media thickness; ankle–brachial index

1. Introduction

Insulin resistance (IR) can be defined as an insufficient tissue response to insulin signaling [1]. The hyperinsulinemic–euglycemic clamp is considered the gold standard method of insulin sensitivity measurement. However, due to its complexity, other methods of quantifying insulin sensitivity are more frequently used in large clinical studies [2]. The homeostasis model assessment of IR (HOMA-IR) may be considered one of the most popular surrogate markers of IR; it also shows a good correlation with the hyperinsulinemic–euglycemic clamp [3].

It is estimated that the insulin-resistant state precedes the onset of type 2 diabetes mellitus (T2DM) by approximately 15 years [4]. Vascular lesions characteristic of atherosclerosis (AS) are often found in newly diagnosed diabetic individuals, which implies that the process of vascular damage begins before the onset of T2DM, during the insulin-resistant state [5,6].

Several mechanisms explaining the influence of IR on the insulin target tissues have recently been described. In the endothelium, IR affects nitric oxide (NO) production, which translates into impaired vasodilatation [7]. Hyperinsulinemia, which occurs in order to compensate for decreased insulin sensitivity, activates the mitogen-activated protein kinase pathway, which leads to increased mitogenic responsiveness to insulin [8]. Impaired vasodilatation, together with enhanced smooth muscle proliferation, contributes to atherogenic lesion formation [7].

In the adipose tissue, IR causes the inhibition of lipoprotein lipase function, which results in an increased release of free fatty acids, promoting the assembly of very low-density lipoproteins (VLDLs). The triglycerides (TGs) contained in the VLDL are transferred to either high-density lipoproteins (HDLs) or low-density lipoproteins (LDLs), forming TG-enriched HDLs or TG-enriched LDLs. The former are rapidly removed from the circulation by the kidneys, while the latter form small dense LDL-cholesterol (sdLDL) particles of enhanced atherogenic activity [7]. In hypertriglyceridemia, decreased levels of HDL cholesterol and the appearance of sdLDL are the key features of diabetic dyslipidemia and are associated with the accelerated development of AS [9].

Additionally, clinical evidence increasingly supports the link between IR and increased sympathetic nervous system activity, with significant implications for AS. IR is strongly associated with increased sympathetic nervous system activity, which contributes to both the development of atherosclerosis and the exacerbation of IR itself. Sympathetic nervous system overdrive leads to sustained hypertension through peripheral vasoconstriction, a key factor in the development and progression of atherosclerosis [10,11].

IR leads to increased plasminogen activator inhibitor 1 and fibrinogen production, enhanced thromboxane excretion, and decreased levels of tissue plasminogen activator, thereby promoting platelet aggregation and thrombosis [12]. Hyperglycemia occurs when beta-cells are no longer able to produce the sufficient quantity of insulin to compensate for impaired insulin sensitivity; in addition, free fatty acids are excessively released from the adipose tissue under the insulin-resistant state and induce oxidative stress and a proinflammatory response [4,8]. The prothrombotic state, oxidative stress, and inflammation are conditions that favor the progression of AS [8,12].

Considering the metabolic alterations caused by IR, it may be speculated that the possible causal relationship between IR and AS is likely to exist. The aim of our study was to investigate whether preclinical AS might be found in insulin-resistant patients and to assess whether IR defined as a HOMA-IR value ≥ 2.5 might predict the development of AS in the future.

2. Materials and Methods

2.1. Study Design

To conduct this study, we retrieved data from the institutional database of the National Medical Institute of the Ministry of the Interior and Administration in Warsaw. We reviewed the medical records of patients admitted to the Department of Internal Medicine, Endocrinology, and Diabetology at the National Medical Institute between 2014 and 2017. Our search specifically focused on records containing the terms: "oral glucose tolerance test", "glucose tolerance test", "OGTT", and "GTT". From these records, we identified 178 patients who met the following eligibility criteria: (1) they had undergone a prolonged (5 h) oral glucose tolerance test, (2) had complete medical records, (3) had no diagnosis of type 2 diabetes mellitus (T2DM), cancer, tumor-induced hypoglycemia, or hyperglycemia, and (4) were not taking lipid-lowering or antidiabetic medications.

At least four years after their initial hospital stay, all 178 patients were invited to participate in a prospective follow-up examination, conducted between August and September 2021. We attempted to contact all 178 patients by telephone. If a patient did not respond after three attempts, they were excluded from the study. Patients who did not attend the follow-up visit or did not provide informed consent were also excluded from further analysis. The final sample included 79 participants (n = 79).

The following examinations were performed both during the hospital stay (baseline) and in 2021 (follow-up visit): (1) estimation of the values of atherogenic indices (AIs), (2) calculation of the body mass index (BMI), (3) collection of blood samples and measurement of the concentration of insulin, glucose, HDL, LDL, total cholesterol, and TG, and (4) calculation of the HOMA-IR. Additionally, in order to estimate the severity of AS, all the patients that participated in the follow-up examination underwent an assessment of the ankle–brachial index (ABI) and carotid intima media thickness (CIMT). Other procedures that were performed only during the follow-up visit included measurement of waist circumference and measurement of the concentration of glycated hemoglobin (HbA1c).

The study cohort was divided into two groups based on the HOMA-IR that was calculated using the results obtained during the hospital stay between 2014 and 2017. Group 1 included patients with a HOMA-IR value lower than 2.5 (n = 59), while the subjects from group 2, who were considered insulin-resistant, were characterized by a HOMA-IR value equal to or higher than 2.5 (n = 20).

Insulin levels were measured using a noncompetitive electrochemiluminescence-based immunoassay, while blood glucose levels were estimated using the hexokinase method. HbA1c values were determined via capillary electrophoresis. The Friedewald formula was used to calculate the LDL-cholesterol levels. The HDL-cholesterol, total cholesterol, and TG levels were assessed with fluorometric–enzymatic assays.

2.2. Definitions

The HOMA-IR was defined as the product of fasting glucose [mg/dL] and fasting insulin concentration [uIU/mL] divided by 405 [13]. In order to recognize IR, we adopted the HOMA-IR cut-off value equal to 2.5.

The severity of subclinical AS was estimated using AIs, CIMT, and the ABI. We calculated the values of the AIs using the following equations: (1) atherogenic index of plasma (AIP): log10(TG/HDL-cholesterol); (2) Castelli's risk index I (CRI-I): total cholesterol/HDL-cholesterol; (3) Castelli's risk index II (CRI-II): LDL-cholesterol/HDL-cholesterol; and (4) atherogenic coefficient (AC): non-HDL-cholesterol/HDL-cholesterol [14].

The ABI is one of the tools that enables the assessment of vascular impairment present in the peripheral arteries [15]. According to the scientific statement from the American

Heart Association, the ABI may be regarded as a good marker of peripheral artery disease (PAD), with acceptable sensitivity and specificity [16]. In our study, the ABI was defined as the highest of the systolic blood pressure (SBP) values measured on the dorsalis pedis and posterior tibial artery divided by the highest of the left and right brachial SBP values [17]. SBP was assessed with the employment of a pocket blood flow detector (Sonomed Doppler MD4, Sonomed Ltd., Warsaw, Poland). An ABI value lower than 0.9 was considered a marker of PAD and preclinical AS [14], while an ABI higher than 1.4 was classified as an indicator of medial arterial calcification [17].

CIMT was assessed following the recommendations of the American Society of Echocardiography [18]. All the study participants were examined with the same Canon Aplio a450 ultrasound scanner, TMS Ltd., Warsaw, Poland and by the same operator. In order to estimate CIMT, B-mode ultrasound images of the distal 10 mm of the distal wall of the common carotid artery were obtained bilaterally. The mean value of CIMT was calculated on the basis of a three-angle CIMT measurement on each side. The higher of the mean right and mean left CIMT values was used in the further analysis. Results higher than 1 mm were considered as abnormal [19].

The following diagnostic criteria for dyslipidemia were applied: TG $\geq$ 150 mg/dL, or TC $\geq$ 190 mg/dL, or LDL-cholesterol $\geq$ 115 mg/dL, or HDL-cholesterol < 40 mg/dL (for men) and <45 mg/dL (for women) [20].

2.3. Statistical Analysis

The descriptive data are shown as means + standard deviation or as medians with interquartile ranges. Categorical variables were compared using the chi-square test. Comparisons between normally distributed continuous variables were performed using the Student's *t*-test. Non-normally distributed continuous data were analyzed using the Mann–Whitney U test. We used multivariate logistic regression to assess the relationship between the HOMA-IR and the markers of preclinical AS, upon the adjustment to a set of the confounding variables of choice. In the time-dependent analysis, the potential of the HOMA-IR, BMI, age, and other selected confounding variables to predict the occurrence of preclinical AS during an observation period of at least four years was estimated using the Cox proportional hazard regression analysis. Both the multivariate and Cox regression analyses were adjusted for the following confounders: age, sex, BMI, smoking (at present and/or in the past), the HOMA-IR, dyslipidemia, and serum concentrations of TG, HDL, LDL, and total cholesterol. The goodness of fit of the logistic regression models showing a significant discrimination between controls and patients was estimated using the Hosmer–Lemeshow test. In some bivariate and multivariate analyses, we used the approach of resampling with replacement (the bootstrap-boosted versions of the tests, with 10,000 iterations) to make sure that the revealed differences were not detected by pure chance. The borderline of the significance level was accepted at $p < 0.05$. The collected data were analyzed using the Statistica 13.3 software (StatSoft Polska Sp. z. o. o. 2022) and R Package Software v. 4.4.

3. Results

3.1. Study Group Characteristics

The clinical and biochemical characteristics of the study participants are given in Table 1. Additionally, a comparison of baseline characteristics between patients included in the follow-up study and those excluded is available in the Supplementary Material (Table S1).

At the baseline, there were no statistical differences between group 1 (the patients without IR) and group 2 (the insulin-resistant group) in terms of age (37.8 $\pm$ 13.4 y vs.

34.4 ± 11.8 y; $p = 0.272$), gender (9 (15.25%) vs. 6 (30%) male patients; $p = 0.167$), prevalence of arterial hypertension (10 (16.95%) vs. 4 (20%) patients; $p = 0.876$), and dyslipidemia (19 (32.2%) vs. 6 (30%) patients; $p = 0.784$). At the baseline, no patient was on lipid-lowering medication or on antihyperglycemic therapy. During the follow-up visit, two patients from group 1 (3.39%) and one patient from group 2 (5%) reported taking statins, while nine subjects from group 1 (15.25%) and nine individuals from group 2 (45%) were taking metformin. No major adverse cardiovascular events defined as an occurrence of myocardial infarction, stroke, or cardiovascular death were reported during the follow-up period. During a four-year observation period, eleven (18.64%) subjects from group 1 developed insulin resistance, while four (20%) patients from group 2 became non-insulin-resistant. Two patients from group 1 and no patients from group 2 developed T2DM.

Table 1. Patient characteristics.

	Baseline			Follow-Up		
Variables	**Group 1 (*n* = 59)**	**Group 2 (*n* = 20)**	***p***	**Group 1 (*n* = 59)**	**Group 2 (*n* = 20)**	***p***
BMI [kg/m^2]	28.5 ± 7.5	32.5 ± 5.6	0.01 *	27.2 ± 6.9	29.9 ± 6.1	0.08
Fasting glucose [mg/dL]	82.7 ± 8.8	88.1 ± 6.1	0.01 *	93.1 ± 15.5	94.2 ± 10.7	0.32
IFG (*n*) [%]	2 (3.39%)	0	0.82	13 (22.03%)	4 (20%)	0.86
Fasting insulin [mIU/L]	6.8 ± 2.95	19.6 ± 9.33	0.000001 *	10.6 ± 7.5	21.9 ± 11.6	0.00002 *
AIP	0.18 ± 0.3	0.5 ± 0.3	0.001 *	0.21 ± 0.3	0.32 ± 0.34	0.3
CRI-I	3.11 ± 1.05	4.25 ± 1.5	0.0009 *	3.2 ± 1.02	3.99 ± 1.75	0.04 *
CRI-II	1.7 ± 0.8	2.52 ± 1.03	0.002 *	1.75 ± 0.76	2.23 ± 0.9	0.03 *
AC	2.11 ± 1.05	3.25 ± 1.5	0.001 *	2.17 ± 1.02	2.99 ± 1.74	0.04 *
Total cholesterol [mg/dL]	180.7 ± 29.2	189.1 ± 37.3	0.44	190.7 ± 31.2	201.2 ± 50.9	0.8
LDL cholesterol [mg/dL]	96.6 ± 26.5	111.2 ± 29.5	0.06	103.4 ± 28.1	114.6 ± 37.8	0.33
HDL cholesterol [mg/dL]	63.1 ± 18.9	47.8 ± 13.6	0.003 *	64.6 ± 18.3	55.7 ± 21.1	0.01 *
Triglycerides [mg/dL]	105.9 ± 63.5	155.8 ± 88.9	0.004 *	117.6 ± 62.7	143.2 ± 146.5	0.72

IFG—impaired fasting glucose; AIP—atherogenic index of plasma; CRI-I—Castelli's risk index I; CRI-II—Castelli's risk index II; AC—atherogenic coefficient; LDL—low-density lipoprotein; HDL—high-density lipoprotein, *—statistically significant.

The laboratory results showed that the patients with insulin resistance had significantly higher baseline markers of glucose metabolism, including fasting glucose levels and mean fasting insulin concentrations, compared to those without insulin resistance. Additionally, the mean fasting insulin concentration remained significantly higher in the insulin-resistant group during the follow-up visit. (Table 1).

There were significant differences between the groups in terms of adiposity markers. The insulin-resistant patients had significantly higher baseline BMIs than the individuals without IR (Table 1). The mean waist circumference measured during the follow-up appointment was also significantly higher in the patients from the insulin-resistant group (94.3 ± 18.9 cm vs. 104 ± 15.6 cm; $p = 0.021$).

No significant difference between the groups was observed in terms of total and LDL cholesterol concentration, regardless of the time when the lipid profile was assessed. Conversely, the mean HDL cholesterol concentration was significantly higher in the first group, both during the first hospitalization and at the follow-up visit (Table 1).

Irrespective of the time when the results were obtained, the values of CRI-I, CRI-II, and AC were significantly higher in the insulin-resistant group. Although the results obtained during hospitalization showed that the value of the AIP was significantly higher in the insulin-resistant group, no significant difference was found between the follow-up results of the group without IR compared to the results of the group with IR (Table 1).

3.2. ABI and CIMT

There was no statistically significant difference between the groups in terms of the mean ABI (Table 2). Similarly, a comparison between the analyzed groups regarding the number of individuals with abnormal ABIs revealed no differences (Table 2). The mean CIMT measured in the non-insulin-resistant subjects was comparable to that measured in the insulin-resistant patients. The prevalence of abnormal CIMT was similar in the two groups (Table 2).

Table 2. Results from the follow-up examination: assessment of the markers of preclinical atherosclerosis.

Variables	Group 1—Follow-Up (n = 59)	Group 2—Follow-Up (n = 20)	p
ABI mean	1.08 ± 0.12	1.18 ± 0.24	0.161
ABI < 0.9 [n (%)]	13 (22.03%)	5 (25%)	0.84
ABI > 1.4 [n (%)]	0	2 (10%)	0.51
Mean CIMT [mm] follow-up	0.75 ± 0.25	0.78 ± 0.21	0.35
CIMT > 0.8 mm [n (%)] follow-up	17 (28.81%)	7 (35%)	0.68
CIMT > 1 mm [n (%)] follow-up	10 (16.95%)	6 (30%)	0.39

ABI—ankle–brachial index; CIMT—carotid intima media thickness.

3.3. Association Between HOMA-IR, BMI, and Markers of Preclinical AS

Bootstrapped multivariate logistic regression showed that the HOMA-IR was associated with preclinical AS defined as an ABI lower than 0.9, independently of age, sex, dyslipidemia, smoking, triglycerides, LDL-, HDL- and total cholesterol levels. Contrary to our expectations, the BMI was found to be associated with a decreased risk of an abnormally low ABI (Table 3). In the crude model, we observed that the BMI was significantly associated with the increased CIMT. This relationship remained significant even after adjusting for other cardiovascular risk factors (Table 4).

The Cox regression analysis revealed that the HOMA-IR was a predictor of preclinical AS determined by either increased CIMT or abnormal ABI values, independently of the analyzed confounding factors (Tables 5 and 6). We found that the BMI was significantly associated with increased CIMT. Interestingly, the patients with a higher BMI were less likely to have an abnormally low ABI (Tables 5 and 6).

Table 3. Relationships between insulin resistance (IR) and the presence of preclinical atherosclerosis determined by abnormally low ankle–brachial index (ABI) in groups of patients showing abnormally low ABI (marked ABI < 0.9) and controls (ABI ≥ 0.9).

Variable/Risk Factor	Control (ABI ≥ 0.9) (*n* = 61)		Low-ABI Patients (ABI < 0.9) (*n* = 18)		Crude OR (95% CI)	*p*	Adjusted OR (95% CI) *	*p*
	Median (IQR) Number/Frequency		Median (IQR) Number/Frequency					
Explanatory variables:								
Insulin resistance (HOMA-IR)	1.66 (1.01–2.50)		1.53 (0.96–2.56)		1.050 (0.789–1.398)	0.739	**1.609 (1.041–2.487)** & **1.697 (1.068–2.696)**	**0.032** **0.025**
BMI [kg/m^2]	31.1 (24.4–36.3)		26.5 (22.5–29.4)		**0.896 (0.812–0.988)** & **0.894 (0.821–0.972)**	**0.027** **0.009**	**0.594 (0.423–0.833)** & **0.578 (0.378–0.884)**	**0.003** **0.011**
Confounding variables:								
Age [yr]	36.0 (26.3–44.8)		31.5 (27.5–41.8)		0.987 (0.945–1.029)	0.534		
Sex [male]	11	18.6	4	22.2	1.247 (0.343–4.529)	0.538		
Smoking [0/1]	10	16.9	4	22.2	1.400 (0.380–5.152)	0.613	1.562 (0.393–6.199)	0.526
Smoking at present [0/1]	13	22.4	3	16.7	0.692 (0.173–2.765)	0.603	0.582 (0.140–2.417)	0.457
Dyslipidemia [0/1]	19	32.2	6	33.3	1.053 (0.343–3.232)	0.929	1.163 (0.352–3.843)	0.805
Total cholesterol [mg/dL]	186 (159–207)		163 (145–210)		0.988 (0.970–1.006)	0.200	0.987 (0.967–1.008)	0.219
LDL cholesterol [mg/dL]	102 (86–129)		91 (61–112)		0.980 (0.959–1.001) & 0.979 (0.955–1.005)	0.058 0.111	0.978 (0.956–1.000) & 0.976 (0.946–1.008)	0.054 0.143
HDL cholesterol [mg/dL]	58 (45–72)		56 (47–71)		0.999 (0.970–1.028)	0.939	1.001 (0.971–1.032)	0.938
Triglycerides [mg/dL]	105 (72–137)		84 (63–166)		1.005 (0.998–1.011)	0.196	0.989 (0.946–1.033)	0.610

Continuous variables given as medians and interquartile ranges; categorical ones—as numbers and frequencies. * OR, presented as OR (±95% CI), calculated with the aid of multiple logistic regression analysis; crude OR values are adjusted for all (presented in the table above) confounding variables in the case of HOMA-IR and BMI, or adjusted for age and sex in the case of all the remaining confounders. $p < 0.05$ and the corresponding ORs are in bold. & The bootstrap-boosted OR values, estimated along with the classical resampling procedure with 10,000 iterations, are given for statistically significant outcomes.

Table 4. Relationships between insulin resistance (IR) and the presence of preclinical atherosclerosis determined by increased carotid intima media thickness (CIMT) in groups of patients showing increased CIMT (marked (CIMT > 1 mm) and controls (CIMT ≤ 1 mm).

Variable/Risk Factor	Control (CIMT ≤ 1 mm) (n = 63) Median (IQR) Number/Frequency	Increased-CIMT Patients (CIMT > 1 mm) (n = 16) Median (IQR) Number/Frequency	Crude OR (95% CI)	p	Adjusted OR (95% CI) *	p
Explanatory variables:						
Insulin resistance (HOMA-IR)	1.46 (0.96–2.42)	2.07 (1.55–2.42)	**1.366 (1.005–1.858)** & 1.390 (0.986–0.960)	**0.047** 0.060	2.492 (0.787–7.893) & 2.348 (0.781–7.057)	0.121 0.129
BMI [kg/m^2]	27.1 (22.7–32.1)	33.5 (28.9–37.9)	**1.129 (1.036–1.230)** & **1.137 (1.035–1.249)**	**0.006** **0.0007**	**1.587 (1.082–2.328)** & **1.616 (1.067–2.449)**	**0.018** **0.024**
Confounding variables:						
Age [yr]	31.0 (25.0–41.0)	51.0 (41.5–59.0)	**1.107 (1.048–1.169)** & **1.113 (1.050–1.179)**	**0.0003** **0.0003**		
Sex [male]	9 14.8	6 37.5	**3.467 (1.008–11.919)** & 3.437 (0.730–16.180	**0.049** 0.118		
Smoking [0/1]	8 13.1	6 37.5	**3.975 (1.132–13.955)** & **3.637 (1.049–12.611)**	**0.031** **0.042**	2.233 (0.526–9.471)	0.276
Smoking at present [0/1]	13 21.7	3 18.8	0.834 (0.206–3.375)	0.800	1.004 (0.202–5.001)	0.996
Dyslipidemia [0/1]	16 26.2	9 56.3	**3.616 (1.156–11.314)** & **3.437 (1.169–10.108**	**0.027** **0.024**	1.788 (0.452–7.077)	0.408
Total cholesterol [mg/dL]	173 (152–204)	206 (193–214)	**1.035 (1.012–1.057)** & **1.037 (1.014–1.060)**	**0.002** **0.001**	1.022 (0.997–1.049)	0.088
LDL cholesterol [mg/dL]	91 (76–113)	125 (106–136)	**1.047 (1.018–1.076)** & 1.049 (1.022–1.077)	**0.001** **0.0004**	**1.040 (1.006–1.075)** & **1.046 (1.003–1.091)**	**0.022** **0.035**
HDL cholesterol [mg/dL]	59 (46–72)	50 (44–63)	0.993 (0.963–1.024)	0.654	0.964 (0.919–1.010)	0.125
Triglycerides [mg/dL]	90 (66–137)	123 (109–144)	1.003 (0.996–1.010)	0.393	1.003 (0.994–1.012)	0.539

Continuous variables given as medians and interquartile ranges; categorical ones—as numbers and frequencies. * OR, presented as OR (±95% CI), calculated with the aid of multiple logistic regression analysis; crude OR values are adjusted for all (presented in the table above) confounding variables in the case of HOMA-IR and BMI, or adjusted for age and sex in the case of all the remaining confounders. $p < 0.05$ and the corresponding ORs are in bold. & The bootstrap-boosted OR values, estimated along with the classical resampling procedure with 10,000 iterations, are given for statistically significant outcomes.

Table 5. Time-dependent relationship between insulin resistance (IR) and the presence of preclinical atherosclerosis determined by abnormally low ankle–brachial index (ABI) in groups of patients showing abnormally low ABI (marked ABI < 0.9) and controls (ABI ≥ 0.9).

Variable/Risk Factor	Crude HR (±95% CI)	p	Adjusted HR (±95% CI) *	p
Explanatory variables:				
Insulin resistance (HOMA-IR)	1.101 (0.885–1.370)	0.387	**1.435 (1.076–1.913)** & **1.417 (1.081–1.857)**	**0.014** **0.011**
BMI [kg/m^2]	0.929 (0.856–1.008)	0.075	**0.701 (0.543–0.904)** & **0.706 (0.549–0.908)**	**0.006** **0.007**
Confounding variables:				
Age [yr]	0.984 (0.948–1.020)	0.371		
Sex [male]	0.788 (0.259–2.393)	0.674		
Smoking [0/1]	0.955 (0.308–2.959)	0.936	0.760 (0.224–2.576)	0.660
Smoking at present [0/1]	1.489 (0.429–5.174)	0.531	1.893 (0.497–7.206)	0.349
Dyslipidemia [0/1]	1.330 (0.489–3.620)	0.576	1.143 (0.382–3.416)	0.811
Total cholesterol [mg/dL]	0.989 (0.973–1.006)	0.207	0.990 (0.972–1.008)	0.287
LDL cholesterol [mg/dL]	0.982 (0.964–0.999) & 0.963 (0.926–1.002)	0.049 0.061	0.981 (0.962–1.001) & 0.983 (0.958–1.008)	0.054 0.178
HDL cholesterol [mg/dL]	1.001 (0.976–1.028)	0.911	1.006 (0.978–1.035)	0.680
Triglycerides [mg/dL]	1.003 (0.998–1.009)	0.214	1.004 (0.998–1.009)	0.205

* HR, presented as HR (±95% CI), calculated with the aid of Cox proportional hazard regression analysis; crude HR values are adjusted for all (presented in the table above) confounding variables in the case of HOMA-IR and BMI, or adjusted for age and sex in the case of all the remaining confounders. $p < 0.05$ and the corresponding HRs are in bold. & The bootstrap-boosted HR values, estimated along with the classical resampling procedure with 10,000 iterations, are given for statistically significant outcomes.

Table 6. Time-dependent relationship between insulin resistance (IR) and the presence of preclinical atherosclerosis determined by increased carotid intima media thickness (CIMT) in groups of patients showing increased CIMT (marked (CIMT > 1 mm) and controls (CIMT ≤ 1 mm).

Variable/Risk Factor	Crude HR (±95% CI)	p	Adjusted HR (±95% CI) *	p
Explanatory variables:				
Insulin resistance (HOMA-IR)	**1.245 (1.052–1.473)** & **1.242 (1.042–1.479)**	**0.011** **0.016**	**1.419 (1.033–1.948)** & **1.421 (1.020–1.981)**	**0.031** **0.038**
BMI [kg/m^2]	**1.091 (1.023–1.164)** & **1.091 (1.006–1.183)**	**0.008** **0.035**	**1.280 (1.078–1.519)** & **1.277 (1.071–1.522)**	**0.005** **0.006**
Confounding variables:				
Age [yr]	**1.049 (1.015–1.085)** & **1.044 (1.005–1.084)**	**0.005** **0.027**		
Sex [male]	0.385 (0.140–1.060)	0.065		
Smoking [0/1]	0.509 (0.176–1.472)	0.213	0.855 (0.266–2.752)	0.793
Smoking at present [0/1]	1.312 (0.371–4.632)	0.673	1.287 (0.341–4.858)	0.710
Dyslipidemia [0/1]	0.601 (0.211–1.713)	0.341	1.068 (0.347–3.287)	0.909
Total cholesterol [mg/dL]	**1.025 (1.007–1.043)** & **1.023 (1.004–1.043)**	**0.006** **0.018**	1.012 (0.993–1.031)	0.227
LDL cholesterol [mg/dL]	**1.032 (1.008–1.056)** & **1.036 (1.006–1.067)**	**0.008** **0.019**	1.021 (0.997–1.045)	0.083

Table 6. *Cont.*

Variable/Risk Factor	Crude HR (±95% CI)	p	Adjusted HR (±95% CI) *	p
HDL cholesterol [mg/dL]	0.999 (0.972–1.026)	0.942	0.983 (0.952–1.015)	0.299
Triglycerides [mg/dL]	1.002 (0.996–1.009)	0.438	1.002 (0.995–1.009)	0.540

* HR, presented as HR (±95% CI), calculated with the aid of Cox proportional hazard regression analysis; crude HR values are adjusted for all (presented in the table above) confounding variables in the case of HOMA-IR and BMI, or adjusted for age and sex in the case of all the remaining confounders. $p < 0.05$ and the corresponding HRs are in bold. & The bootstrap-boosted HR values, estimated along with the classical resampling procedure with 10,000 iterations, are given for statistically significant outcomes.

4. Discussion

It is well established that there is an association between atherosclerosis (AS) and metabolic syndrome, yet the specific role of individual factors involved in the shared pathophysiology of these conditions remains challenging to determine [21]. Insulin resistance (IR) is a key component of metabolic syndrome, and several mechanisms may explain its link to AS [22]. One major mechanism involves the insulin resistance-induced reduction in nitric oxide (NO) bioavailability, which is essential for maintaining endothelial function [23]. Reduced NO levels contribute to atherosclerotic plaque formation by promoting platelet aggregation, enhancing monocyte adhesion, and increasing the infiltration of vascular smooth muscle cells into the endothelium, all of which play a central role in AS development [24]. Clinical evidence suggests that targeting asymmetric dimethylarginine, an endogenous inhibitor of NO, may offer a promising therapeutic strategy for cardiovascular disease, as NO deficiency is implicated in its pathogenesis [25].

Additionally, the sympathetic nervous system has been shown to contribute to the pathophysiology of both AS and IR. Studies suggest that hyperinsulinemia, a key marker of IR, activates the sympathetic nervous system, while recent research proposes that sympathetic nervous system overstimulation may actually drive hyperinsulinemia through reduced blood flow to muscles [10]. This increased sympathetic activity contributes to hypertension, which is an established risk factor for AS [11]. Emerging clinical reports on multi-organ denervation demonstrate its ability to reduce sympathetic nerve activity, decrease atheroma size, and improve insulin sensitivity. These findings underscore the potential benefits of targeting both IR and AS in the same therapeutic intervention [26,27]. A deeper understanding of the relationship between AS and IR could offer significant clinical benefits, including the development of more effective treatments and improved outcomes for patients with these interconnected conditions. Providing new evidence on the clinical significance of the IR-AS relationship could help determine whether there is a rationale for intensifying clinical interventions to detect and treat IR.

Our results revealed that compared to the non-insulin-resistant subjects, the patients with IR had significantly higher markers of adiposity, namely the baseline BMI and follow-up BMI (Table 1). The authors of the ESC guidelines on cardiovascular disease (CVD) prevention enlisted adiposity as one of the major modifiable AS CVD risk factors. A meta-analysis of 58 prospective studies on the association of adiposity measures with CVD demonstrated that both BMI and waist circumference were strongly and similarly associated with AS CVD [21]. In our study, the patients with IR were characterized by significantly higher baseline BMIs and body mass values and significantly higher waist circumference than the individuals without IR. Similar findings were reported by Caporaso et al., who investigated a relationship between IR and health-related outcomes in a large cohort of generally heathy subjects. They found that waist circumference and BMI values increased across the increasing quartiles of the HOMA-IR. This trend persisted even after adjusting for confounding variables, such as age, social status, ethnicity, gender, and smoking and drinking habits, irrespective of the way the HOMA-IR was estimated (as the median, quartiles, or a continuous variable) [22].

In our study, patients with IR had significantly lower baseline and follow-up HDL cholesterol levels and significantly higher baseline TG levels than the individuals without IR, with the mean TG levels exceeding the threshold of 150 mg/dL (Table 1). TG level assessment is recommended to identify individuals in whom LDL cholesterol levels may underestimate the AS CVD risk and is to be performed routinely during the standard lipid profile assessment [20]. While TG levels higher than 150 mg/dL were shown to be associated with AS development, high HDL cholesterol levels were inversely associated with CVD risk [20]. Our results suggest that the patients with IR were characterized by a combination of lipid abnormalities, which are also regarded AS risk factors. Such findings are not surprising provided that multiple studies demonstrated that diabetic dyslipidemia, defined as increased TG and sdLDL cholesterol levels and reduced HDL cholesterol levels, is commonly confirmed in insulin-resistant patients [23,28]. IR is considered a major trigger for diabetic dyslipidemia as it facilitates an increased secretion and decreased clearance of VLDL, which results in hypertriglyceridemia [7]. Furthermore, IR is associated with increased hepatic lipase activity and an enhanced production of TG-enriched HDL particles, which leads to increased HDL catabolism and, thus, decreased HDL levels, which we observed in the insulin-resistant group [7,23].

Numerous authors reported that AIs were strongly associated with AS and might represent a useful tool for AS risk stratification [14,29,30]. Our results (Table 1) suggest that insulin-resistant patients were characterized by significantly higher AI values than the non-insulin-resistant subjects (Table 1). Similar findings were reported by Du et al., who found that insulin-resistant patients were more likely to have significantly higher values of CRI-I, CRI-II, AC, and the TG/HDL ratio than the subjects without IR. Furthermore, they demonstrated a strong association between each of the lipid ratios and IR [31]. The adjusted analysis conducted by Caporaso et al. revealed that the TG to HDL cholesterol ratio tended to increase along with increasing HOMA-IR quartiles [22]. Instead of the crude TG/HDL ratio, we measured AIP, which is a logarithmically transformed TG/HDL ratio. Nevertheless, our results are consistent with both of the aforementioned studies and indicate that patients with IR have significantly higher AIs, which may be regarded as a marker of preclinical AS [29,30].

Our results indicate that the HOMA-IR was associated with markers of preclinical AS independently of cardiovascular risk factors and may be regarded as an independent predictor of abnormal CIMT (Table 4). These findings are consistent with the results of the IRAS study (the Insulin Resistance Atherosclerosis Study), which was the first large, epidemiologic study on the association between insulin sensitivity and prevalent CVD. The IRAS study revealed an inverse association between insulin sensitivity and AS, as estimated by CIMT in the group of Caucasian individuals, which persisted even after adjustment for the established CVD risk factors [32]. In contrast, the results of the MESA study revealed that the relationship between IR and CIMT could not be considered independent as it lost its significance after adjusting for the metabolic syndrome components. Based on those findings, the authors of the MESA study did not recommend the use of the HOMA-IR as an additional AS risk assessment tool as it did not seem to improve CV risk stratification [33]. Like the results of the IRAS study, a meta-analysis by Gast et al., and the Bruneck Study, our results are in opposition to those conclusions and support the hypothesis that the inclusion of the HOMA-IR in the AS risk prediction model may be beneficial [32,34,35].

While numerous authors reported on the association between the ABI and DM, CVD, and metabolic syndrome, little is known about the relationship between the ABI and IR [36]. Britton et al. were the first authors to conduct a prospective analysis of the association between IR and PAD, defined as either an ABI < 0.9 or the development of clinical PAD during the time of observation [36]. They confirmed an independent association between the HOMA-IR and the ABI, and the correlation remained significant even after diabetic patients were excluded from the analysis [36]. Despite the fact that our study was conducted only in Caucasian individuals with a mean age of 36.9 years old, we observed associations (Tables 3 and 5) that were similar to those reported by Britton et al. in 2012 (85% Caucasian patients, mean age: 72.3 years old).

Recent studies regarding the relationship between BMI and CIMT have brought contradictory results. Our findings (Table 6), which are similar to those of Bretton et al. (2011), revealed that BMI was significantly associated with CIMT [37]. As demonstrated by Landecho et al. (2018) and Ge et al. (2014), other markers of obesity, such as high body fat percentage and increased waist circumference, tended to present a higher magnitude of association with CIMT than BMI [38,39].

Although obesity is considered a major risk factor for PAD, we found that BMI was inversely associated with an abnormally low ABI (Tables 3 and 5) [40]. The positive association between BMI and arterial stiffness and, thus, a falsely high ABI, could explain our results [41]. However, considering the recently published studies reporting divergent results regarding the association between obesity and arterial stiffness, this relationship seems to be more complex [42]. Therefore, further research in this field is needed.

Our study has several limitations. In the present study, the method of IR estimation was different from the gold standard method, i.e., the glucose clamp test [3]. As we were aware that it is not used as frequently as other IR assessment tools due to its invasiveness and complexity, we decided to employ the HOMA-IR [3]. Although the HOMA-IR is a surrogate marker of IR, it shows a good correlation with the glucose clamp test [3]. Regrettably, no definite guidelines on how to diagnose IR using indirect IR indices have been introduced yet, nor have any cut-off values been established [3]. The threshold of 2.5 that was applied in this study is also that which is most frequently used in the literature [3]. Since our study was of a cross-sectional nature, no cause–effect relationship could be determined.

5. Conclusions

In conclusion, we found that patients with IR, defined as a HOMA-IR value ≥ 2.5, were characterized by significantly higher AI values and TG levels and significantly lower HDL cholesterol levels than the individuals without IR. Using both the multivariate logistic regression model and Cox regression analysis, we demonstrated that the HOMA-IR can be considered as an independent predictor of an abnormal ABI. Furthermore, we found that the HOMA-IR was significantly associated with increased CIMT, independently of age, sex, arterial, dyslipidemia, smoking, LDL-, HDL- and total cholesterol and triglyceride levels. Therefore, our results suggest that the HOMA-IR can be regarded as an independent predictor of preclinical AS. Further research is necessary to determine whether there are implications for a more aggressive approach towards AS prevention in patients with IR. Large-cohort, longitudinal studies are needed to establish whether IR may be considered an AS risk factor.

Supplementary Materials: The following supporting information can be downloaded at: https://www.mdpi.com/article/10.3390/jcm14030969/s1, Table S1: A comparison between the population included in the follow-up study (group 2) and the patients excluded from the follow-up (group 1).

Author Contributions: B.K., E.F. and M.L. developed the design of the study; M.L., B.K., E.B., A.Ż.-Ł., K.W., A.K., J.J., T.K. and M.C.-B. contributed to the data collection. B.K. and C.W. performed the data analysis. B.K., C.W. and M.L. interpreted the results. M.L. and B.K. prepared the draft of the manuscript. E.F., C.W. and B.K. provided supervision for the project. All authors have read and agreed to the published version of the manuscript.

Funding: This study was funded by the Polish Ministry of Education and Science from state budget resources as part of the "Student science clubs create innovations" program [grant number: SKN/SP/496715/2021].

Institutional Review Board Statement: The study was conducted in accordance with the Declaration of Helsinki and approved by the Bioethics Committee at the Medical University of Warsaw (approval No. KB/108/2021, date 30 July 2021).

Informed Consent Statement: Informed consent was obtained from all subjects involved in the study.

Data Availability Statement: The datasets used and analyzed during the current study are available from the corresponding author on reasonable request.

Conflicts of Interest: The authors declare no conflicts of interest.

Abbreviations

ABI, ankle–brachial index; AC, atherogenic coefficient; AIs, atherogenic indices; AIP, atherogenic index of plasma; AS, atherosclerosis; BMI, body mass index; CI, confidence interval; CIMT, carotid intima media thickness; CRI-I, Castelli's risk index I; CRI-II, Castelli's risk index II; CVD, cardiovascular disease; HbA1c, glycated hemoglobin; HDL, high-density lipoprotein; HOMA-IR, homeostasis model assessment of IR; HR, hazard ratio; IFG, impaired fasting glucose; IR, insulin resistance; LDL, low-density lipoprotein; NO, nitric oxide; OR, odds ratio; PAD, peripheral artery disease; sdLDL, small dense LDL-cholesterol; SBP, systolic blood pressure; T2DM, type 2 diabetes mellitus; TG, triglycerides; VLDL, very low-density lipoproteins

References

1. Freeman, A.M.; Acevedo, L.A.; Pennings, N. Insulin Resistance. In *StatPearls*; StatPearls Publishing: Treasure Island, FL, USA, 2024.
2. Mastrototaro, L.; Roden, M. Insulin resistance and insulin sensitizing agents. In *Metabolism—Clinical and Experimental*; Elsevier: Amsterdam, The Netherlands, 2021; Volume 125. [CrossRef]
3. Placzkowska, S.; Pawlik-Sobecka, L.; Kokot, I.; Piwowar, A. Indirect insulin resistance detection: Current clinical trends and laboratory limitations. *Biomed. Pap. Med. Fac. Univ. Palacky Olomouc Czechoslov.* **2019**, *163*, 187–199. [CrossRef] [PubMed]
4. Zaccardi, F.; Webb, D.R.; Yates, T.; Davies, M.J. Pathophysiology of type 1 and type 2 diabetes mellitus: A 90-year perspective. *Postgrad. Med. J.* **2016**, *92*, 63–69. [CrossRef]
5. Adeva-Andany, M.M.; Ameneiros-Rodríguez, E.; Fernández-Fernández, C.; Domínguez-Montero, A.; Funcasta-Calderón, R. Insulin resistance is associated with subclinical vascular disease in humans. *World J. Diabetes* **2019**, *10*, 63–77. [CrossRef] [PubMed]
6. Weng, W.; Liang, Y.; Brett, J.; Hobbs, T.; Baeres, F.M.M. Longitudinal analysis of atherosclerotic cardiovascular disease risk and healthcare costs in newly diagnosed type 2 diabetes in a real-world setting. *J. Diabetes Its Complicat.* **2020**, *34*, 107500. [CrossRef]
7. Ormazabal, V.; Nair, S.; Elfeky, O.; Aguayo, C.; Salomon, C.; Zuñiga, F.A. Association between insulin resistance and the development of cardiovascular disease. *Cardiovasc. Diabetol.* **2018**, *17*, 122. [CrossRef]
8. Kim, J.-a.; Montagnani, M.; Koh, K.K.; Quon, M.J. Reciprocal Relationships Between Insulin Resistance and Endothelial Dysfunction. *Circulation* **2006**, *113*, 1888–1904. [CrossRef]

9. Arca, M.; Pigna, G.; Favoccia, C. Mechanisms of diabetic dyslipidemia: Relevance for atherogenesis. *Curr. Vasc. Pharmacol.* **2012**, *10*, 684–686. [CrossRef]
10. Esler, M.; Straznicky, N.; Eikelis, N.; Masuo, K.; Lambert, G.; Lambert, E. Mechanisms of Sympathetic Activation in Obesity-Related Hypertension. *Hypertension* **2006**, *48*, 787–796. [CrossRef]
11. Amiya, E.; Watanabe, M.; Komuro, I. The Relationship between Vascular Function and the Autonomic Nervous System. *Ann. Vasc. Dis.* **2014**, *7*, 109–119. [CrossRef]
12. Paneni, F.; Beckman, J.A.; Creager, M.A.; Cosentino, F. Diabetes and vascular disease: Pathophysiology, clinical consequences, and medical therapy: Part I. *Eur. Heart J.* **2013**, *34*, 2436–2443. [CrossRef]
13. Vardeny, O.; Gupta, D.K.; Claggett, B.; Burke, S.; Shah, A.; Loehr, L.; Rasmussen-Torvik, L.; Selvin, E.; Chang, P.P.; Aguilar, D.; et al. Insulin resistance and incident heart failure the ARIC study (Atherosclerosis Risk in Communities). *JACC Heart Fail.* **2013**, *1*, 531–536. [CrossRef] [PubMed]
14. Guo, J.; Wang, A.; Wang, Y.; Liu, X.; Zhang, X.; Wu, S.; Zhao, X. Non-traditional Lipid Parameters as Potential Predictors of Asymptomatic Intracranial Arterial Stenosis. *Front. Neurol.* **2021**, *12*, 679415. [CrossRef] [PubMed]
15. Nixdorff, U.; Achenbach, S.; Bengel, F.; Faggiano, P.; Fernández, S.; Heiss, C.; Mengden, T.; Mureddu, G.; Nagel, E.; Puntmann, V.; et al. *Imaging in Cardiovascular Prevention*; ESC: Huntsville, AL, USA, 2015; pp. 54–76. [CrossRef]
16. Criqui, M.H.; Matsushita, K.; Aboyans, V.; Hess, C.N.; Hicks, C.W.; Kwan, T.W.; McDermott, M.M.; Misra, S.; Ujueta, F. Lower Extremity Peripheral Artery Disease: Contemporary Epidemiology, Management Gaps, and Future Directions: A Scientific Statement From the American Heart Association. *Circulation* **2021**, *144*, e171–e191. [CrossRef] [PubMed]
17. Casey, S.L.; Lanting, S.M.; Chuter, V.H. The ankle brachial index in people with and without diabetes: Intra-tester reliability. *J. Foot Ankle Res.* **2020**, *13*, 21. [CrossRef]
18. Stein, J.H.; Korcarz, C.E.; Hurst, R.T.; Lonn, E.; Kendall, C.B.; Mohler, E.R.; Najjar, S.S.; Rembold, C.M.; Post, W.S. Use of carotid ultrasound to identify subclinical vascular disease and evaluate cardiovascular disease risk: A consensus statement from the American Society of Echocardiography Carotid Intima-Media Thickness Task Force. Endorsed by the Society for Vascular Medicine. *J. Am. Soc. Echocardiogr.* **2008**, *21*, 93–111; quiz 189–190. [CrossRef]
19. Kawnayn, G.; Kabir, H.; Huq, M.R.; Chowdhury, M.I.; Shahidullah, M.; Hoque, B.S.; Anwar, M.B. The Association of Carotid Plaque Size, Carotid Intima-Media Thickness, Resistive Index, and Pulsatility Index With Acute Ischemic Stroke. *Cureus* **2023**, *15*, e41384. [CrossRef]
20. Mach, F.; Baigent, C.; Catapano, A.L.; Koskinas, K.C.; Casula, M.; Badimon, L.; Chapman, M.J.; De Backer, G.G.; Delgado, V.; Ference, B.A.; et al. 2019 ESC/EAS Guidelines for the management of dyslipidaemias: Lipid modification to reduce cardiovascular risk. *Eur. Heart J.* **2020**, *41*, 111–188. [CrossRef]
21. Wormser, D.; Kaptoge, S.; Di Angelantonio, E.; Wood, A.M.; Pennells, L.; Thompson, A.; Sarwar, N.; Kizer, J.R.; Lawlor, D.A.; Nordestgaard, B.G.; et al. Separate and combined associations of body-mass index and abdominal adiposity with cardiovascular disease: Collaborative analysis of 58 prospective studies. *Lancet* **2011**, *377*, 1085–1095. [CrossRef]
22. Caporaso, N.E.; Jones, R.R.; Stolzenberg-Solomon, R.Z.; Medgyesi, D.N.; Kahle, L.L.; Graubard, B.I. Insulin Resistance in Healthy U.S. Adults: Findings from the National Health and Nutrition Examination Survey (NHANES). *Cancer Epidemiol. Biomark. Prev.* **2020**, *29*, 157–168. [CrossRef]
23. Bjornstad, P.; Eckel, R.H. Pathogenesis of Lipid Disorders in Insulin Resistance: A Brief Review. *Curr. Diabetes Rep.* **2018**, *18*, 127. [CrossRef]
24. Cheyou, E.R.S.; Srivastava, A.K. *Vascular Endothelial Dysfunction and Atherosclerosis: Role of Nitric Oxide System*; Springer: Berlin/Heidelberg, Germany, 2015.
25. Leiper, J.; Nandi, M. The therapeutic potential of targeting endogenous inhibitors of nitric oxide synthesis. *Nat. Rev. Drug Discov.* **2011**, *10*, 277–291. [CrossRef] [PubMed]
26. Wang, Y.; Anesi, J.; Maier, M.C.; Myers, M.A.; Oqueli, E.; Sobey, C.G.; Drummond, G.R.; Denton, K.M. Sympathetic Nervous System and Atherosclerosis. *Int. J. Mol. Sci.* **2023**, *24*, 13132. [CrossRef] [PubMed]
27. Dimitriadis, K.; Iliakis, P.; Vakka, A.; Pyrpyris, N.; Pitsillidi, A.; Tsioufis, P.; Fragkoulis, C.; Hering, D.; Weil, J.; Kollias, A.; et al. Effects of Sympathetic Denervation in Metabolism Regulation: A Novel Approach for the Treatment of MASLD? *Cardiol. Rev.* **2025**. [CrossRef] [PubMed]
28. Goldberg, I.J. Clinical review 124: Diabetic dyslipidemia: Causes and consequences. *J. Clin. Endocrinol. Metab.* **2001**, *86*, 965–971. [CrossRef] [PubMed]
29. Won, K.B.; Heo, R.; Park, H.B.; Lee, B.K.; Lin, F.Y.; Hadamitzky, M.; Kim, Y.J.; Sung, J.M.; Conte, E.; Andreini, D.; et al. Atherogenic index of plasma and the risk of rapid progression of coronary atherosclerosis beyond traditional risk factors. *Atherosclerosis* **2021**, *324*, 46–51. [CrossRef] [PubMed]

30. Paramsothy, P.; Katz, R.; Owens, D.S.; Burke, G.L.; Probstfield, J.L.; O'Brien, K.D. Age modification of the association of lipoprotein, lipid, and lipoprotein ratio with carotid intima-media thickness (from the Multi-Ethnic Study of Atherosclerosis [MESA]). *Am. J. Cardiol.* **2012**, *109*, 658–664. [CrossRef]
31. Du, T.; Yuan, G.; Zhang, M.; Zhou, X.; Sun, X.; Yu, X. Clinical usefulness of lipid ratios, visceral adiposity indicators, and the triglycerides and glucose index as risk markers of insulin resistance. *Cardiovasc. Diabetol.* **2014**, *13*, 146. [CrossRef]
32. Howard, G.; O'Leary, D.H.; Zaccaro, D.; Haffner, S.; Rewers, M.; Hamman, R.; Selby, J.V.; Saad, M.F.; Savage, P.; Bergman, R. Insulin sensitivity and atherosclerosis. The Insulin Resistance Atherosclerosis Study (IRAS) Investigators. *Circulation* **1996**, *93*, 1809–1817. [CrossRef]
33. Bertoni, A.G.; Wong, N.D.; Shea, S.; Ma, S.; Liu, K.; Preethi, S.; Jacobs, D.R., Jr.; Wu, C.; Saad, M.F.; Szklo, M. Insulin resistance, metabolic syndrome, and subclinical atherosclerosis: The Multi-Ethnic Study of Atherosclerosis (MESA). *Diabetes Care* **2007**, *30*, 2951–2956. [CrossRef]
34. Gast, K.B.; Tjeerdema, N.; Stijnen, T.; Smit, J.W.; Dekkers, O.M. Insulin resistance and risk of incident cardiovascular events in adults without diabetes: Meta-analysis. *PLoS ONE* **2012**, *7*, e52036. [CrossRef]
35. Bonora, E.; Kiechl, S.; Willeit, J.; Oberhollenzer, F.; Egger, G.; Meigs, J.B.; Bonadonna, R.C.; Muggeo, M. Insulin resistance as estimated by homeostasis model assessment predicts incident symptomatic cardiovascular disease in caucasian subjects from the general population: The Bruneck study. *Diabetes Care* **2007**, *30*, 318–324. [CrossRef] [PubMed]
36. Britton, K.A.; Mukamal, K.J.; Ix, J.H.; Siscovick, D.S.; Newman, A.B.; de Boer, I.H.; Thacker, E.L.; Biggs, M.L.; Gaziano, J.M.; Djoussé, L. Insulin resistance and incident peripheral artery disease in the Cardiovascular Health Study. *Vasc. Med.* **2012**, *17*, 85–93. [CrossRef] [PubMed]
37. Breton, C.V.; Wang, X.; Mack, W.J.; Berhane, K.; Lopez, M.; Islam, T.S.; Feng, M.; Hodis, H.N.; Künzli, N.; Avol, E. Carotid artery intima-media thickness in college students: Race/ethnicity matters. *Atherosclerosis* **2011**, *217*, 441–446. [CrossRef] [PubMed]
38. Ge, W.; Parvez, F.; Wu, F.; Islam, T.; Ahmed, A.; Shaheen, I.; Sarwar, G.; Demmer, R.T.; Desvarieux, M.; Ahsan, H.; et al. Association between anthropometric measures of obesity and subclinical atherosclerosis in Bangladesh. *Atherosclerosis* **2014**, *232*, 234–241. [CrossRef]
39. Landecho, M.; Colina, I.; Sunsundegui, P.; Camarero, B.; Núñez-Córdoba, J.; Beloqui, O. Comparison of correlations of equation-derived body fat percentage and body mass index with carotid intima-media thickness. *Acta Diabetol.* **2018**, *56*, 373–375. [CrossRef]
40. Huang, Y.; Xu, M.; Xie, L.; Wang, T.; Huang, X.; Lv, X.; Chen, Y.; Ding, L.; Lin, L.; Wang, W.; et al. Obesity and peripheral arterial disease: A Mendelian Randomization analysis. *Atherosclerosis* **2016**, *247*, 218–224. [CrossRef]
41. Wildman, R.P.; Mackey, R.H.; Bostom, A.; Thompson, T.; Sutton-Tyrrell, K. Measures of obesity are associated with vascular stiffness in young and older adults. *Hypertension* **2003**, *42*, 468–473. [CrossRef]
42. Kim, H.-L.; Ahn, D.-W.; Kim, S.H.; Lee, D.S.; Yoon, S.H.; Zo, J.-H.; Kim, M.-A.; Jeong, J.B. Association between body fat parameters and arterial stiffness. *Sci. Rep.* **2021**, *11*, 20536. [CrossRef]

MDPI AG
Grosspeteranlage 5
4052 Basel
Switzerland
Tel.: +41 61 683 77 34

Journal of Clinical Medicine Editorial Office
E-mail: jcm@mdpi.com
www.mdpi.com/journal/jcm

www.ingramcontent.com/pod-product-compliance
Lightning Source LLC
Chambersburg PA
CBHW062048220926
51850CB00010B/2694